Anaesthesia: Review 4

Squire's Ether Inhaler
The anesthetic apparatus used for the demonstration by Robert Liston at University College Hospital, London, on 21 December 1846 of the use of ether in a surgical operation. (Courtesy of the Wellcome Institute Library London).

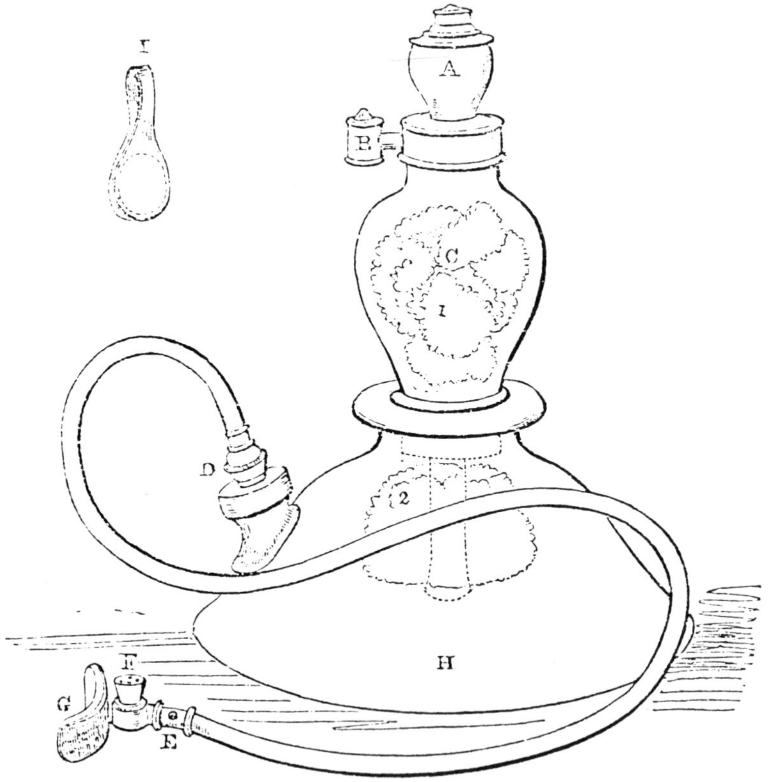

A. The Urn with its stopper, into which the ether is poured.
B. Valve which admits the air.
C. Contains sponge saturated with ether.
D. Valve which opens at each inspiration, and closes at each expiration.
E. Ferule for regulating the quantity of atmospheric air admitted.
F. Valve for the escape of expired air.
G. Mouth-piece.
H. Lower vase.
I. Spring for closing the nose.

Anaesthesia:
Review 4

Edited by

Leon Kaufman
MD, FFARCS
Consultant Anaesthetist, University College Hospital, London;
Consultant Anaesthetist, St Mark's Hospital, London;
Honorary Senior Lecturer, Faculty of Clinical Sciences,
University College London, UK

CHURCHILL LIVINGSTONE
EDINBURGH LONDON MELBOURNE AND NEW YORK 1987

CHURCHILL LIVINGSTONE
Medical Division of Longman Group UK Limited

Distributed in the United States of America by
Churchill Livingstone Inc., 1560 Broadway, New York,
N.Y. 10036, and by associated companies, branches and
representatives throughout the world.

First published 1987

ISBN 0-443-03450-8
ISSN 0263-1512

British Library Cataloguing in Publication Data
Anaesthesia. —— Review 4.
1. Anaesthesia —— Periodicals
617'.96'05 RD78.3

Printed in Great Britain by Bell and Bain Ltd., Glasgow

Preface

The publication of Review 4 has been planned to coincide with the 140th anniversary of the first public demonstration of ether anaesthesia, which took place at University College Hospital, London, on 21st December 1846. To commemorate the use of ether by Morton in Boston two months earlier, we have invited contributions for the first time from our transatlantic colleagues.

The details of the first surgical operation under anaesthesia are set out in the first chapter and it is worth recalling that on this historic occasion the anaesthetist was a medical student. An early anaesthetic text of the 19th century sounded warnings about possible perils and stressed the need for having more than one anaesthetist present at operation. The hazards of anaesthesia are emphasised in the medico-legal section, noting the need to maintain high standards of safety and care as well as the necessity for keeping accurate records.

As in previous volumes there is a distinct emphasis on medicine which could be applied to anaesthetic practice. There are chapters on the asthmatic patient, followed by an account of high frequency ventilation. Many detailed aspects of the cardiovascular system are included, with sections on drug therapy in hypertension, the production of induced hypotension, the management of cardiac arrhythmias, and anaesthesia for cardiac surgery and post-operative care.

We have the benefit of one of our transatlantic colleagues of his experience in trauma emergency care, while another section deals with many of the problems involved in anaesthesia for laser surgery. The section on paediatric anaesthesia and intensive care has been updated and now occupies two chapters. The use of narcotics in general anaesthesia is considered, as well as studies on the recovery from neuromuscular blockade.

Early anaesthesia was concerned with providing insensibility during operation, whereas at present we are also concerned with the management of post-operative and chronic pain relief as well as debating the benefits of supressing the endocrine response to surgery. The productivity of the 'literature' continues unabated so that the updated material now occupies two chapters. This is indeed a far cry from the medical articles that were available 140 years ago.

My colleagues have presented their chapters with enthusiasm and punctuality. Miss S. Wiggins has again borne the task of coordinating the whole volume with cheerful efficiency, assisted by Miss J. Rowan and Mr T. Wells.

London, 1986 L.K.

Contributors

Beverley Astley MB BS, FFARCS
Consultant Anaesthetist, University College Hospital and The Middlesex Hospital, London, UK

P. M. Bailey MB BS, FFARCS
Consultant Anaesthetist, Bloomsbury Hospital Group, London, UK

W. F. Bynum MD, PhD
Reader in History of Medicine, University of London; Head, Academic Unit, Wellcome Institute for the History of Medicine, London, UK

A. John Camm BSc, MD, FRCP
Professor of Cardiovascular Medicine, St Bartholomew's Medical College, London, UK

Christopher S. B. Child MB BS, FFARCS
Consultant Anaesthetist, The Royal Sussex County Hospital, Eastern Road, Brighton, UK

D. Wyn Davies MB, MRCP
Honorary Senior Registrar in Cardiology, St Bartholomew's Hospital, London, UK

G. Farnsworth MB, ChB, DRCOG, FFARCS
Consultant Anaesthetist, St George's Hospital, London, UK

Stanley P. Galant MD
Clinical Professor of Pediatrics and Acting Director, Allegy/Immunology Division, Department of Pediatrics, University of California, Irvine Medical Center, Orange County, California, USA

Ronald Green MA, MB, BChir, FFARCS
Honorary Consultant Anaesthetist, The Royal Free Hospital and St George's Hospital, London, UK

E. M. Grundy RD, BSc, MRCP, FFARCS
Consultant Anaesthetist, The Middlesex Hospital and University College Hospital, London, UK

Charles R. K. Hind BSc, MD, MRCP
Consultant Physician, Royal Liverpool Hospital, Prescott Street, Liverpool, UK

C. W. Howell MB, FFARCS
Consultant Anaesthetist, King's College Hospital, London, UK

Ian G. James MB, Ch, FFARCS
Consultant Anaesthetist, The Hospital for Sick Children, Great Ormond Street, London, UK

Leon Kaufman MD, FFARCS
Consultant Anaesthetist, University College Hospital and St Mark's Hospital, London; Honorary Senior Lecturer, Faculty of Clinical Sciences, University College London, UK

William A. Littler MD, FRCP
Professor of Cardiovascular Medicine, The University of Birmingham, UK

Colin F. Mackenzie MB, ChB, FFARCS
Associate Professor of Anesthesiology, University of Maryland School of Medicine, Baltimore, Maryland; Formerly Senior Attending Anesthesiologist, Maryland Institute for Emergency Medical Services Systems, Maryland, USA

Margaret J. S. Robertson MB, ChB, FRCP(Glas), FFARCS
Consultant Anaesthetist, Islington District Hospital, London, UK

Stephen Andrew Smith MB, ChB, MRCP (UK)
Research Fellow and Honorary Registrar, Department of Cardiology, University of Birmingham and East Birmingham District General Hospital, Birmingham, UK

Edward Sumner MA, BM, BCh, FFARCS
Consultant in Paediatric Anaesthesia and Intensive Care, The Hospital for Sick Children, Great Ormond Street, London, UK

A. C. Wainwright MB BS, FFARCS
Consultant Anesthetist, Southampton General Hospital, Southampton, UK

David White MB BS, FFARCS
Consultant Anaesthetist, Northwick Park Hospital, Harrow, Middlesex, and Division of Anaesthesia, Clinical Research Centre, Harrow, Middlesex, UK

Contents

1 *W. F. Bynum*

Ether at University College Hospital, 1846

INTRODUCTION

The difficulty of controlling pain adequately during both minor and major surgical procedures had long influenced the way these operations were performed.

Speed was at a premium and the conscious patient was generally a witness to whatever was done to his body, although his subsequent testimony might well have been clouded by the pain itself, as well as by the alcohol, opium, cold or other measures often employed to deaden the discomfort or blunt the memory of the traumatic event. The production of unconsciousness by these traditional means could not be achieved without serious risk to the patient, and as long as consciousness remained, pain control was not complete. The capacity of nitrous oxide ('laughing gas') to block the memory of pain in the conscious subject was known since the very beginning of the nineteenth century (Cartwright 1952), but its medical implications were not exploited for several decades.

Mesmerism was occasionally helpful but often unreliable, and Henry Hill Hickman's (1800–1830) experiments in the 1820s with carbon dioxide provided a vision but no practicable results. Like nitrous oxide, ether, too, had a social history ('ether frolics') before being appropriated into medicine and surgery as an anaesthetic (the root word being coined by Oliver Wendell Holmes (1809–1894)). During the 1840s, however, both nitrous oxide and ether were employed by dentists and surgeons deliberately to alter consciousness and hence to control pain during operations (Cartwright 1967). Beyond their obvious significance, these developments have two noteworthy resonances: they derived from the United States and thus represent the first major American contribution to medicine (Davison 1965), and both substances were simple, laboratory-manufactured compounds, thus providing an undeniable chemical triumph and so stimulating the growth of experimental pharmacology and the systematic application of chemistry to medicine (Bynum 1970). Despite earlier instances, as far as the public was concerned, the first major operation using an anaesthetic occurred in the Massachusetts General Hospital on 16 October 1844, with John Collins Warren (1778–1856) operating on a patient rendered unconscious by William Thomas Green Morton (1819–1868), administering ether. Warren is reported to have said at the conclusion of the painless operation, 'Gentlemen, this is no humbug. We have seen something today that will go round the whole world'.

UNIVERSITY COLLEGE HOSPITAL, 21 DECEMBER 1846

Warren was correct. The news did travel, not only throughout the United States, where it provoked various acrimonious priority disputes, but also to Europe, where in London the anaesthetic properties of ether were demonstrated at a meeting of the Medico-Chirurgical Society in London on 11 November 1846. During the following weeks, ether was used more than once in Britain, in the house of an American doctor, Francis Boott, practising at 24 Gower Street, London, and at the Dumfries and Galloway Royal Infirmary. Nevertheless, the analogous operation to Warren's at the Massachusetts General Hospital took place at the University College Hospital on 21 December. It was public, attended by numerous important medical men and widely reported and discussed, for example, in the pages of the Lancet and the London Medical Gazette. The episode is almost as famous as the one that had taken place two months earlier on the other side of the Atlantic.

The surgeon was Robert Liston (1794–1847), professor of clinical surgery at the medical school and senior surgeon to the hospital. Liston knew Boott, who had received a letter describing the Boston operation, and between Saturday 19 December and Monday 21 December, Liston discussed the matter with Boott, with Mr Robinson, the dentist who had used ether for a tooth extraction in Boott's house, with William Squire, a medical student at UCH, and with Squire's uncle, Peter Squire (1798–1884), a successful Oxford Street chemist (Todd 1984). The uncle prepared the ether which his nephew administered to a Harley Street butler named Frederick Churchill, whose chronic disease of the knee joint made amputation necessary. Liston had already operated on him on 25 November in an attempt to save the leg, but post-operative infection had supervened and Churchill agreed to amputation (Cock 1911). Liston's dresser recorded the following note in the case book, describing the historic occasion:

'Dec. 21. It having been decided to remove the limb today, at 25 minutes past 2 p.m., the patient was taken into the operating theatre. Prior to the operation ether vapour was given to breathe for between 2 and 3 minutes, the effect of this was so far to stupefy as to cause complete insensibility to pain although consciousness was retained and questions were answered. Professor Liston finished the complete removal of the limb in 25 seconds — not the slightest groan was heard from the patient nor was the countenance at all expressive of pain. This is the first capital operation which has been performed in this country under the narcotizing influence of ether vapour, and it was perfectly successful. The patient did not know that the limb was removed ... ' (Merrington 1976).

Churchill had a relatively uneventful course and was discharged from the hospital as 'cured' on 11 February 1847. It had taken Liston under half a minute to remove his leg. Forty years later, Squire remembered the patient as saying, when regaining consciousness, 'Take me away. I can't have it off, I must die as I am.' (Squire 1888). Liston was supposed to have said, 'This Yankee dodge, Gentlemen, beats Mesmerism hollow'. To prove his point, he evulsed both sides of a great toe-nail of another etherized patient.

The apparatus used by Peter Squire to administer the ether had been devised by his uncle and was described in an eye witness account:

'In these cases the ether vapour was administered by means of an ingenious apparatus extemporaneously contrived by Mr Squire of Oxford Street. It consisted of the bottom part of a Nooth's Apparatus, having a glass funnel filled with sponge soaked in pure washed ether, in the upper orifice, and one of Read's flexible inhaling tubes in the lower. [This tube was fitted with an expiratory valve and a mouthpiece. By turning a ferrule placed behind the mouthpiece the supply of fresh air which the patient received could be regulated.] As the ether fell through the neck of the funnel it became vaporized, and the vapour being heavy descended to the bottom of the vase, and was thence inspired through the flexible tube. No heat was applied to the apparatus or the ether.' (Duncum 1947).

Liston and all others present were conscious of the historical significance of the occasion and on the same day the surgeon wrote to Dr Boott, who had been unable to attend, 'It is a very great matter thus to destroy sensibility to such an extent, and without, apparently, any bad result'(Duncum 1947). At supper that night, Liston's excitement was such that he could hardly contain himself. As he had reason to believe, the medical press picked up the story immediately, and the journals for 1847 are filled with discussions of the new possibilities. Within months, the use of anaesthesia was no longer a novelty.

AFTERMATH

The operating theatre where Liston performed the surgery had been crowded and we know the names of a number of witnesses. There is, however, no conclusive evidence that two medical students popularly believed to have been there were actually present: Joseph Lister (1827–1912) and Joseph Thomas Clover (1825–1882) (Calverley 1985). Clover did witness an unsuccessful attempt by Squire ten days later (1 January 1847) to anaesthetize two patients, and he went on to become the leading anaesthetist of his generation (Thomas 1972). Curiously, Squire did not keep up his early interest in the field, becoming instead a consultant physician and a Fellow of the Royal College of Physicians. Liston did not live long to enjoy his acclaim: he died suddenly of a dissecting aortic aneurysm less than a year later, on 7 December 1847. The butler Frederick Churchill hobbled off the stage of history when he left UCH in February 1847.

REFERENCES

Bynum W F 1970 Chemical structure and pharmacological action: a chapter in the history of 19th century molecular pharmacology. Bulletin of the History of Medicine 44: 518–538

Calverley R K 1985 J. T. Clover: A giant of Victorian anaesthesia. In: Ruprecht J, Lieburg M J V, Lee J A, Erdmann W (eds) Anaesthesia, essays on its history. Springer Verlag, Berlin

Cartwright F F 1952 The English pioneers of anaesthesia. John Wright, Bristol

Cartwright F F 1967 The development of modern surgery from 1830. Arthur Barker Ltd, London

Cock F W 1911 The first operation under ether in Europe — the story of three days. University College Hospital Magazine 1: 127–144

Davison M H Armstrong 1965 The evolution of anaesthesia. John Sherratt, Altrincham

Duncum B M 1974 The development of inhalation anaesthesia. Oxford University Press for Wellcome Historical Medical Museum, London

Merrington W R 1976 University College Hospital and its medical school: a history. Heinemann, London

Squire W 1888 On the introduction of ether inhalation as an anaesthetic in London. Lancet ii: 1220–1221

Thomas K B 1972 The Clover/Snow Collection. Papers of Joseph Clover and John Snow in the Woodward Biomedical Library, University of British Columbia, Vancouver. Anaesthesia 27: 436–449
Todd R 1984 Peter Squire: 1798–1884. The Pharmaceutical Journal April 7: 419–424

Medicine relevant to anaesthesia

RESPIRATION

Pulmonary oedema

Pulmonary oedema is known to occur in climbers at high altitude and may be fatal. Treatment has consisted of oxygen therapy by mask until the climbers descend to lower altitudes. Larson (1985) reported on the use of a tightly fitting mask with spring loaded valves to obtain a positive expiratory pressure of 10 cm of water: oxygenation improved by 20%.

Sudden infant death syndrome

In a prospective study Wilson et al (1985) studied the respiratory and heart rate patterns in infants destined to be victims of sudden death syndrome. They found that the respiratory variables were of little value although the heart rate was higher in the affected group.

An analysis of the carotid-bodies from infants dying of sudden infant death syndrome showed that the dopamine content had a 10-fold increase and a three-fold increase for noradrenaline compared with controls (Perrin et al 1984). They suggested that these amines inhibited respiration and that infants were unable to respond to hypoxia.

Another mechanism for sudden unexplained infant death is that there is defective surfactant during lung development so that large areas of the lungs may collapse producing a right to left shunt, affecting control of breathing. The situation may be reversed with large changes in intrathoracic pressure. These episodes may be repeated but sudden death may occur if the infant fails to respond (Talbert & Southall 1985).

Respiratory distress syndrome

In a retrospective study it has been shown that the ventilation of neonates has improved the outcome in respiratory distress syndrome. The commonest cause of death was intraventricular haemorrhage. Pneumothorax developed in a third of the babies irrespective of age. The presence of a patent ductus arteriosus did not affect the survival rate but increased the need for prolonged artificial ventilation (Greenough & Roberton 1985).

Laryngeal obstruction

In acute epiglottitis complete laryngeal obstruction may occur during procedures which precipitate crying in children. Tarnow-Mordi et al (1985) described such an episode when the setting up of an intravenous infusion caused a child to cry resulting in respiratory arrest from laryngeal obstruction. Intubation was unsuccessful and oxygen had to be administered via a cannula inserted through the cricothyroid membrane.

Scoliosis

Respiratory function has been studied by Cooper et al (1984) showing that scoliosis of less than 60° had a decreased maximum inspiratory pressure but the expiratory pressure was normal suggesting that the inspiratory muscles work at a mechanical disadvantage. The vital capacity is still a useful guide to assessment as well as the arterial PO_2 during sleep. Guilleminault et al (1981) found that respiratory failure occurred at night during REM sleep.

Quadriplegia

Quadriplegia with respiratory paralysis due to cervical trauma was treated with phrenic nerve continuous electrical pacing. The hemidiaphragms were stimulated simultaneously. The pulse frequency of stimulation ranged from 7.1–8.3 Hz and the respiratory rate from 5–9 per min in the supine position (Glenn et al 1984).

Haemophilia

Pulmonary function has been studied in haemophiliac patients as it was thought that repeated infusions of commercial factor VII concentrates might affect lung function. It had been recommended that factor VII concentrate should only be infused through a filter (40 μm) but Chediak et al (1984) were unable to confirm that lung diffusing capacity for carbon monoxide was affected in non-smokers. As expected diffusing capacity was reduced in smokers.

Heroin addicts

Respiratory function is impaired in heroin addicts. Recently Itkonen et al (1984) demonstrated a decrease in lung diffusing capacity for carbon monoxide following the use of pentazocine and tripelennamine, an antihistamine (known as 'Ts and Blues'). The mechanisms for this abnormality may be due to arteriolar-capillary obstruction granuloma leading to fibrosis. There may also be a decrease in ventilation–perfusion ratio.

Post-operative pulmonary function

Simonneau et al (1983) suggested that the reduction in pulmonary function following upper abdominal surgery was due to diaphragmatic dysfunction. They found that there was pulmonary collapse with elevation of the diaphragm with a reduction in vital capacity (VC) and functional residual capacity (FRC). This persisted for 7 days and was not relieved by post-operative analgesia provided by epidural fentanyl. The use of dry gases may be a factor as studies on the hyperpnoea with fully saturated air at 37°C did not cause heat or water loss or coughing (Blanner et al 1984). Attempts to prevent pulmonary collapse by deep breathing may result in a significant rise in blood lactic acid (Freedman et al 1983).

The effect of acute changes in arterial CO_2 have been studied in normal men post-operatively and when the end-tidal CO_2 reached 7.5%, diaphragmatic contractility was reduced which predisposed to fatigue. This might also explain the acute episodes of respiratory failure seen in patients with chronic obstructive respiratory disease (Juan et al 1984).

Theophylline has a potent and long lasting effect on diaphragmatic strength and fatigue in patients with fixed airway obstruction (Merciano et al 1984). Theophylline was administered, 30 mg per kg body weight in two doses per day, and transdiaphragmatic pressure increased by 16% after 7 days and persisted even after 30 days. The benefits of theophylline are not only due to the bronchodilation but possibly due to an action on skeletal muscle or possibly by increasing calcium influx through the slow calcium channel of the sarcolemma. This could be mediated by adenosine receptors.

Extrapyramidal disorders

Vicken et al (1984) studied lung function (in particular airflow) in patients with extrapyramidal disorders and found evidence of upper airway obstruction due to the involvement of the upper airway musculature. This may cause severe limitation of airflow although it has always been supposed that the respiratory muscles have been compromised. Laryngeal stridor was a feature in patients with Parkinson's disease and emergency intubation may be necessary to prevent the retention of secretions, lung collapse and associated respiratory infection.

Asthma

Circulating catecholamines in acute asthma have been studied by Ind et al (1985). Plasma noradrenaline concentration was increased two to three times normal but plasma adrenaline surprisingly did not increase even during the acute attack. They suggested that there was impairment of adrenaline secretion though the mechanism was still unknown. β_2-Agonists cause hypokalaemia. The inhalation of fenoterol was found to reduce the plasma potassium level to 2.9 mmol/l. (Haalboom et al 1985)

Severe asthmatics may fail to respond to conventional treatment with hydrocortisone, salbutamol and mechanical ventilation. Ether has recently been shown again to have a place in life-threatening acute severe asthma (Robertson et al 1985). They reported two cases in whom ether produced a dramatic fall in airway pressure and an improvement in clinical condition as well as in blood gases.

The view that adrenoceptor agonists act by increasing cyclic AMP and decreasing calcium ions has suggested that calcium-channel blocking agents may have a place in the treatment of asthma. The effect of drugs, such as verapamil and nifedipine on airway smooth muscle has recently been reviewed by Barnes (1983), and although results seemed initially disappointing it seems that they may inhibit bronchio-constriction without causing bronchodilation.

Eschenbacher et al (1984) have shown that morphine can inhibit broncho-constriction in mild asthmatics and this effect can be reversed by naloxone. There is a positive correlation between the inhibiting effects of morphine and atropine. 0.15 ml per kg of morphine does not appear to have a bronchoconstrictive effect in mild asthmatics, although there may still be histamine release and respiratory depression. Gross & Skorodin (1984) suggested that the parasympathetic system played a major part in the bronchoconstriction in emphysema. Bronchodilatation was obtained using either an adrenergic agent such as salbutamol or atropine mathonitrate (1.5 mg by inhalation). The dominant reversible component of airway obstruction in emphysema is parasympathetic activity and this is reversed by atropine.

Shock lung — adult respiratory distress syndrome

Wardle (1984) has reviewed the aetiology, pathology and treatment of adult respiratory distress syndrome (ARDS) but the type of intravenous fluid for therapy has always remained controversial in view of the problems associated with extravasation of fluids from the pulmonary capillaries. Metildi et al (1984) in a study of 46 patients with an intrapulmonary shunt greater than 20% found that clinically there was no advantage in promoting colloid solutions (albumin) in preferance to crystalloid (a Ringer lactate solution).

CARDIOVASCULAR SYSTEM

Cardiac Disorders

In asymptomatic healthy patients with ventricular ectopic beats a longterm follow-up study failed to find an increased risk of sudden cardiac death compared with a control group (Kennedy et al 1985).

The mechanism underlying multifocal atrial tachycardia is often unknown and may be associated with hypoxaemia, beta adrenergic stimulation, hypokalaemia, acidaemia or due to an overdose of digoxin. Verapamil given intravenously in the dose of 1 mg followed by 4 mg over a 5 minute period reduced atrial and ventricular rates and even converted the atrial tachycardia to normal sinus rhythm (Levine et al 1985a).

Multifocal atrial tachycardia may be caused by theophylline, the mechanism being thought to be due to abnormal atrial automaticity and calcium-channel blockers have also been recommended for treatment (Levine et al 1985b).

Maisel et al (1985) described three patients who became hypotensive after receiving oral quinidine and intravenous verapamil. They suggested that the hypotension was due to alpha-receptor blockade as well as the other known actions of quinidine and verapamil.

The pathology in sudden ischemic cardiac death has been investigated by Davies & Thomas (1984). In a study of 100 deaths the incidence of coronary thrombi was 74%: the right coronary artery which supplies the conducting system was commonly affected. 'Plaque fissuring' was present in most of the remaining cases post-operatively. Plaque Fissuring is described as the development of an opening of the lumen of the vessel into the intima (dissection haemorrhage: plaque haemorrhage).

Heart block following the onset of bacterial endocarditis is often an indication for surgical intervention. Dinubile (1984) successfully treated a patient with aortic and mitral endocarditis with first degree heart block with medical therapy alone which prompted him to suggest the following guidelines for selecting patients for operation. These are: progressive heart block; aortic valve involvement; no improvement in heart block, despite a week of antibiotics; no obvious other causes of the conduction defect.

Wolfson & Swartz (1985) commented that despite many years of measurement of serum bactericidal activity there was very little data on whether it assisted in the management of patients with bacterial endocarditis. In an addendum they reported that the test could predict bacteriological cure but not clinical outcome.

Coriat et al (1982) felt they were able to predict the incidence of myocardial ischemia in patients with known coronary artery disease about to undergo vascular surgery. If the pre-operative resting ECG revealed ST abnormalities irrespective of whether the patients had angina or not, the chances of developing perioperative myocardial ischaemia were increased. Induction of anaesthesia in particular appeared to be hazardous.

A recent study of patients who have had myocardial revascularization suggests that patients who have had significant coronary artery disease and have had myocardial surgery can tolerate general surgical procedures satisfactorily. In a study of 73 patients cardiac complications including signs of myocardial infarct and pulmonary embolus, developed in one patient while another had complete heart block with congestive heart failure, requiring a permanent cardiac pacemaker (Prorok & Trostle 1984).

Sick sinus syndrome

This syndrome in which there are alternating periods of bradycardia and tachycardia is thought to be due to a defect not only in the sinoatrial node but also in other pacemakers in the heart. Watt (1985) postulated that there was increased sensitivity to adenosine and that treatment might include phosphodiesterase inhibitors such as theophylline. As the bradycardia has been regarded as an impending Stokes-Adams attack, treatment with a cardiac pacemaker has been recommended. Mazuz & Friedman (1983) found that the survival rate was not improved by the insertion of a permanent pacemaker. The severity of the bradycardia was not related to the degree of symptoms and a pacemaker was only indicated when symptoms occurred.

Belic & Talano (1985) advocated the use of intravenous hydralazine before resorting to pacemaker therapy. The complications of permanent transvenous pacing are discussed by Phibbs & Marriott (1985).

Anaesthesia and the circulation

There have been some recent studies on the effect of halogenated anaesthetics on the heart. Trigt et al (1984a) proposed the use of an index to quantify the amount of anaesthesia to depress the inotropic state of the heart by 20% (ID_{20}). Halothane appears to have a greater myocardial depressant effect than enflurane but when the ID_{20} is related to the minimum alveolar concentrations (MAC of each agent) the myocardial depressant effects are of the same degree. The addition of nitrous oxide did not further depress the myocardium. Halothane caused no change in diastolic compliance (Trigt et al 1984b). In further animal experiments Manohar & Parks (1984) noted that the addition of nitrous oxide to enflurane anaesthesia increased cerebral blood flow.

The mechanism of arrhythmias produced by hydrocarbon anaesthetic agents have been studied by Reynolds (1984) showing that superventricular arrhythmias occur when the pacemaker moves from S–A node to the A–V node which is more resistant to anaesthetic agents. Ventricular arrhythmias occur because of impaired conduction across the A–V node leading to ventricular ectopic foci or reentrent excitation. Hydrocarbon anaesthetics and adrenaline create conditions favourable to both these mechanisms. Increased intraventricular pressure may trigger off latent pacemakers leading to ectopic beats. Ectopic beats may also arise if there is a reduction in duration of the Purkinje fibre action potentials. The study also reiterates some practical applications from previous literature. Three times more adrenaline is required to produce ventricular ectopic beats when isoflurane is administered compared with halothane. Lignocaine when administered with adrenaline increases the safety dose of adrenaline during halothane anaesthesia.

Antiarrhythmic drugs

The importance of metabolites of drugs is often forgotten and recently Kates et al (1984) have drawn attention to the problems associated with some of the newer anti-arrhythmic drugs. One of the metabolites of encainide has a half life of 5 hours in contrast to the 1.5–3.5 hours of the parent drug. It is nine times more potent than encainide. Lorcainide is dealkylated to norlorcainide which is just as active as the original drug.

The degree of metabolism of these drugs may influence the duration of action when encainide patients metabolize the drug poorly. The half life will vary from 7–22 hours while in those in whom metabolism is rapid the half life will vary from 1.5–4 hours but as the metabolites are active the drug action may persist.

Amiodarone, a class III anti-arrhythmic drug may give rise to interactions with other agents such as warfarin (see Marcus 1983). The plasma concentrations of warfarin rise after even 3 to 4 days of amiodarone therapy but the onset may be delayed for as long as 3 weeks. It affects other drugs used in the management of cardiac disease such as digoxin. The elimination of digoxin is decreased. There are also interactions with quinidine, disopyramide, mexiletine and procainamide. Cardiac arrest has been reported following the use of amiodarone with β-blockers such as propranolol and calcium antagonists such as verapamil. Hypotension has also been reported during anaesthesia (Gallagher et al 1981). (See Aronson 1985.)

MYOTONIA CONGENITA

In dystrophia myotonia there is wasting of muscles as well as the inability to relax. There is an increase in morbidity and mortality following operations associated with respiratory failure (Kaufman 1960). In myotonia congenita, myotonia is usually elicited in the limb muscles and wasting is absent. Lung function tests may be within normal limits. Myotonia may occur in the respiratory muscles including the diaphragm leading to the inability of respiratory muscles to relax during expiration (Estenne et al 1984).

DYSTROPHIA MYOTONICA

A survey of patients with this dystrophy revealed that the mortality was often as high as 25% and the cause of death was respiratory failure due to muscle weakness and associated with respiratory infection (Kaufman 1960). Perusal of case notes of a recent death suggested that the cause of death was pulmonary oedema. Perloff et al (1984) in a detailed study of 25 patients found that the dystrophic process affected the His-Purkinje system rather than the cardiac muscle and although cardiac failure was not often present there was a high incidence of atrial and ventricular arrhythmias. Damage to the conduction system may result in death due to AV block or ventricular tachycardia. Cardiac arrhythmias have deleterious effects in the presence of pre-existing cardiac disease (Naito et al 1983).

DIABETES

Diabetes should be regarded as a multi-system disease. There is even an increased sensitivity to platelet aggregation when the blood sugar is elevated (Mustard & Packham 1984).

The incidence of bundle branch block is significantly higher in diabetics when compared with hypertensives in whom left bundle branch block is not an uncommon feature. The myocardial damage is believed to be due to a microangiopathic cause rather than arteriosclerotic disease (Blandford & Burden 1984).

Williams et al (1984) studied 52 patients and found that 25% had impaired sensitivity to hypoxia with a reduction in ventilation in response to hypercapnia. Seven per cent of the patients had an abnormal pattern of respiration during exercise, some of whom had evidence of autonomic neuropathy as judged by the small pupil size. Abnormal patterns of breathing with central or obstructive apnea occurred during sleep in type 1 diabetes with autonomic neuropathy (Mondini & Guilleminault 1985).

Autonomic neuropathy is known to affect cardiac function and oesophageal emptying may also be affected. In a study of insulin dependent diabetics with autonomic neuropathy it has been shown that domperidone, a potent peripheral dopamine antagonist did not improve oesophageal emptying of solids and will therefore be ineffectual in these patients (Maddern et al 1985).

There are hazards associated with the addition of insulin to intravenous infusion bags. It has been suggested that the insulin may adhere to the plastic of the infusion bag. Talbot (1984) has shown that in many instances when the insulin is being injected into the infusion bag the needle may fail to penetrate the inner seal of the injection port and be made into the port dead space. This may explain some of the instances of so called insulin resistance.

Wiseman et al (1985) found that in early insulin dependent diabetes there was an increase in glomerular filtration rate and an increase in kidney size. When the blood glucose level was brought under control the glomerular filtration rate fell but the kidney did not decrease in size.

The problems associated with continuous subcutaneous insulin infusion were reviewed by Watkins (1985) who found that ketoacidosis occurred more frequently than in those treated by conventional means and the method did not appear to be suitable for the 'brittle' diabetic. Other mishaps occurring during insulin pump therapy include infection, technical problems with the siting of the needle, pump failure, blocked infusion lines, loose connections and pump malfunction. There also appears to be an increased incidence of hyperkalaemia. In addition hypoglycaemia may occur following decreased food intake, vigorous exercise or the pump delivering too much insulin ('pump runaway') (Leading Article, Lancet 1985a).

Continuous infusion therapy is not recommended during pregnancy as pump failure may lead to ketoacidosis with a high incidence of intrauterine death. The reduction in perinatal mortality appears to be associated with good blood glucose monitoring maintaining the levels between 5–7 mmol/l (Leading Article, Lancet 1985b). Intranasal insulin has been tried by Salzman et al (1985) using an aerosol preparation which also contained surfactant. Their results suggested that intranasal insulin might be used in association with conventional treatment. Schade and Eaton (1985) were critical of the study in that subcutaneous insulin appeared to give better glycosylated haemoglobin concentrations than with intranasal insulin. There are also possible problems as to whether nasal mucosal absorption would be effective during influenza or even the common cold.

In type 1 diabetes being treated with insulin propranolol may cause hypoglycaemia. However in type II diabetes it had no effect when administered alone but it potentiated the hyperglycaemic action of hydrochlorothiazide. This effect was unrelated to the serum potassium level or insulin secretion. The diuretic may act directly on hepatic glucose production whereas the propranolol may inhibit glucose uptake (Dornhorst et al 1985).

Alberti & Thomas (1979) introduced a regime for the management of diabetics during surgery which involved the infusion of a solution containing 10% dextrose, potassium and insulin. This had subsequently been modified by Bowen et al (1984) but in their series of 27 patients 2 developed hypoglycaemia and the surgical procedures were mostly of a minor nature. Thomas et al (1984) claimed good results in the management of diabetics at operation using their original regime but this failed to convince Hall (1984) who suggested that there were too many variables in the study including the endocrine and metabolic response to the surgical stimulus. Regimes involving intravenous insulin also require separate infusion lines.

NEUROLEPT MALIGNANT SYNDROME

Malignant hyperthermia is a hazard which may occur during the course of anaesthesia and may be triggered by various anaesthetic agents. There is an increase of the calcium ion concentration in the sarcoplasm in muscle. The condition has recently been reviewed by Nelson & Flewellen (1983) and Ellis (1985). The earliest physiological change that might be detected is a rapid increase in the end-tidal CO_2 (Verburg et al 1984). Treatment is with intravenous dantrolene.

There have been suggestions that the malignant hyperthermia syndrome might be related to the neurolept malignant syndrome (NMS) which is characterized by muscle rigidity, hyperthermia, autonomic instability and stupor or coma. NMS is associated with the major tranquillizers particularly butyrophenones and pheonthiazines suggesting there is dopamine receptor blockade in the basal ganglia and hypothalamus. The onset may be gradual but may develop within 24–72 hours with muscle rigidity and increased temperature up to 40°C. There is tachycardia, fluctuations in blood pressure and sweating. There may be rigidity with opisthotonos or involuntary movement such as tremor and even oculogyric crisis. There may be dyspnoea due to rigidity of the chest wall. Damage of skeletal muscle may lead to myoglobin release with acute renal failure. The condition may be precipitated by drugs such as haloperidol, chlorpromazine or prochlorperazine. Mortality is high due to hypoventilation, cardiovascular collapse, renal failure and aspiration pneumonia.

The major difference between NMS and malignant hyperthermia is that the muscular rigidity in the former is central (presynaptic) whereas in the latter it is peripheral (postsynaptic). In NMS neuromuscular blocking drugs can produce flaccid paralysis whereas in malignant hyperthermia they are ineffectual. (See Leading Article, Lancet 1984, Szabadi 1984.) However this has been disputed by Downey et al (1984) who reported one case of NMS in whom the muscle biopsy response was similar to that seen in malignant hyperthermia.

Treatment is to stop the offending drug and to treat the symptoms such as hyperthermia as they arise. Intravenous dantrolene appears to be effective (Ritchie 1983) while oral doses appear to be effective in less acute cases. Dantrolene was ineffectual in the case described by Downey (1984). Bromocriptine, a dopamine agonist has been successfully used to treat NMS (Mueller et al 1983).

DIURETICS

The clinical pharmacology and therapeutic use of diuretics have been reviewed by Lant (1985a,b). The 'loop' diuretics may be administered during anaesthesia and these include frusemide or bumetanide which is 40–60 times more potent. Renal blood flow is temporarily reduced and then increased following intravenous frusemide, effects which can be blocked by indomethacin.

There have also been studies postulating that diuretics including frusemide and the less efficient thiazides reduce blood pressure not only by their diuretic effect but also by a direct vasodilator action. Longterm treatment does lead to a decrease in total peripheral vascular resistance (Freis 1983). Materson (1983) also concluded that the mechanism of action of diuretics in reducing blood pressure was unknown. However Schuster et al (1984) were able to demonstrate that frusemide was able to expand blood volume irrespective of its diuretic properties. They suggested that frusemide decreased the resistance of the capacitance vessels leading to a lowering of capillary hydrostatic pressure while there was also an increase in osmotic pressure. Both these factors assist in the reabsorption of oedema fluid and may account for the effectiveness of the drug in the treatment of pulmonary oedema.

Other studies have shown that in congestive cardiac failure frusemide causes venous dilatation and venous pooling before the onset of diuresis (Dikshit et al 1973). This effect is related to renin release and angiotension formation. These vascular effects are blocked by captopril (Johnson et al 1983) and by propranolol which also prevents an increase in plasma aldosterone (Johnson et al 1985).

Aldosterone secretion is stimulated by ACTH, renin, a rise in potassium or a fall in plasma sodium. Renin acts on circulating globulins to form angiotension I which is converted into angiotension II which acts on the adrenal cortex causing secretion of aldosterone. In animal experiments plasma aldosterone initially increased and then returned to base levels despite increased plasma renin during repeated injections of frusemide. The plasma aldosterone levels closely followed those of the serum potassium. The addition of potassium supplement to prevent hypokalaemia still resulted in elevated levels of renin and aldosterone. It appeared that serum potassium modulates the synthesis of aldosterone induced by angiotension II and ACTH (Fujimaki et al 1984). Captopril also abolished the rise in plasma aldosterone induced by frusemide.

The effect of frusemide on potassium loss depends on fluid and salt intake and that potassium balance is maintained if there is a liberal sodium intake (Wilcox et al 1984). Frusemide also has an effect on the cerebrospinal fluid composition resulting in a fall in CSF sodium in normocapnia and a reduction in CSF chloride during hypercapnia (Johnson et al 1984).

Kaplan et al (1985) treated hypertensive patients with diuretic-induced hypokalaemia. The diuretic was not specified but they showed that when patients whose serum potassium was below 3.5 mmol/l the addition of 60 mmol/d of potassium chloride led to a fall in blood pressure which correlated with the fall in plasma renin activity (PRA) but was not related to plasma aldosterone. Kassirer & Harrington (1985) however urged caution in their interpretation of these results.

An attempt has been made to evaluate the possible role of adrenergic mechanisms in the release of renin following frusemide. Cannella et al (1983) found that in patients with mild essential hypertension frusemide (1 mg/kg intravenously) produced a prompt and long-lasting increase in PRA. The increase within the first half-hour was closely related to the peak increase in urinary output and sodium loss. There was a significant decrease in plasma volume and central venous pressure. Plasma catecholamines were unchanged initially but the noradrenaline level increased significantly after 1 hour and the adrenaline level at 1.5 hours — times at which there was a marked loss of body fluid. The excretion of water and sodium returned to normal after 2.5 hours. There were no changes in blood pressure but the pulse rate rose significantly after 1.5 hours. Their findings suggested that adrenergic mechanisms are only involved in response to loss of body fluid.

Fieldman et al (1985) found that plasma arginine vasopressin (AVP) rose markedly within an hour of the onset of surgery with levels well above that necessary to produce a maximum antidiuresis. Kaufman & Bailey (1986) confirmed that ADH levels rose rapidly during the first half-hour of surgery and continued to rise throughout the surgical procedure. If bumetanide was given early during the operation the rise in ADH levels were suppressed and a diuresis initiated.

Cardiac receptors and vagal afferent pathways may be involved in the ADH response to volume depletion (Grimaldi et al 1985). In a study of diabetic patients 50% were considered to have cardiac autonomic neuropathy. Volume depletion was assessed after intravenous administration of frusemide. In those with autonomic dysfunction the mean blood pressure fell and there was no increase in ADH. PRA and plasma aldosterone were elevated in both the patients with autonomic dysfunction and the controls.

The factors affecting plasma levels of aldosterone have been already outlined but Gilchrist et al (1984) have shown that metoclopramide (10 mg i.v.), a dopamine blocking agent, caused a significant increase in plasma aldosterone within 10 minutes without any effect on plasma ACTH, plasma renin, angiotension II or potassium. At 20 minutes the level had increased to a peak of three-fold. Metoclopramide also caused a rise in plasma vasopressin after 15 minutes with further peaks at 90 and 120 minutes accompanied by a slight but significant drop in blood pressure (Nomura et al 1984).

Thus it can be seen that diuretics and the interaction between the various hormones and electrolytes produce results which are complex and difficult to interpret.

REFERENCES

Alberti K G M M, Thomas D J B 1979 The management of diabetes during surgery. British Journal of Anaesthesia 51: 693–710

Aronson J K 1985 Cardiac arrhythmias: theory and practice. British Medical Journal 290: 487–488

Banner A S, Green J, O'Conner M 1984 Relation of respiratory water loss to coughing after exercise. New England Journal of Medicine 311: 883

Barnes P J 1983 Calcium-channels blockers in asthma. Thorax 38: 481–485

Belic N, Talano J V 1985 Current concepts in sick sinus syndrome. II. ECG manifestation and diagnostic and therapeutic approaches. Archives of Internal Medicine 145: 722–726

Blandford R L, Burden A C 1984 Abnormalities of cardiac conduction in diabetes. British Medical Journal 289: 1659

Bowen D J, Daykin A P, Nancekieveill M L, Norman J 1984 Insulin-dependent diabetic patients during surgery and labour. Use of continuous intravenous insulin-glucose-potassium infusions. Anaesthesia 39: 407–411

Cannella G, Galva M D, Campanini M, Cesura A M, De Marinis S, Picotti G B 1983 Sequential changes in plasma renin activity and plasma catecholamines in mildly hypertensive patients during acute, furosemide-induced body-fluid loss. European Journal of Pharmacology 25: 299–302

Chediak J, Chausow A, Solarski A, Telfer M C 1984 Pulmonary function in hemophiliac patients treated with commerical factor VIII concentrates. The American Journal of Medicine 77: 293–295

Cooper D M, Rojas J V, Mellins R B, Keim H A, Mansell A L 1984 Respiratory mechanics in adolescents with idiopathic scoliosis. American Review of Respiratory Disease 130: 16–22

Coriat P, Harari A, Daloz M, Viars P 1982 Clinical predictors of intraoperative myocardial ischemia in patients with coronary artery disease undergoing non-cardiac surgery. Acta Anaesthesiologica Scandinavica 26: 287–290

Davies M J, Thomas A 1984 Thrombosis and acute coronary-artery lesions in sudden cardiac ischemic death. New England Journal of Medicine 310: 1137–1140

Dikshit K, Vyden J K, Forrester J S, Chatterjee K, Prakash R, Swan H J C 1973 Renal and extra renal haemodynamic effects of frusemide in congestive heart failure after acute myocardial infarction. New England Journal of Medicine 228: 1087–1090

Dinubile M J 1984 Heart block during bacterial endocarditis: a review of the literature and guidelines for surgical intervention. American Journal of the Medical Sciences 287: 30–32

Dornhorst A, Powell S H, Pensky J 1985 Aggravation by propranolol of hyperglycaemic efect of hydrochlorothiazide in type II diabetics without alteration of insulin secretion. Lancet 1: 123–126

Downey G P, Rosenberg M, Caroff S et al 1984 Neuroleptic maligant syndrome. Patient with unique clinical and physiologic features. American Journal of Medicine 77: 338–340

Ellis F R, Heffron J J A 1985 Clinical and biochemical aspects of malignant hyperpyrexia. Recent Advances in Anaesthesia. In: Atkinson R S, Adams A P (eds) Churchill Livingstone, Edinburgh, 173–207

Eschenbacher W L, Bethel R A, Boushey H A, Sheppard D 1984 Morphine sulfate inhibits bronchoconstriction in subjects with mild asthma whose responses are inhibited by atropine. American Review of Respiratory Disease 130: 363–367
Estenne M, Borenstein S, De Troyer A 1984 Respiratory muscle dysfunction in myotonia congenita. American Review of Respiratory Disorders 130: 681–684
Fieldman N R, Forsling M L, Le Quesne L P 1985 The effect of vasopressin on solute and water excretion during and after surgical operations. Annals of Surgery 201: 383–390
Freedman S, Cooke N T, Moxham J 1983 Production of lactic acid by respiratory muscles. Thorax 38: 50–54
Freis E D 1983 How duiretics lower blood pressure. American Heart Journal 106: 185–187
Fujimaki M, Nagahama S, Suzuki H, Saito I, Saruta T 1984 Modulation of aldosterone secretion in frusemide-induced hypokalaemia. Acta Endocrinologica 107: 91–96
Gallagher J D, Lieberman R W, Meranze J, Spielman S R, Ellison N 1981 Amiodarone-induced complications during coronary artery surgery. Anesthesiology 55: 186
Gilchrist N L, Espiner E A, Nicholls M G, Donald R A 1984 Effect of metoclopramide on aldosterone and regulatory factors in man. Clinical Endocrinology 21: 1–7
Glenn W W L, Hogan J F, Loke J S O, Ciesielski T E, Phelps M L, Rowedder R 1984 Ventilatory support by pacing of the conditioned diaphragm in quadriplegia. New England Journal of Medicine 311: 1150–1155
Greenough A, Roberton N R C 1985 Morbidity and survival in neonates ventilated for respiratory distress syndrome. British Medical Journal 290: 597–600
Grimaldi A, Pruszczynski W, Thervet F, Ardaillou R 1985 Antidiuretic hormone response to volume depletion in diabetic patients with cardiac autonomic dysfunction. Clinical Science 68: 545–552
Gross N J, Skorodin M S 1984 Role of the parasympathetic system in airway obstruction due to emphysema. New England Journal of Medicine 311: 421
Guilleminault C, Kurland G, Winkle R, Miles L E 1981 Severe kyphoscoliosis, breathing, and sleep. 'Quasimodo' syndrome during sleep. Chest 79: 626–630
Haalboom J R E, Deenstra M, Struyvenberg A 1985 Hypokalaemia induced by inhalation of fenoterol. Lancet 1: 1125–1127
Hall G M 1984 Diabetes in Anaesthesia — a promise unfulfilled. Anaesthesia 39: 627–628
Heatley R V, Thomas P, Prokipchuk E J, Gauldie J, Sieniewicz D J, Bienenstock J 1982 Pulmonary function abnormalities in patients with inflammatory bowel disease. Quarterly Journal of Medicine, new series 203: 241–250
Ind P W, Causon R C, Brown M J, Barnes P J 1985 Circulating catecholamines in acute asthma. British Medical Journal 290: 267–269
Itkonen J, Schnoll S, Daghestani A, Glassroth J 1984 Accelerated development of pulmonry complications due to illict intravenous use of pentazocine and tripelennamine. The American Journal of Medicine 76: 617–622
Johnson D C, Frankel H M, Kazemi H 1984 Effect of furosemide on cerebrospinal fluid composition. Respiration Physiology 56: 301–308
Johnson G D, Nicholls D P, Leahey W J, Finch M B 1983 The effects of captopril on the acute vascular responses to frusemide in man. Clinical Science 65: 359–363
Johnson G D, O'Connor P C, Nicholls D P, Leahey W J, Finch M B 1985 The effects of propranolol and digoxin on the acute vascular responses to frusemide in normal man. British Journal of Clinical Pharmacology 19: 417–421
Juan G, Calverley P, Talamo C, Schnader J, Roussos C 1984 Effect of carbon dioxide on diaphragmatic function in human beings. New England Journal of Medicine 310: 874–879
Kaplan N M, Carnegie A, Raskin P, Heller J A, Simmons M 1985 Potassium supplementation in hypertensive patients with diuretic-induced hypokalemia. New England Journal of Medicine 312. 746–749
Kassirer J P, Harrington J T 1985 Fending off the potassium pushers. New England Journal of Medicine 312: 785–787
Kates R E, Woosley R L, Harrison D C 1984 Clinical importance of metabolites of antiarrhythmic drugs. The American Journal of Cardiology 53: 248–251
Kaufman L 1960 Anaesthesia in dystrophia myotonica. A review of the hazards of anaesthesia. Proceedings of the Royal Society of Medicine 53: 183–187
Kaufman L, Bailey P M 1986 (in press)
Lant A 1985 Diuretics. Clinical pharmacology and therapeutic use (pt I). Drugs 29: 57–87
Lant A 1985 Diuretics. Clinical, pharmacology and therapeutic use (Pt II), Drugs 29: 162–88
Larson E B 1985 Positive airway pressure for high-altitude pulmonary oedema. Lancet 1: 371–373
Leading Article 1984 Neuroleptic Maligant Syndome. Lancet 1: 545–546
Leading Article 1985a Acute mishaps during insulin pump treatment. Lancet 1: 911–912

Leading Article 1985b Diabetes in pregnancy. Lancet 1: 961–962
Levine J H, Michael J R, Guarnieri T 1985a Treatment of multifocal artrial tachycardia with verapamil. New England Journal of Medicine 312: 21–25
Levine J H, Michael J R, Guarnieri T 1985b Multifocal atrial tachycardia: a toxic effect of theophylline. Lancet 1: 12–14
Maddern G J, Horowitz M, Jamieson G G 1985 The effect of domperidone on oesophageal emptying in diabetic autonomic neuropathy. British Journal of Clinical Pharmacology 19: 441–444
Maisel A S, Jotulsky H J, Insel P A 1985 Hypotension after quinidine plus verapamil: possible additive competition at alpha-adrenergic receptors. New England Journal of Medicine 312: 167–170
Manohar M, Parks C M 1984 Porcine brain myocardial perfusion during enflurane anaesthesia without and with nitrous oxide. Journal of Cardiovascular Pharmacology 6: 1092–1101
Marcus F I 1983 Drug interactions with amiodarone. American Heart Journal 106: 924–929
Materson B J 1983 Insights into intrarenal sites and mechanisms of action of diuretic agents. American Heart Journal 106: 188–208
Mazuz M, Friedman H S 1983 Significance of prolonged electrocardiographic pauses in sinoatrial disease: sick sinus syndrome. American Journal of Cardiology 52: 485–489
Metildi L A, Shackford S R, Virgilio R W, Peters R M 1984 Crystalloid versus colloid in fluid resuscitation of patients with severe pulmonary insufficiency. Surgery Gynecology and Obstetrics 158: 207–212
Mondini S, Guilleminault C 1985 Abnormal breathing patterns during sleep in diabetes. Annals of Neurology 17: 391–395
Mueller P S, Vester J W, Fermaglich J 1983 Neuroleptic malignant syndrome. Journal of the American Medical Association 249: 386–388
Murciano D, Aubier M, Lecocguic Y, Pariente R 1984 Effects of theophylline on diaphragmatic strength and fatigue in patients with chronic obstructive pulmonary disease. New England Journal of Medicine 311: 349–353
Mustard J F, Packham M A 1984 Platelets and diabetes mellitus. New England Journal of Medicine 311: 665–667
Naito M, David D, Michelson E L, Schaffenburg M, Dreifus L S 1983 The hemodynamic consequences of cardiac arrhythmias: evaluation of the relative roles of abnormal atrioventricular sequencing, irregularity of ventricular rhythm and atrial fibrillation in a canine model. American Heart Journal 106: 284–291
Nelson T E, Flewellen E H 1983 Current concepts: the malignant hyperthermia syndrome. New England Journal of Medicine 309: 416–418
Nomura K, Kurimoto F, Demura H et al 1984 Effect of metoclopramide on plasma vasopressin in man. Clinical Endocrinology 21: 117–121
Perloff J K, Stevenson W G, Roberts N K, Cabeen W, Weiss J 1984 Cardiac involvement in myotonic muscular dystropy (Steinert's Disease): a prospective study of 25 patients. American Journal of Cardiology 54: 1074–1081
Perrin D G, Becker L E, Madapallimatum A, Cutz E, Bryan A C, Sole M J 1984 Sudden infant death syndrome: increased carotidbody dopamine and noradrenaline content. Lancet 2: 535–537
Phibbs B, Marriott H J L 1985 Complications of permanent transvenous pacing. New England Journal of Medicine 312: 1428–1432
Prorok J J, Trostle D 1984 Operative risk of general surgical procedures in patients with previous myocardial revascularization. Surgery, Gynecology and Obstetrics 159: 214–216
Reynolds A K 1984 On the mechanism of myocardial sensitization to catecholamines by hydrocarbon anesthetics. Canadian Journal of Physiology and Pharmacology 62: 183–198
Ritchie P 1983 Neuroleptic malignant syndrome. British Medical Journal 287: 560
Robertson C E, Sinclair C J, Steedman D, Brown D, Malcom-Smith N 1985 Use of ether in life-threatening acute severe asthma. Lancet 1: 187–188
Salzman R, Manson J E, Griffing G T et al 1985 Intranasal aerosolized insulin: mixed-meal studies and long-term use in type-1 diabetes. New England Journal of Medicine 312: 1078–1084
Schade S D, Eaton R P 1985 Insulin delivery: how, when and where. New England Journal of Medicine 312: 1120–1121
Schuster C J, Weil M H, Bsso J, Carpio M, Henning R J 1984 Blood volume following diuresis induced by furosemide. American Journal of Medicine 76: 585–592
Simonneau G, Vivien A, Sartene R et al 1983 Diaphragm dysfunction induced by upper abdominal surgery. American Review of Respiratory Diseases 128: 899–903
Szabadi E 1984 Neuroleptic malignant syndrome. British Medical Journal 288: 1399–1400
Talbot E M 1984 Dangers of adding insulin to intravenous infusion bags with fixed needle syringes. British Medical Journal 289: 678–680

Talbert D G, Southall D P 1985 A bimodal form of alveolar behaviour induced by a defect in lung surfactant - a possible mechanism for sudden infant death syndrome. Lancet 1: 727–728
Tarnow-Mordi W O, Berril A M, Darby C W, Davis P, Pook J 1985 Precipitation of laryngeal obstruction in acute epiglottitis. British Medical Journal 290: 629
Trigt P Van, Christian C C, Fagraeus L et al 1984a Myocardial depression by anesthetic agents (halothane, enflurane and nitrous oxide): quantitation based on end-systolic pressure-dimension relations. American Journal of Cardiology 53: 243–247
Trigt P Van, Spray T L, Pasque M K, Peyton R B, Wechsler A S 1984b Anesthesia-induced myocardial depression: quantitation of effects on systolic and diastolic function. Surgery 96: 368–374
Verburg M P, Oerlemans F T J J, Van Bennekom C A, Gielen M J M, De Bruyn C H M M, Crul J F 1984 In vivo induced malignant hyperthermia in pigs. 1. Physiological and biochemical changes and the influence of dantrolene sodium. Acta Anaesthesiologica Scandinavica 28: 1–8
Vicken W G, Gauthier S G, Dollfus R E, Hanson R E, Darauay C M, Cosio M G 1984 Involvement of upper-airway muscles in extrapyramidal disorders. A cause of airflow limitation. New England Journal of Medicine 311: 438
Wardle E N 1984 Shock lungs: the post-traumatic respiratory distress syndrome. Quarterly Journal of Medicine, New Series LIII 211: 317–329
Watkins P J 1985 Pros and cons of continuous subcutaneous insulin infusion. British Medical Journal 290: 655–656
Watt A H 1985 Sick sinus syndrome: an adenosine-mediated disease Lancet 1: 786–788
Wilcox C S, Mitch W E, Kelly R A et al 1984 Factors affecting potassium balance during frusemide administration. Clinical Science 67: 195–203
Williams J G, Morris A I, Hayter R C, Ogilvie C M 1984 Respiratory responses of diabetics to hypoxia, hypercapnia, and exercise. Thorax 39: 529–530
Wilson A J, Stevens V, Franks C I, Alexander J, Southall D P 1985 Respiratory and heart rate patterns in infants destined to be victims of sudden infant death syndrome: average rates and their variability measured over 24 hours. British Medical Journal 290: 499–501
Wiseman M J, Saunders A J 1985 Effect of blood glucose control on increased glomerular filtration rate and kidney size in insulin-dependent diabetes. New England Journal of Medicine 312: 617–621
Wolfson J S, Swartz M N 1985 Drug therapy: serum bactericidal activity as a monitor of antibiotic therapy. New England Journal of Medicine 312: 968–975

3

S. P. Galant

Anaesthesia and asthma

INTRODUCTION

Asthma is a common disease thought to be present in approximately 5–10% of the population with a higher prevalence in children (Cropp 1985). Dundee et al (1978) reported that 3.5% of 10 000 patients presenting for surgery had bronchial asthma. The asthmatic individual faced with the prospect of surgery presents an increased risk of cardiorespiratory complications to the surgeon and anaesthetist compared to the non asthmatic patient. Approximately 75% of these complications are pulmonary, including some previously asymptomatic asthmatics who develop intra-operative bronchospasm (Shnider & Papper 1961). Stein et al (1962) found that the frequency of post-operative pulmonary complications in patients who present with broncho-pulmonary disease to be 70% as opposed to 3% in patients with normal pre-operative pulmonary status. Thus, careful pre- and post-operative care can reduce complications in these patients.

PATHOPHYSIOLOGY OF ASTHMA

In order to understand more clearly the asthmatic state, the response to anaesthesia and therapeutic strategies, the current concepts of the pathophysiology of asthma are described. Bronchial asthma is a disease of hyperirritable airways manifested by reversible airway obstruction associated with the following pathologic changes: bronchospasm, mucosal oedema, cellular infiltrates, mucus secretion, desquamation of surface epithelial cells, basement membrane thickening and globlet cell hyperplasia (Kaliner 1980). These changes have been attributed to the action of the chemical mediators of anaphylaxis released by lung mast cells.

Histamine and the products of arachidonic acid metabolism, now known as leukotrienes (LT), are thought to be the most important mediators contributing to bronchial airway obstruction (Lewis et al 1982). The pharmacology of LT and histamine is briefly described. (See also Casale & Kaliner 1984.)

Histamine

Histamine causes its pharmacological response by combining with surface cellular membrane receptors designated H_1 and H_2. Histamine causes bronchoconstriction by directly reacting with H_1 receptors on smooth muscle cells and may cause reflex bronchoconstriction by stimulating H_1 vagal afferent irritant receptors. In addition, H_1 receptors mediate increased vascular permeability, PGE_1 and $PGF_{2\alpha}$ generation from human lung and increases in cyclic guanosine monophosphate (CGMP) (Wasserman 1980). H_2 receptor stimulation results in gastric acid secretion, increases in cyclic adenosine monophosphate (CAMP), inhibition of mast cell histamine release, and eosinophilic migration. Vasodilation (hypotension), flush and headache are mediated by both H_1 and H_2 receptors.

Leukotrienes (LT)

The other major mediator in asthma is the biologically active moiety previously referred to as slow reacting substance of anaphylaxis (SRS-A) and now knowm as LT C, D and E metabolites of the lipoxygenase pathway. Studies in human bronchial muscle (Dahlen et al 1980) indicate that LTC and LTD are 1000 times more potent bronchoconstrictors than histamine on a molar basis.

Autonomic Activity

Finally, all normal bronchial tone is mediated by vagal constrictor influence. In asthmatics, the inhalation of muscarinic blocking agents (e.g. atropine) causes bronchodilation which suggests that acetylcholine release might be contributing to the bronchostriction (Storms et al 1975). The potential mechanisms by which cholinergic efferent discharge may be induced in asthma include both mediator stimulated reflex discharges and increased cholinergic hyperreactivity as a reflection of disturbed autonomic balance in asthma (Kaliner et al 1982). This imbalance consists of hypersensitivity to cholinergic and alpha adrenergic stimuli, both of which predispose to increased airway muscle tone, and hyporesponsiveness to beta adrenergic stimuli, which might make the asthmatic less responsive to normal bronchodilator influence. These influences taken as a whole facilitate hyperreactivity of the asthmatic tracheobronchial tree to a variety of immunological and non-immunological stimuli which could result in airway obstruction.

PRE-OPERATIVE ASSESSMENT

Prior to surgery the patient's asthma must be evaluated as to the severity and activity. One must inquire into the duration of the disease, the frequency of coughing and wheezing, both at rest and with exercise, the necessity for medication and the frequency of emergency visits and hospitalization. Sputum, if present, should be characterized as to quantity and quality. A careful smoking history might indicate the degree of bronchitic component. A medication history includes the dosage and frequency of administered theophylline, β adrenergic drugs, sodium cromoglycate (cromolyn sodium) and corticosteroids in addition to a history of drug allergy. Particular attention should be noted to abuse of adrenergic inhalers, which could sensitize the myocardium to arrhythmias during anaesthesia. Steroid coverage will be necessary during the peri-operative period in order to prevent potential adrenal insufficiency if the patient had received corticosteroids in the year prior to surgery (Spark 1975).

Table 3.1 Considerations in use of asthma medication

Drug	Comment
Sympathomimetics Epinephrine and β adrenergic agents	Severe arrhythmias are possible particularly when hypoxaemia and acidosis are present. Halothane increases arrhythmia potential.
Anticholinergics Atropine and glycopyrrolate	Not dangerous to asthmatic if patient adequately hydrated.
Theophylline Aminophylline	Halothane, sympathomimetics and pancuronium increase arrhythmia potential. Monitor theophylline levels since surgery can alter clearance. High dose can antagonize neuromuscular effect of pancuronium.
Corticosteroids	Corticosteroid supplementation recommended in patients receiving suppressive doses within 1 year of surgery. Give hydrocortisol (Solucortef) 125 mg/m^2 1 h before induction, then as continuous infusion over first 24 h. Rapidly taper over next 24–48 h to pre-operative dosage or discontinue.

The physical examination provides an opportunity to rule out infection and assess vital signs, heart and lungs. The patient should be examined in both upright and supine position and asked to breathe out forcibly through the mouth to rule out bronchial obstruction.

In addition to the usual pre-operative laboratory tests, one should examine the sputum, chest radiograph and pulmonary function (PFT) by simple spirometry. The forced expiration volume in one second (FEV_1) and minute ventilatory volume (MVV) give good predictive information regarding the ability to sustain respiratory stress (Geiger & Hedley-Whyte 1985). Response to bronchodilators and arterial blood gases may also be useful indicators particularly if the PFTs are abnormal initially.

PRE-OPERATIVE MANAGEMENT

Certain factors increase the risk of anaesthesia. Smoking or smoke exposure should be discontinued at least 1 week prior to surgery. In addition, active respiratory infection should be treated with physiotherapy (USA = chest therapy) and antibiotics where appropriate. No elective surgery should be scheduled if the asthma is unstable. Appropriate bronchodilators, steroids, if necessary, and physiotherapy may be required to reduce intra-operative and post-operative pulmonary complications. An attempt should be made to correct airway obstruction in the asthmatic patient even prior to emergency surgery. If the FEV_1/FVC ratio is less than 40% ventilatory failure should be anticipated in the post-operative period (Weiss & Faling 1968).

Pre-operative medication

The asthmatic patient may be particularly anxious before operation so that a patient and sympathetic pre-operative visit is advisable to allay the patient's fears. Sedation with diazepam may be prescribed. Antihistamines have also been recommended for sedation and drying secretions in the upper airways. [Promethazine (phenergan) in the UK: hydroxyzine (activax) in the US.] Anticholinergic drugs are not contra-indicated provided the patient is adequately hydrated.

Opiates should be avoided as they depress respiration and are potential releasers of histamine which can result in bronchoconstriction and hypotension. Philbin et al (1981) have shown that H_1 and H_2 blockers given prophylactically can inhibit the cardiovascular effects. Pethidine (meperidine) appears surprisingly to be a more potent histamine releaser than morphine: fentanyl is less likely to release histamine (Moss 1985).

INDUCTION

A smooth induction of anaesthesia may prevent an attack of bronchospasm. Methohexitone has been preferred to thiopentone for induction but both drugs can cause histamine release and also fail to suppress bronchial reflexes. Ketamine prevents antigen-induced bronchospasm in 'asthmatic dogs' (Hirshman et al 1979) but prolonged recovery, as well as the cardiovascular and hallucinatory effects limit its use.

The most common single precipitating factor of intra-operative asthma is intubation. Pre-oxygenation is advisable while inhalation of topical anaesthetic agents, beta receptor stimulants (e.g. salbutamol) or anticholinergic agents may be required.

MAINTENANCE ANAESTHESIA

Inhalation

Although diethylether has traditionally been recommended for use in the asthmatic it does increase bronchial secretions and causes laryngeal irritation (see p. 7). In contrast halothane is non-irritant and is a bronchodilator. Deep levels of anaesthesia can be rapidly attained which is a distinct advantage as bronchospasm appears more frequently during light levels of anaesthesia (Hirshman 1983). Unfortunately deep halothane anaesthesia may produce profound cardiovascular effects, sensitizing the myocardium to β adrenergic stimulation and to the effects of aminophylline. The pulmonary vascular response to hypoxia is abolished leading to ventilation perfusion imbalance. Isoflurane and enflurane are equally effective in reducing bronchoconstriction and have less effects on the myocardium (Hirshman & Bergman 1978).

Intravenous Agents

During operation incremental doses of fentanyl or alfentanil provide analgesia without inducing bronchospasm. The use of intravenous morphine is not recommended.

Neuromuscular blocking agents

There are few controlled studies regarding the effects of neuromuscular blocking agents on airway tone. Crago et al (1972) found that respiratory resistance increased in man following the administration of D-tubocurarine but not pancuronium. Moss et al (1981) showed that D-tubocurarine caused a dose dependent increase in histamine release, a property not shared by pancuronium. However, care should be used with aminophylline in the presence of pancuronium as cardiac arrhythmias may ensue especially if pre-existing cardiac disease exists (Belani et al 1982).

Bronchospasm may be induced by neostigmine given to reverse the action of nondepolarizing relaxants especially if insufficient atropine has been given to block its muscarinic actions. The use of atracurium avoids the necessity for neostigmine and although histamine may be released locally the incidence of bronchospasm however appears to be low.

Conduction of regional anaesthesia

Although theoretically conduction anaesthesia is the technique of choice in patients with hyperreactive airways it is associated with a high incidence of complications including intra-operative wheezing (Chen & Horton 1978). Spinal anaesthesia may give rise to bronchoconstriction by blocking the sympathetic innervation to the adrenal glands with concomitant reduction of catecholamine release (Barnes et al 1980). The attitude of the patient to being awake and the site of operation may limit the use of local anaesthetic techniques.

Intra-operative asthma

Although bronchospasm is the most frequent complication in the asthmatic it is not the only cause of wheezing. The differential diagnosis should include pulmonary oedema, endobronchial intubation, mechanical obstruction of the endotracheal tube, tension pneumothorax, anaphylactoid reaction and aspiration of gastric contents. The diagnosis of bronchospasm in the nonventilated patient is suggested by the presence of laboured breathing, intercostal retraction and predominantly expiratory wheezing. In the ventilated patient wheezing is a less reliable sign and airway obstruction should be suspected when there is a rise in inspiratory delivery pressure with a rapidly decreasing compliance.

Intra-operative bronchospasm frequently develops in patients who are lightly anaesthetized and follows procedures such as intubation or surgical stimulation. The level of anaesthesia may need to be deepened with halothane and further measures may include the use of nebuliser lignocaine (lidocaine), atropine, aerolized β adrenergic agents or the use of intravenous aminophylline or corticosteroids. The use of aminophylline and sympathomimetic drugs may cause cardiac arrhythmias. Prolonged mechanical ventilation with muscle relaxants may be necessary with high inspiratory pressures.

Post-operative considerations

The changes in pulmonary function following anaesthesia and surgery are determined in large part by the site of incision. The most significant changes follow upper abdominal and thoracic surgery. Pain is important in decreasing the vital capacity and effective cough, but the proximity of operative site to the diaphragm (responsible for 60% of normal ventilation) is equally important. In addition, the asthmatic has a decreased ventilatory response to isocapnic hypoxaemia and hypercapnea (Hudgel & Weil 1975). During this period narcotics and sedatives must be used very cautiously or respiratory failure may develop.

Atelectasis is a common complication in the asthmatic because of decreased cough, respiratory depression and the tendency to develop viscous mucus. Airway obstruction can be minimized by administering warmed and humidified air while the patient should be adequately hydrated. The inhalation of a bronchodilator may relieve symptoms (UK = salbutamol, USA = metaproterenol). The physiotherapist should encourage the patient to take slow, deep breaths to ensure uniform distribution of gas throughout the lung.

Asthmatic patients require careful observation at night especially during the early morning hours when sudden death from ventilatory arrest has been reported (Hetzel et al 1977). Deterioration in pulmonary status can be detected by changes in vital signs including pulsus paradoxus, arterial blood gases and spirometry. Thus, tachycardia greater than 110/min, pulsus paradoxus $>$ 30 mm Hg, $FEV_1 < 1L$, FVC $< 1.5L$ and FEV_1/PVC ratio $< 30\%$, MVV $< 50\%$ of predicted and a rising Pa_{CO_2} suggest exhaustion and impending respiratory failure and the need for ventilatory support.

REFERENCES

Barnes P, FitzGerald G, Brown M, Dollery C 1980 Nocturnal asthma and changes in circulating epinephrine, histamine and cortisol. New England Journal of Medicine 303: 263–267

Belani K G, Anderson W W, Buckley J J 1982 Adverse drug interaction involving pancuronium and aminophylline. Anesthesia and Analgesia 61: 473–474

Casale T B, Kaliner M 1984 Allergic reactions in the respiratory tract. In: Bienenstock J (ed) Immunology of the Lung and Upper Respiratory Tract. McGraw Hill, New York, ch 16, p 326–344

Chen W Y, Horton D J 1978 Airways obstruction in asthmatics induced by body cooling. Scandinavian Journal of Respiratory Disease 59: 13–20

Crago R R, Bryan A C, Laws A K, Winestock A E 1972 Respiratory flow resistance after curare and pancuronium measured by forced oscillations. Canadian Anaesthesiology Society Journal 19: 607–614

Cropp G J A 1985 Special features of asthma in children. Chest 87: 55S–62S

Dahlen S E, Hedqvist P, Hammarström S, Samuelsson B 1980 Leukotrienes are potent constrictors of human bronchi. Nature 288: 484–486

Dundee J W, Fee J P, McDonald J R, Clarke R S 1978 Frequency of atopy and allergy in an anesthetic patient population. British Journal of Anaesthesiology 50: 793–798

Geiger K, Hedley-Whyte J 1985 Preoperative and postoperative considerations. In: Weiss E B, Segal M J, Stein M (ed) Bronchial Asthma, 2nd edn. Little Brown, Boston, ch 75, p 892–907

Hetzel M R, Clark T J H, Branthwaite M A 1977 Asthma analysis of sudden deaths and ventilatory arrests in hospital. British Medical Journal 1: 808–811

Hirshman C A 1983 Airway reactivity in humans, anesthetic implications. Anesthesiology 58: 170–177

Hirshman C A, Dunes H, Farbood A, Bergman N A 1979 Ketamine block of bronchospasm in experimental canine asthma. British Journal of Anaesthesia 51: 713–718

Hirshman C A and Bergman N A 1978 Halothane and enflurane protect against bronchospasm in asthma dog model. Anesthesia and Analgesia 57: 629–633

Hudgel D W, Weil J V 1975 Depression of hypoxic and hypercapnic ventilatory drive in severe asthma. Chest 68: 493–497

Kaliner M A 1980 Mast cell-derived mediators and bronchial asthma. In: Hargreave F E (ed) Airway Reactivity. Astra Pharmaceuticals Canada Ltd, Mississauga, Ontario, p 175

Kaliner M, Shelhamer J H, Davis P B, Smith L J, Venter J C 1982 Autonomic nervous system abnormalities and allergy. Annals of Internal Medicine 96: 349–357

Lewis R D, Levine L, Austen K F, Corey E J 1982 Radioimmunoassays (RIA) of the slow reacting substance of anaphylaxis (SRS-A) leukotrienes. Journal of Allergy and Clinical Immunology (supplement) 69: 93

Moss J 1985 Histamine release in anesthesia and surgery. New England and Regional Allergy Proceedings 6: 28–36
Moss J, Rosow C E, Savarese J J, Philbin D M, Kniffen K J 1981 Role of histamine in the hypotensive action of d-tubocurarine in humans. Anesthesiology 55: 19–25
Philbin D M. Moss J, Atkins C W et al 1981 The use of H_1 and H_2 histamine antagonists with morphine anesthesia: A double blind study. Anesthesiology 55: 292–296
Shnider S M, Papper E M 1961 Anesthesia for the asthmatic patient. Anesthesiology 22: 886–892
Spark R F 1975 Hypothalemic-pituitary-adrenal axis in surgery. In: Skillman J J (ed) Intensive Care Little Brown, Boston, p 311
Stein M, Koota G M, Simon M, Frank H A 1962 Pulmonary evaluation of surgical patients. Journal of American Medical Association 181: 765–770
Storms W W, Do Pico G A, Reed C E 1975 Aerosol SCH 1000 — an anticholinergic bronchodilator. American Review of Respiratory Disease 111: 419–422
Wasserman S I 1980 The lung mast cell: its physiology and potential relevance to defense of lung. Environmental Health Perspectives 35: 153–164
Weiss E B, Faling L J 1968 Clinical significance of Pa_{CO_2} during status asthmaticus: the cross-over point. Annals of Allergy 26: 545–551

4 *C. R. K Hind, S. Robertson*

Treatment of acute severe asthma

Asthma is a common and potentially lethal disease which affects 2–4% of the British population (Gregg 1983). Although individual doctors will rarely see death as the outcome of an acute asthmatic attack, over 1200 asthmatics die of their disease each year (about 2 in every 1000 British asthmatics). It is a sobering thought that despite the many recent advances made in the treatment of this disorder, there has been no improvement in the standardized mortality rates associated with asthma since the introduction of adrenaline in the late 1890s (Clark 1983). In fact this mortality rate increased dramatically in the 1960s due to overreliance on the newly introduced isoprenaline pressurized aerosols (Inman & Adelstein 1969), and more recently there has been a further increase in deaths in New Zealand (Jackson et al 1982) and a lesser trend in Great Britain (Khot & Burn 1984). This latest epidemic is thought to be related to a combination of high dose nebulized β_2-sympathomimetic agents and sustained-release theophylline preparations (Grant 1985). A survey of home nebulizer use in the UK showed that 25% of patients had never received any formal medical instructions on the use of the nebulizer, and some patients were using 50 mg salbutamol a day which is 250 times the manufacturer's recommended dose for this drug (Laroche et al 1985).

ACUTE SEVERE ASTHMA

Retrospective studies of the circumstances surrounding asthma deaths both inside and outside hospital have suggested a number of possible causes (Table 4.1) (Cochrane & Clark 1975, British Thoracic Association 1982). The rate of evolution of a severe attack is characteristically over 24 or more hours, and at post-mortem such patients' lungs have mucosal oedema and airways plugged with tenacious mucus. However some patients die within 30 minutes of an acute attack, and at post-mortem the lungs appear macroscopically and microscopically normal, suggesting that death was due to overwhelming bronchoconstriction. This is one reason why the rather vague term 'status asthmaticus' is no longer used to describe this medical emergency (Clark 1983). The term implied an asthmatic attack which was 'prolonged' (though clearly death can occur early) and unresponsive to treatment (though this was not clearly defined). As a result more clinicians now use the more straightforward term 'acute severe asthma' to describe an episode which is increasing in severity over a short period of time and which does not respond to the patient's usual treatment, or even to an increase in treatment.

Table 4.1 Factors associated with a fatal outcome from acute severe asthma

1.	Lack of patient or doctor awareness of the severity of the attack
2.	Inadequate or inappropriate treatment: e.g. underuse of corticosteroids; use of sedatives
3.	Rapid speed of onset of the terminal attack
4.	Failure of diagnosis during life e.g. labelled as a chronic bronchitic

Assessment of severity

Analysis of the records of those asthmatics who died in hospital has pointed to inadequate assessment of the asthmatic attack by the doctor which in turn led to undertreatment and, perhaps, inappropriate placement of the patient within the hospital (Ormerod & Stableforth 1980, Cochrane & Clark 1985). No single clinical feature has been shown to be a reliable gauge of severity. The most effective means of assessment involves the use of as many objective measures as possible, which should always be clearly documented. These are summarized below (Clark 1983, Cochrane 1984, Tatham & Gellert 1985).

History

The cardinal features of severe asthma are a history of decreasing exercise tolerance, sleep disturbance due to early morning attacks of wheezing, and failure to obtain relief from the usual (or an increase in) bronchodilator treatment. Patients who have an excessive diurnal variation in airway calibre are known as 'morning dippers' as they tend to have increased bronchospasm between 2–4 a.m. They and patients with brittle disease, i.e. intractable persisting asthma which is resistant to conventional therapy, are thought to be particularly at risk of catastrophically rapid attacks, with the possibility of death within minutes of the onset of the attack (MacDonald et al 1976, Hetzel et al 1977).

Examination

The signs which indicate a severe attack and which must be documented are:

1. Difficulty in speaking a sentence without a pause for breath. In severe cases the patient may be too breathless to be able to say even a single word.

2. Tachypnoea, with the use of accessory muscles.

3. Pulse rate over 110/min. Over 140/min implies severe hypoxia.

4. Pulsus paradoxus more than 10 mm Hg (i.e. an exaggeration of thc normal 5-10 mm Hg difference in systolic arterial pressure between inspiration and expiration). The mechanism of this remains uncertain. One theory is that pooling of blood within the lungs, due to dilatation of the pulmonary veins during expiration, leads to a fall in left atrial and thus left ventricular stroke volume. Even this sign may be absent, even in severe asthma, and its disappearance indicates decreasing inspiratory effect caused by exhaustion or improvement.

5. Quiet breath sounds and absent wheezes indicate that the rate of expiratory flow is very slow which is a dangerous sign. It may also mean a pneumothorax is present.

6. Cyanosis and signs of carbon dioxide retention are very late signs, and indicate an impending cardiorespiratory arrest.

Investigations

1. Measure airflow obstruction by recording the peak expiratory flow rate (PEFR) or forced expiratory volume in 1 s (FEV_1). This is the most important single observation to make, as it provides the simplest and best guide to severity. The FEV_1 and FVC are measured on a spirometer, either the conventional water-sealed type or else a 'dry' machine (e.g. Vitalograph). The PEFR is a measure of the maximum speed averaged over 10 ms, as recorded using the Wright peak flow meter. The best of three readings is taken for all of these tests of forced expiration. In a severe attack the PEFR is less than 100 l/min and FEV_1 less than 1 litre (or 30% of the predicted normal) in adults. Some patients with acute severe asthma are too breathless to perform these tests. Serial measurement (i.e. 6 hourly, before and after nebulized brochodilator treatment) is the most useful way of monitoring subsequent progress of the disease.

2. Arterial blood gas analysis should be performed in all patients admitted to hospital. The Pa_{CO_2} correlates well with severity. Any elevation of Pa_{CO_2} (i.e. above 35 mm Hg) indicates that ventilation is proving inadequate and more vigorous treatment is required.

3. A chest X-ray should be performed daily to look for evidence of collapse or infection or the presence of a pneumothorax or pneumomediastinum.

4. An electrocardiogram may reveal changes of acute pulmonary hypertension which should return to normal when the attack improves.

5. Hypokalaemia may occur during acute severe asthma , due in part to the high levels of circulating catecholamines and the renal response to stress (Webb et al 1979). This may be further aggravated by the use of nebulized β-sympathomimetic agents and oral/intravenous corticosteroids.

Treatment of Acute Severe Asthma

There is no simple formula. Every asthmatic demands careful appraisal and choice of treatment, and the clinician must always assess the response to treatment by serial PEFR (or FEV_1) measurements and blood gas analyses, and be on the lookout for associated dangers (e.g. hypokalaemia, pneumothorax). The therapy includes specific treatment to reverse airflow obstruction (Table 4.2) and general measures (Table 4.3).

Specific treatment of reverse airflow obstruction

Step 1. The initial treatment of an acute severe attack should consist of a *bronchodilator* inhaled by a nebulizer.

1. Nebulized selective *β_2-adrenergic stimulant*: e.g. salbutamol 5 mg or terbutaline 10 mg in a simple nebulizer (e.g. Inspiron 'mini-neb'). Use half these doses if there is a past history of ischaemic heart disease. Peak improvement is reached after 15 minutes and effects last up to 6 hours. This treatment may be repeated 2–4 hourly, as necessary.

Table 4.2 Acute adult severe asthma: specific treatment to reverse airflow obstruction

Step 1	
Nebulized B_2-agonist	(e.g. salbutamol 5 mg, terbutaline 10 mg)
AND	
Nebulized ipratropium bromide (500 mg)	
	If no response in 30–60 min repeat once
	If still no response — Step 2
Step 2	
Corticosteroids:	hydrocortisone 250 mg i.v. 6 hourly AND
	prednisolone 30–60 mg each morning
AND	
i.v. aminophylline:	bolus
	infusion 0.5 mg/kg/h
	monitor plasma levels 8–12 hourly

There are a number of practical points to remember. This simple nebulizer has a dead space of 0.6 ml, so the aerosol should be diluted in normal saline or water to make at least 5 ml of solution. The nebulizer must be driven by oxygen at a flow rate of at least 8 l/min, which will deliver the drug in 10–15 minutes. There is no apparent advantage to delivering the drug through an intermittent positive pressure breathing device (e.g. Bird or Bennett ventilator) (Campbell et al 1978). Intravenous administration (5 mg in 500 ml normal saline, 3–20 mg/min) has no advantages even in unconscious patients (nebulizers can be given via a ventilator), and causes more unwanted effects (e.g. tachycardia, hypokalaemia) (Lawford et al 1978, Bloomfield et al 1979).

2. Nebulized *ipratropium bromide* (500 mg–1 mg) gives additional benefit to that provided by nebulized β_2-sympathomimetic drugs (Ward et al 1981, Leahy et al 1983). Ipratropium is an atropine derivative that is a powerful anticholinergic inhibitor of vagally mediated bronchomotor tone. Peak effects are reached after 30–45 minutes, and last 3–5 hours. There are no systemic atropine-like effects (e.g. glaucoma, urinary retention) and no inhibition of mucociliary clearance (Paterson et al 1979). It has been suggested that ipratropium and the β_2-agonists may act preferentially on different parts of the bronchial tree (e.g. large conducting airways — ipratropium; small airways — β_2-agonists) but the evidence is conflicting (Ingram et al 1977, Partridge & Saunders 1981). It is important to remember to dilute the drug in 5 ml N saline and not water, as hypotonic solutions can cause bronchoconstriction.

Table 4.3 Acute adult severe asthma: general measures

Routinely used	Continuous oxygen Intravenous rehydration Monitor serum potassium
Rarely used	Antibiotics Chest physiotherapy
Never used	Sedation Bronchial lavage, unless on a ventilator (rarely)

Step 2. This is reserved for those patients who show no improvement in PEFR within 1–2 hours after 10 mg salbutamol (20 mg terbutaline) and 500 mg ipratropium by nebulizer, or for those whose initial assessment indicates that no delay in starting maximal therapy can be contemplated.

1. *Corticosteroids.* An intravenous loading dose of 200–250 mg hydrocortisone (3–4 mg/kg body weight) is given and repeated 6 hourly for 24 hours, and at the same time start oral prednisolone or increase present dose to 30–60 mg each morning. The intravenous steroid will take 4–6 hours to act, and the oral, 12–24 hours. Regular urinalysis to detect diabetes is important. The action of steroids in acute severe asthma is not understood. Certainly in vitro glucocorticoids can effect almost every stage of inflammatory and immunological activity, but only by using often supra-pharmacological doses (Kay 1983). Similarly studies of their use in acute severe asthma have produced contradictory results (Pierson et al 1974, Luksza 1982). At present, however, no firm evidence is available to show that steroids should be withheld and most clinicians feel they are safe and may be life-saving (Grant 1982).

2. *Intravenous aminophylline.* A loading dose of 5.6 mg/kg body weight is given over 15 minutes (i.e. 250–500 mg) followed by a continuous infusion of 0.5 mg/kg body weight/hour with 8–12 hourly estimations of plasma theophylline concentrations to guide dosage. A loading dose must *not* be given to patients already receiving oral sustained-release theophylline preparations (e.g. phyllocontin, uniphylline) unless the result of a plasma theophylline measurement is available. Techniques are now available for on the spot measurements (Cuss et al 1985). These sustained released theophylline preparations are reviewed in Drugs and Theraputics Bulletin 1985.

This drug has an extremely narrow therapeutic range 10–20 mg/l and potentially lethal effects (e.g. dysrythmias, general seizures, cardiac arrests) have been seen with levels as low as 25 mg/l. Such effects are not necessarily preceded by nausea, headache and vomiting (Woodcock et al 1983).

It is not possible to predict with confidence the ideal dose for a particular patient. As a result, estimation of plasma concentration is mandatory if intravenous treatment is contemplated for more than 24 hours (Conway et al 1984).

General Measures (Table 4.3)

Continuous hummidified oxygen (40%) should be given to keep the Pa_{O_2} at least above 8 KPa (when 90% of the haemoglobin is saturated), whilst monitoring the Pa_{CO_2}. If there is concern about possible CO_2 retention, start at 28% oxygen.

Intravenous hydration is necessary both to replace the excessive water losses through the lungs and because the patient may be too breathless to drink (e.g. 1–1.5 l/24h). It will also help preserve an adequate circulating volume and may help mobilize secretions. Routine antibiotic treatment is no longer given, unless there are strong indications of bacterial infection (e.g. lobar pulmonary infiltrate) (Graham et al 1982). Fever may occur in a viral or bacterial infection, and sputum which looks mucopurulent in most cases contains predominantly eosinophils rather than neutrophils. Similarly chest physiotherapy is not indicated unless the chest X-ray indicates lung collapse associated with mucus impaction, or the patient needs help with the use of nebulizers. However severely affected and exhausted patients will not be able to co-operate with the physiotherapist.

Artificial Ventilation

A small number of patients do not improve in spite of maximal therapy and require ventilation. In a 9 year period 1% of all hospital admissions for asthma in one series required ventilation. 40% of these died (Scoggin et al 1977). Other reports have an approximate 10% death rate (Westerman et al; Sheehy et al 1972). The indications for ventilation were surprisingly uniform and were:

1. Drowsiness and confusion
2. CO_2 retention
3. Morbidity in casualty or
4. A cardiac arrest

Table 4.4 outlines a suggested criteria for ventilation. Acute asthmatics have hyperinflated lungs and have to exert a lot of energy in expiration. During an asthmatic attack the mechanical work of ventilation is two to nine times greater than normal and peak airway pressures up to 70 cm of water may be generated (Dacosta & Hedstrand 1970). Expiration is prolonged in an effort to expel the total tidal volume. With artificial ventilation it is important to lengthen the expiratory cycle so as to give a long enough period for inspiration as well as a long expiratory time otherwise inflation pressures will be unacceptably high for the necessary tidal volume. If all the tidal volume is not expired then air trapping will occur giving further lung distension causing lung damage with stretching and distortion of lung capillaries. This causes an increase in pulmonary resistance which will result in a low cardiac output and lead to right heart failure. Thus in the acute asthmatic patient it is important to choose a low minute volume with a slow rate (Branthwaite 1978). The Pa_{CO_2} may well rise from underventilation but the patient will not come to harm unless there is a gross acidosis which can be corrected by sodium bicarbonate (Menitove et al 1983). The hypercarbia will make the patient fight the ventilator so it is important to keep the patient well sedated and if necessary paralysed. Positive end expiratory pressure has no place in asthma as it will cause overdistension of the lungs as the air has greater difficulty in escaping during the expiratory phase time.

Induction of these distressed and hypoxic patients can be difficult and dangerous. A semi-elective procedure should be anticipated before the patient becomes

Table 4.4 Suggested indications for ventilation based on sequential observations

1.	Exhaustion, intolerable distress
2.	Evidence of deterioration in pulmonary function $Pa_{O_2} < 6.7$ KPa (50 mmHg) and falling $Pa_{CO_2} > 6.7$ KPa (50 mmHg) and rising
3.	Evidence of deterioration in cardiac function hypotension, cardiac dysrhythmia
4.	Emergency indications cardiac or respiratory arrest irreversible respiratory depression due to drugs (e.g. sedatives) lung collapse, acute pneumothorax, acute pneumomediastinum

moribund. Webb et al (1979) suggested a gas induction in the semi-recumbent position with the bronchodilating agent halothane (Schnider & Papper 1961, Hirshman et al 1978a). However careful monitoring of the heart must be carried out as halothane sensitizes the myocardium to the dysrhythmic effects of catecholamines (Wood et al 1968). Ether also relieves bronchospasm and is useful in experienced hands but it has been generally replaced by newer agents with fewer side effects. Enflurane and isoflurane are known to be bronchodilators in the non-asthmatic (Wood et al 1968) and reported clinical experience with these agents is awaited. They are less likely to give arrythmias in the presence of adrenaline or aminophylline (Stirt et al 1981, 1983). It is important not to intubate too early as reflex bronchospasm may occur with instrumentation or as the endotracheal tube enters the trachea. Webb et al (1979) suggested using a lignocaine spray to prevent reflex (irritant) bronchospasm. Downes & Hirshman (1981) suggest it may not prevent bronchoconstriction. Intravenous lignocaine has been found useful in treating bronchospasm (Brandus et al 1970) but its effect on the myocardium and brain should temper its usage.

Some anaesthetists prefer an intravenous induction with a relaxant. Ketamine has been shown by several workers to improve bronchospasm and be a useful induction agent (Betts & Parkin 1971, Corssen et al 1972). Convulsive-like movements have been noted when an aminophylline infusion has been used at the same time (Hirshman et al 1982b). Suxamethonium is the most frequently used rapidly acting muscle relaxant. There are very few reports of bronchospasm following suxamethonium (Fellini et al 1963, Eustace 1967) so it would appear to be a safe agent.

Once intubation has occurred, total paralysis by a long acting muscle relaxant must be achieved and control of respiration obtained by manual ventilation. D-Tubocurarine is associated with histamine release (Salem et al 1968, Moss & Roscow 1983) and for this reason it is considered to be contra-indicated in asthma. Fung (1985) points out there is no real evidence of D-tubocurarine being associated with worsening of bronchospasm. Pancuronium has been the choice of relaxant for many years because of its low potential for the release of histamine and appears to be a safe agent (Nana et al 1972) but there has been a report of bronchospasm in an asthmatic (Heath 1973). Because of expense and shortness of action there would seem to be no place for vecuronium and atracurium in the long term ventilation of an asthmatic.

Ventilator The ventilator used should be capable of giving a preset volume in the face of increased airways resistance and the facility to increase the expiratory time. Minute volumes should be low, i.e. 6–8 litres in an average adult with a rate of 10–14 breaths per minute. The expiratory phase should be 50% of the respiratory cycle (Branthwaite 1978). The required inspired O_2 level should be determined from several blood gas estimations to keep the $P\text{O}_2$ above 8 kPa. Although oxygen toxicity may be a clinical entity it is vital the patient does not become brain damaged from hypoxia. By accurately measuring the chest wall at regular intervals with a tape measure an increase in diameter by one centimetre or more will suggest air trapping and the minute volume will have to be decreased. On listening to the expiratory ventilator tubing detached from the ventilator it should be possible to hear the end of expiration before the next cycle starts. If this does not happen air trapping will occur.

After the start of artificial ventilation it is not uncommon for the blood pressure to drop to low levels. This may be due to right-sided heart failure but it is more likely to be due to a relative hypovolaemia caused by dehydration giving a low filling pressure. The patient may have a normal or high central venous pressure because of the increased pulmonary vascular pressure from distortion and stretching of the capillaries. The giving of aliquots of colloid such as 4% human albumin solution (plasma protein fraction) or gelatine solutions in 200 ml boluses every 10 minutes should bring the blood pressure to acceptable levels, i.e. high enough to produce a urinary output (Webb et al 1979). Cardiac failure will ensue if too much fluid is given. If possible the patient's low circulating volume should be corrected before intubation.

Opiates are commonly used to maintain sedation and respiratory depression in ventilated patients. Morphine is capable of releasing histamine and has been shown to have a bronchoconstrictive effect in asthma (Blumberg 1973). However morphine (Pontoppidan et al 1972) and phenoperidine (Webb et al 1979) have been used successfully. Fentanyl does not release histamine (Moss & Roscow 1983) and is relatively cardiac stable. Pethidine in spite of its bronchial spasmolytic effect has produced bronchospasm in asthmatics. Diazepam has been shown not to aggravate bronchospasm in asthmatics (Heinonen & Muittari 1972) but it must be remembered it has a long duration of action and active metabolites. Reports are awaited on the usefulness of midazolam. Most clinicians find the combination of a muscle relaxant such as pancuronium and small doses of opiate satisfactory. It is necessary to give the drugs in adequate doses and regularly to prevent 'fighting' and accidents on the ventilator.

Care must be taken to humidify the inspired gases. Mucus plugging associated with atelectasis and poor oxygenation is often a problem before and during ventilation. Bronchial lavage in the hypoxic patient is dangerous as it can give further hypoxia leading to life threatening arrythmias and brain damage. In adults the instillation of 2 ml of normal saline via the endotracheal tube every half hour will, in less than 24 hours, and with the aid of skilled physiotherapy, bring up large amounts of secretions. Bromhexine was used routinely by Webb et al (1979).

Artificial ventilation is only supportive therapy and it is important to continue bronchodilator and steroid treatment at maximal doses. Bronchodilating agents can be given by nebulizers inserted in the ventilator tubing circuit. Antibiotics should not be given unless there is very good evidence of a chest infection or septicaemia. There must be careful attention to cumulative fluid balance as chronic fluid overload will make it difficult to wean the patient off the ventilator. If heart failure develops inotrophic agents will be required.

The complications for artificial ventilation of asthmatics include pneumothorax pneumomediastinum cardiac arrythmias, right-sided heart failure, atelectasis and pneumonia, and accidents with the apparatus. These complications were common to most of the series reviewed including children (Wood et al 1968).

Patients can be classified according to the time they spend on a ventilator into two main groups:

1. Those patients who are ventilated for exhaustion, who have little or no lung damage and respond quickly to therapy usually only require 24–72 hours. These patients have powerful muscles of respiration and weaning is not necessary. Unfortunately extubation is not always easy due to reflex bronchospasm from the

endotracheal tube. Small doses of diazepam and extubation with experienced supervision may be successful. Extubation can be tried with the patient anaesthetized with halothane.

2. The second group are often older, have some degree of pulmonary or cardiac failure, have a poor response to bronchodilator drugs or considerable atelectasis. These patients usually require to be ventilated for 2 weeks or more. Tracheostomy should be carried out if ventilation is predicted to last more than 3 weeks as it makes nursing and weaning (which can be protracted) easier. It must be remembered that these patients may require artificial ventilation again at a later date so the decision to do a tracheostomy should be made with considerable thought.

Lenggenhager (1985) suggests the use of a low pressure chamber with 100% oxygen in the treatment of acute bronchospasm. Clinical observation that the resistance of airways is reduced at high altitudes is supported by model experiments, by theoretical considerations and by measurement of the maximal breathing capacity at low barometric pressures. He has tried the low pressure chamber in acute asthma with some success.

Acute severe asthma is a frightening, complex and difficult condition to treat and the adverse effects of the drugs used are as dangerous as the disease itself. It is important to recognize the danger signs of a severe attack (Table 4.4) and institute artificial ventilation before mucus plugging and atelectasis is widespread or a cardiac arrest has occurred. The significant mortality of the past should now improve with the greater understanding of the disease and its therapy.

Anaesthesia for the asthmatic patient has not been reviewed in this article but is considered by Galant in Chapter 3. See also review articles by Fury (1985) and Kingston & Hirshman (1985).

REFERENCES

Betts E K, Parkin C E 1971 Use of ketamine in an asthmatic child. A case report. Anesthesia and Analgesia 50: 420

Bloomfield P, Charmichael J, Petrie G R, Jewell N P, Crompton G K 1979 Comparison of salbutamol given intravenously and by intermittent positive-pressure breathing in life threatening asthma. British Medical Journal 1: 848–850

Blumberg M Z 1973 Morphine for severe asthma? New England Journal of Medicine 288: 50

Brandus V, Jotte S, Benoit C V, Wolff W I 1970 Bronchial spasm during general anaesthesia. Canadian Anaesthetists Society Journal 17: 269–274

Branthwaite M A 1978 Artificial ventilation for pulmonary disease. Private printing for Brompton Hospital, p 9–11 (Available £2)

British Thoracic Association 1982 Death from asthma in two regions of England. British Medical Journal 285: 1251–1255

Campbell I A, Hill A, Middleton H, Momen M, Prescott R J 1978 Intermittent positive pressure breathing. British Medical Journal 1: 1186–1189

Clark T J H 1983 Acute severe asthma. In: Clark T J H, Godfrey S (eds) Asthma, 2nd edn. Chapman and Hall, London, ch 17, p 393–414

Cochrane G M 1984 The role of bronchodilators in severe acute asthma. In: Clark T J H (ed) Bronchodilator therapy. Adis, New Zealand, Ch 10, p 167–187

Cochrane G H, Clark T J H 1975 A survey of asthma mortality in patients between ages 35 and 64 in the Greater London Hospitals in 1971 Thorax 30: 300–305

Conway S P, Gillies D R N, Littlewood J N 1984 Intravenous aminophylline in acutely ill patients receiving theophylline. British Medical Journal 288: 715–716

Corssen G, Gutierrez J, Reves J G, Huber F C 1972 Ketamine in the anaesthetic management of asthmatic patients. Anesthesia and Analgesia 51: 588–596

Cuss F M, Palmer J B, Barnes P J 1985 Rapid estimation of plasma theophylline concentrations. British Medical Journal 291: 384

Dacosta J, Hedstrand U 1970 The mechanical work of breathing during controlled ventilation in normal subjects and patients with bronchial asthma. Acta Societatis Medicorum Upsaliensis 75: 110–118
Downes H, Hirshman C A 1981 Lidocaine aerosols do not prevent allergic bronchoconstriction. Anesthesia and Analgesia 60: 28–32
Drugs and Therapeutics Bulletin 1985 Sustained release theophylline preparations. 23: 33–36
Eustace B R 1967 Case Report. Suxamethonium induced bronchospasm. Anaesthesia 22: 638–641
Fellini A A, Bernstein R L, Zauder H L 1963 Bronchospasm due to suxamethonium. Report of a case. British Journal of Anaesthesia 35: 657–659
Fung D L 1985 Emergency anaesthesia for asthma patients. Clinical Reviews in Allergy 3: 127–141
Graham V A L, Milton A F, Knowles G K, Davies R J 1982 Routine antibiotics in hospital management of acute asthma. Lancet 1: 418–421
Grant I W B 1985 Asthma in New Zealand. British Medical Journal 286: 374–377
Grant I W B 1982 Are corticosteroids necessary in the treatment of severe acute asthma. British Journal of Diseases of the Chest 76: 125–129
Greenberger P A, Patterson R 1985 Management of asthma during pregnancy. New England Journal of Medicine 312: 897–902
Gregg I 1983 Epidemiology. In: Clark T J H, Godfrey S (eds) Asthma. Chapman and Hall, London, ch 11: p 242–284
Heath M L 1973 Case Report. Bronchospasm in an asthmatic patient following pancuronium. Anaesthesia 28: 437–440
Heinonen J, Muittari A 1972 The effect of diazepam on airways resistance in asthmatics. Anaesthesia 27: 37–40
Hetzel M R, Clark T J H 1983 Adult asthma. In: Clark T J H, Godfrey S (eds) Asthma, 2nd edn. Chapman and Hall, London, ch 19, p 457–489
Hetzel M R, Clark T J H, Branthwaite M A 1977 Asthma: analysis of sudden deaths and ventilatory arrest in hospital. British Medical Journal 1: 808–811
Hirshman C A, Edelstein G, Peetz A, Wayne R, Downes H 1982a Mechanisms of action of inhalation anaesthesia on airways. Anesthesiology 56: 107–111
Hirshman C A, Kreiger W, Littlejohn G, Lee R, Julien R 1982b Ketamine aminophilline induced decrease in seizure threshold. Anesthesiology 56: 464–467
Ingram R H, Wellman J J, McFadden E R, Mead J 1977 Relative contributions of large and small airways to flow limitation in normal subjects and after atropine and isoprenaline. Journal of Clinical Investigation 59: 696–703
Inman W H W, Adelstein A M 1969 Rise and fall of asthma mortality in England and Wales in relation to use of pressurised aerosols. Lancet ii: 279–285
Isles A F, MacLeod S M, Levison H 1982 Theophylline — new thoughts about an old drug. Chest 82: 495–511
Jackson R T, Beaglehole R, Rea H H 1982 Mortality from asthma: a new epidemic in New Zealand. British Medical Journal 285: 771–774
Kay A B 1983 The immunological basis of asthma. In: Clark T J H (ed) Steroids in Asthma. Adis, London, ch 3, p 46–48
Khot A, Burn R 1984 Deaths from asthma. British Medical Journal 289: 557
Kingston R, Hirshman C A 1984 Perioperatic management of asthma. Anesthesia and Analgesia 63: 844–855
Laroche C M, Harries A Y K, Weston R C F, Britton M G 1985 Domicilary nebulisers in asthma: a district survey. British Medical Journal 290: 1611–1613
Lawford P, Jones B J M, Milledge J S 1978 Comparison of intravenous and nebulised salbutamol in initial treatment of severe asthma. British Medical Journal 1: 84
Leahy B C, Gomm S A, Allen S C 1983 Comparison of nebulised salbutamol with nebulised ipratropium bromide in acute asthma. British Journal of Diseases of the Chest 77: 159–163
Lenggenhager K 1985 Treatment of severe bronchial asthma with a low pressure chamber and 100% O_2. Anesthesia and Analgesia 64: 551–553
Luksza A R 1982 Acute severe asthma treated without steroids. British Journal of Diseases of the Chest 76: 15–19
MacDonald J B, Seaton A, Williams D A 1976 Asthma deaths in Cardiff 1963–1974: 90 deaths outside hospital. British Medical Journal 1: 1493–1495
Menitove S M, Goldring R M 1983 Combined ventilator and bicarbonate strategy in the management of status asthmaticus. American Journal of Medicine. 74: 398–901
Moss J, Roscow C E 1983 Histamine release by narcotics and muscle relaxants in humans. Anesthesiology 59: 330–339

Nana A, Cardan E, Leittersdorfer T 1972 Pancuronium bromide: its use in asthmatics and patients with liver disease. Anaesthesia 27: 154–158
Ormerod L P, Stableforth D E 1980 Asthma mentality in Birmingham. British Medical Journal 1: 687–690
Partridge M R, Saunders K B 1981 Site of action of ipratropium bromide and clinical and physiological determinants of response in patients with asthma. Thorax 36: 530–533
Paterson J W, Woolcock A J, Shenfield G M 1979 Bronchodilator drugs. American Review of Respiratory Disease 120: 1149–1188
Pierson W E, Bierman C W, Kelley V C 1974 A double-blind trial of corticosteroid therapy in status asthmaticus. Paediatrics 54: 282–287
Pontoppidan H, Geffin B, Lowenstein E 1972 Acute respiratory failure in the adult. New England Journal of Medicine 287: 743–752
Salem M R, El Kim Y, Etr A A 1968 Histamine release following intravenous injection of d-tubocurarine. Anesthesiology 29: 380–382
Scoggin C H, Shalin S A, Petty T L 1977 Status asthmaticus: a nine year experience. Journal of the American Medical Association 283: 1158–1162
Sheehy A F, Di Benedetto R, Lefrak S, Lyons H A 1972 Treatment of status asthmatacus. A report of 70 episodes. Archives of Internal Medicine 130: 37–42
Shnider S M, Papper E M 1961 Anaesthesia for the asthmatic patient. Anesthesiology 22: 886–892
Stirt J A, Berger J M, Roe S D, Ricker S M, Sullivan S F 1981 Safety of enflurane following the administration of aminophyline in experimental animals. Anesthesia and Analgesia 60: 871–873
Stirt J A, Berger J M, Sullivan S F 1983 Lack of arrythmogenicity of isoflurane following the administration of aminophyline in dogs. Anesthesia and Analgesia 62: 586–671
Tatham M E, Gellert A R 1985 The management of acute asthma. Postgraduate Medical Journal 61: 599–606
Ward M J, Fentem P H, Smith R W H, Davies D 1981 Ipratropium bromide in acute asthma. British Medical Journal 282: 598–600
Ward M J, MacFarlane J T, Davies P 1982 Treatment of acute severe asthma with intravenous aminophylline and nebulised ipratropium after salbutamol. Thorax 37: 785
Webb A K, Bilton A H, Hanson G C 1979 Severe bronchial asthma requiring ventilation. A review of 20 cases and advice on management. Postgraduate Medical Journal 55: 161–170
Westerman D E, Benatar S R, Potgieter P D, Ferguson A D 1979 Identification of the high risk asthmatic patient, experience of 39 patients undergoing ventilation for status asthmaticus. American Journal of Medicine 66: 565–572
Wood D W, Downes J J, Lecks H I 1968 The management of respiratory failure in childhood status asthmaticus. Experience with 30 episodes and evaluation of a technique. Journal of Allergy 42: 261–267
Woodcock A A, Johnson M A, Geddes D M 1983 Theophylline prescribing, serum concentrations and toxicity. Lancet ii: 610–612

5 *E. Grundy*

High frequency ventilation

INTRODUCTION

Effective gas exchange in the lung requires the presention of fresh gas to the alveolus and the removal of used gas from the alveolus. The size and metabolic state of the patient determines the amount of gas required per minute. Conventional artificial ventilation uses rates and tidal volumes within the physiological range. However, recently the idea of using small tidal volumes appeared attractive as this was seen to be associated with a lower peak inspiratory airway pressure and less fluctuation in intrathoracic pressure. This inevitably meant the use of higher ventilatory frequencies.

Ventilation with tidal volumes of less than anatomical dead space volume can provide adequate gas exchange. The giraffe and swan (with their long necks and long tracheas) manage this routinely and it has been known for some time that carbon dioxide removal can be achieved in man with tidal volumes of considerably less than anatomic dead space (Briscoe et al 1954). However, the mechanisms of achieving this are not immediately obvious and have been recently reviewed by Drazen et al (1984).

SMALL TIDAL VOLUME

Traditional

The conventional model of ventilation has fresh gas being presented at pressure at the airway opening; this gas then flows turbulently through the anatomical dead space and 'flushes it out', before appearing at the level of the alveolus. This bulk convection thus takes gas from the airway opening to the alveolar zone. At the alveolus the fresh gas forms an interface with the alveolar gas, further onward movement is then by molecular diffusion, and this takes the gas across the alveolar zone, across the alveolar-capillary membrane and into the pulmonary capillaries. In man molecular diffusion probably takes less than 10 ms. This model works well for larger tidal volumes producing turbulent flow, as can be seen for tidal volumes of above 400 ml in Fig. 5.1. However, at lower tidal volumes more gas gets through to take part in gas exchange than this conventional model predicts.

Nearby alveoli

The transition from the conducting airways, with no gas exchanging function, to the alveolar sacs where only gas exchange takes place, is not sharply demarcated

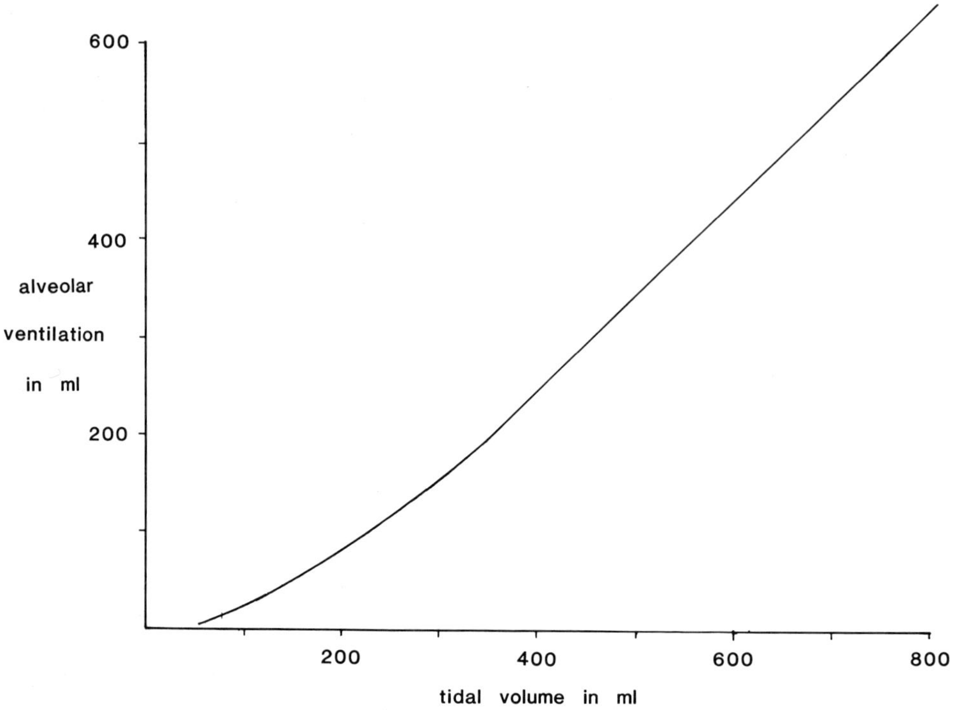

Fig. 5.1

anatomically. The respiratory bronchioles (17th–19th generation) are predominantly conducting airways but do have alveolar sacs opening off them. The alveolar ducts (20th–22nd generation) have gas exchanging epithelium throughout and in addition conduct gas to the alveolar sacs (23rd generation).

Thus any gas that penetrates to the 17th generation air passage by bulk convection will take part in gas exchange and, whereas a small tidal volume will only do this, a normal tidal volume will penetrate right through to the 23rd generation air passages.

Asymmetric velocity profiles

If the flow profiles during inspiration and expiration are different, bulk convection occurs (Haselton & Scherer 1980). If inspiratory flow is laminar, a given block of gas takes up a parobilic profile, and if this is then followed by a turbulent expiratory flow, a square wave pushes the parabolic profile back en bloc. Thus, although the overall result is no net gas movement, in fact there has been axial convection of gas towards the lung periphery and the peripheral gas has moved towards the airway opening. Measurement of velocity profiles in models of the human central airways have shown that inspiratory and expiratory velocity profiles are significantly different from each other, and so this mechanism contributes to bulk convection at small tidal volumes.

Pendelluft

Within the lung differing areas of lung have different time constants. Thus some areas of the lung are fast fillers with short time constants, whereas other areas are slow fillers with long time constants. During early inspiration the fast filling areas become full and during late inspiration are actually emptying into the slow fillers. This is Pendelluft, where the sum of gas movement within the lung is greater than the gas flow down the trachea, i.e. there is gas movement between areas of the lung without gas movement in the trachea. It is apparent that with high frequency ventilation, a slow filler could still be filling from a fast filler which at the same time is providing gas for expiration up the trachea (Lehr 1980).

Taylor dispersion

This is probably the major mechanism of gas movement at small tidal volume and involves augmented axial convection. If the volume of gas entering the airway is small and the flow is laminar the velocity profile in the airway will be parabolic and therefore the gas in the axis of the airway will penetrate much more deeply. The longer the duration of inspiration the more accentuated this spike of augmented axial convection becomes: e.g. over 3 units of time, the gas at the peripheral ring remains stationary whereas the axial gas has travelled three times the distance. As this axial spike of gas penetrates into the gas exchanging units of the lung periphery, the spike of fresh gas exposes a large area of interface with alveolar gas (vide infra).

Molecular diffusion

As we have seen earlier with conventional ventilation, fresh gas is presented at the alveolus and molecular diffusion across the alveolar zone is complete within less than 10 ms. Even with high frequency ventilation, inspiratory times are considerably in excess of 10 ms (see Table 5.2). Thus there is the potential for molecular diffusion to take on a considerably greater role in the movement of gas across the alveoli. It can be appreciated that with Taylor dispersion the spike of augmented axial convection produces a dramatic increase in the interface between fresh gas and alveolar gas thus allowing molecular diffusion an enhanced role in the movement of gas. Slutsky et al (1980) have produced a theroretical model on these assumptions and compared it convincingly with an experimental preparation.

Summary

These mechanisms can explain adequately how, with a small tidal volume, there is bulk convection of gas from the airway opening to the region of the alveolar zone, where an enhanced role for molecular diffusion permits adequate alveolar gas exchange. Now we must consider the influence of high frequency ventilation on gas exchange.

HIGH VENTILATORY FREQUENCY

Time constant

Our conventional model of ventilation has a mass of gas presented at the airway opening under pressure. This potential energy is converted to kinetic energy to allow the gas to flow along the airway. However, by the end of inspiration this gas is static, the kinetic energy having become potential energy again, stored by distension of the alveoli in the lung units. The time course for this change is determined by the 'time constant' for the lung (the product of total lung compliance and airways resistance). Representative values for time constants can be seen in Table 5.1. It is known that

Table 5.1 Representative values of respiratory parameters for adults in various situations

	Total lung compliance (ml cm H_2 0^{-1})	Airway resistance (cm H_2 0.1^{-1} s)	Time constant (ms)
Normal adult	100	1	100
Anaesthetized adult	50	5	250
Adult respiratory distress syndrome	20	20	400

95% of change has occured within three time constants, and the inspiratory time available with increasing respiratory frequency can be seen from Table 5.2. It can be appreciated rapidly that with higher frequencies, especially with lung pathology (and hence longer time constants) there will be insufficient time for inspiration to go to completion, that is with static gas distending alveoli. It therefore follows that with higher ventilatory frequencies either a reduced tidal volume is delivered to the lung periphery or a higher peak inspiratory pressure is required in order to force the gas to the lung periphery within the available time (two-thirds of the gas will enter within one time constant).

Table 5.2 Duration of inspiration at increasing ventilatory frequency assuming that inspiration occurs over 25% of the ventilatory cycle

Ventilatory min^{-1}	Frequency Hz	Duration of inspiration ms
15	0.25	1000
30	0.5	500
60	1	250
120	2	125
240	4	62
480	8	31
960	16	16
1920	32	8

Airway resistance

This is unfortunately not a constant value and alters as flow changes from laminar to turbulent. Fortunately within the flow range used with conventional ventilation the magnitude of change is small: the assumption of a constant value for airways resistance introduces only minimal error. However, without this flow range a significant error is introduced.

Gas inertia

Of increasing relevance is the kinetic energy of the molecules of gas undergoing bulk convection — as ventilation cycles from inspiration to expiration they will still retain their foreward kinetic energy and continue to progress peripherally into the lung until this kinetic energy has become dissipated. This inertia of the gas molecules is not present with conventional ventilation (where end inpiration is a static state) but obviously will become increasingly important with higher ventilatory frequencies with their shorter inspiratory times, higher inspiratory flow rates and hence higher kinetic energy of gas molecules.

Impedance

The pressure–flow relationships at conventional ventilatory frequencies are adequately expressed by airways resistance. With higher ventilator frequencies airways resistance can no longer be assumed to be constant and inertia makes an increasing contribution — impedance is the parameter used to express the pressure–flow relationships at high ventilatory frequency and it is dependant on both frequency and flow rate.

It has been shown (Gavriely et al 1985) that the largest component of impedance to a high frequency generator lies in the endotracheal tube. This impedance was greatest with a wide bore endotracheal tube and high gas flow rates (large tidal volumes at high frequency). These are the conditions under which the influence of gas inertance would be maximal thus supporting the position of Taylor dispersion with augmented axial convection as the major mechanism of bulk gas movement during high frequency ventilation.

Distribution

Effective respiration, i.e. gas exchange, requires that regional ventilation and perfusion be matched. With conventional respiratory rates, regional ventilation is determined by regional compliance. However, with higher respiratory rates airways resistance and gas inertance have an increasing influence over the distribution of ventilation. Potentially this will result in a change in the distribution of ventilation from areas of high compliance to areas of low impedance. One assumes there is no corresponding change in regional lung perfusion and to date there is no evidence to the contrary, i.e. perfusion remains gravity dependant.

Path length

Another aspect of the higher ventilatory frequencies used is the time available for the bulk convection of gas during inspiration and expiration and the path length it must travel. This is some 20–25 cm from the laryngeal inlet in adult man, but much less in the neonate and most experimental animals. Thus the tidal volume presented at the airway opening will progressively distend the major conducting airways, then the nearby fast alveoli and finally the peripheral slow alveoli. With progressive shortening of inspiration a situation will arise when there is not enough time for the tidal volume to get past the major conducting airways (non gas exchanging units) which therefore act in a way analogous to a capacitor. By implication this also means that the pressure at the airway opening is not transmitted through to the lung periphery and hence the pleural space. However the reverse will also occur during expiration, namely there will not be enough time for intra-alveolar pressure to empty the alveoli. Thus there will be continuous positive airway pressure in the peripheral lung units — the very units where small airway closure is most likely to occur.

EXPERIMENTAL

Delivery system

One cannot look at the experimental results without being aware of the mechanism used to deliver the low tidal volume high frequency ventilation. This area is largely technical: however an appreciation of the delivery systems and their inherent limitations allows a fuller insight into high frequency ventilation.

For adult man it is generally accepted that high frequency ventilation is any rate greater than 1 Hz. It should be noted that the range of ventilatory frequencies given below is arbitary and mostly determined by the technical considerations of the ventilator.

High frequency positive pressure ventilation (HFPPV) (1–2 Hz)

Conventional ventilators deliver a volume of gas during inspiration by occlusion of a relatively wide bore expiratory limb. The mechanical device used to occlude the expiratory limb must function rapidly. It will have a certain mass and hence inertia — the more rapidly it is moved the shorter the response time and the more likely valve bounce is to occur. This is a fundamental problem that means that conventional ventilators are inappropriate for rates above 2 Hz; however they have the advantage of delivering a known volume of gas of known composition.

High frequency jet ventilation (HFJV) (2–6 Hz)

These ventilators allow a high pressure gas source to flow into the airway during part of the respiratory cycle — empirically inspiratory times of 20–35% of the respiratory cycle time have been found most efficient. With a jet ventilator the inspiratory flow is delivered through a narrow (1–2 mm diameter) tube usually at tracheal level. A variant is the flow interrupter type of ventilator when the entire cross section of the airway is utilized for inspiratory flow. These systems require no pneumatic seal of the expiratory limb and hence this is open to atmosphere throughout the cycle. This potentially results in the entrainment of an unknown volume of air (ambient gas): thus the volume and composition of the tidal volume are unknown. However, this open system has the inherent advantage of allowing the patient to take a spontaneous breath at any time during the respiratory cycle which is a major safety feature and of great advantage when weaning a patient.

High frequency oscillation (HFO) (6–40 Hz)

Oscillator type ventilators tend to be used for the higher frequencies. They consist of either a piston driven by a motor or a diaphragm driven electronically at the airway opening generating a to and fro motion of the gas within the airways. The tidal volume is determined by the volume displaced by the piston or diaphragm. This type of ventilator generates a negative pressure during expiration which is thus an active phase of ventilation. Fresh gas is fed in at the airway opening and a low pass filter exhaust port allows excess gas to exit the system (i.e. the low pass filter offers high impedance to high frequencies; thus the tidal volume generated tends to pass down the lower impedance offered by the airway opening rather than be lost through the exhaust port).

External

Certain experimental models have applied high frequency oscillations on the pleural surface of the lung or the chest wall. This latter method can cause damage to the underlying lung. The future of this approach is uncertain.

Carbon dioxide elimination

Low tidal volume

Ventilation with conventional ventilators at low tidal volumes has revealed carbon dioxide in the expired gases with tidal volumes as low as 50–75 ml. However, there does appear to be a cut off point below which no carbon dioxide is detectable in the expiratory gas and conversely all studies have shown increasing carbon dioxide elimination with increasing tidal volume.

High frequency

On theoretical grounds one could anticipate that ventilation with a fixed tidal volume would show a linear relationship between carbon dioxide removal and ventilatory frequency until a time is reached when the duration of inspiration is not long enough to permit the gas to penetrate the conducting airways and reach the gas exchanging areas of the lung. It has been shown in both human adult volunteers (Goldstein et al 1981) and adult patients (Rossing et al 1981) that there was a critical ventilatory frequency of between 3–6 Hz at which carbon dioxide elimination reached a plateau. Above this frequency carbon dioxide elimination was a function of the applied tidal volume and independant of the ventilatory frequency. (NB This critical frequency is undoubtedly dependent on the anatomy of the lung and is certainly higher in dogs and neonates.)

Airway resistance

Goldstein et al (1981) showed that carbon dioxide elimination was dependent on lung volume, being increased at higher lung volume. They also showed increased carbon dioxide elimination after the inhalation of isoprenaline. The presumption is that a reduction in airways' resistance associated with both of these manoeuvres has allowed more effective penetration of the delivered tidal volume to the alveolar zone.

Oxygen delivery

One of the original hopes for high frequency ventilation was that a change from compliance/airway resistance distribution of ventilation to one determined by airway resistance/gas inertia would result in a redistribution and improvement in ventilation. However, it is now accepted that, at equivalent lung volumes, there is no improvement in arterial oxygen tension.

CLINICAL

Introduction

The indiscriminate use of high frequency ventilation offers no theoretical advantage over conventional mechanical ventilation and is not currently recommended (Crawford & Rehder 1985). However, there are a number of special situations where high frequency ventilation may have a role to play.

Endoscopy of the airway

The use of a jet ventilator for airway endoscopy permits near unobstructed access to the surgical field, and the use of high frequency reduces respiratory movement of the surgical field and is enthusiastically used in some centres. (Borg et al 1980). However, ventilation with such an open system denies the anaesthetist accurate information about the tidal volume and the inspiratory gases (vide infra).

Bronchopleural fistula

There are now a number of cases reporting effective ventilation by high frequency jet ventilation after failure of conventional ventilatory techniques. The assumption must be that the distribution of ventilation shifts from compliance determined to airway resistance/gas inertance determined. These patients represent a group where high frequency ventilation offers a lifeline in what was previously often a hopeless situation.

Weaning from ventilator

The majority of patients wean rapidly and readily from ventilatory support on a T-piece circuit. Failure of conventional T-piece weaning can present a clinical problem. The open circuit of the high frequency jet ventilator offers many advantages — it is in essence a circuit which allows the patient to take a breath of fresh gas whenever he will, whilst in addition the jet ventilator can cycle away offering respiratory support and carbon dioxide elimination. Progressive reduction of the high frequency contribution to ventilation will permit progressive weaning. The early literature suggested that high frequency ventilation produced reflexogenic central apnoea per se: however this has now been shown to be secondary to lung distension by the PEEP effect.

Adult respiratory distress syndrome (ARDS)

The adult respiratory distress syndrome patient can be notoriously difficult to achieve good respiratory gas exchange at acceptable airway pressures. The theoretical advantages of high frequency ventilation are: (1) reduced pulmonary barotrauma as small tidal volume ventilation achieves effective minute ventilation at a lower peak and mean airway pressure; (2) less cardiovascular impairment, also because of the lower airway pressure; and (3) a distribution of ventilation less dependent on regional compliance. All three factors should be to the patients advantage in this syndrome: however the hope that high frequency ventilation would revolutionize ventilatory support for these patients has yet to be realized.

Humidification

Several of the early reports of high frequency ventilation reported the problem of profuse secretions shortly after the initiation of high frequency ventilation. This was probably a consequence of the use of dry gases, and more recent reports do not mention this problem. The desirability of humidifying the inspired gases is obvious, but it is often a difficult technical problem with high frequency ventilators.

Monitoring

Conventional ventilators, with their controlled and isolated inspiratory phase, offer many parameters to monitor such as inspiratory tidal volume, $F\text{I}_{O_2}$, airway pressure, or expiratory volume, $F\text{E}_{CO_2}$. With the open system of the high frequency jet ventilator the tidal volume, $F\text{I}_{O_2}$, $F\text{E}_{CO_2}$ and airway pressure are not measureable. In addition, with a tidal volume of 100 ml the chest expansion is only of the order of 2–3 mm and barely detectable.

Thus the monitoring of high frequency ventilation on a breath to breath basis is not possible, and one must rely on intermittent measurements, such as arterial blood gases or occasional large tidal volumes to generate an end tidal CO_2. It is possible that future developments with transcutaneous or intravascular electrodes may solve this problem.

CONCLUSION

There are sound theoretical reasons to explain why low volume high frequency ventilation should achieve adequate gas exchange. In adult man tidal volumes as low as 50–75 ml can be used but ventilatory frequencies above 3–6 Hz do not appear to offer any advantage (higher frequencies may be appropriate for a neonate). Consequently the place of high frequency oscillation in adults is unclear.

Clinically the required frequencies can be supplied by a jet ventilator which has the safety advantage of utilizing an open system. The technique has become established for airway endoscopy in the operating theatre. In intensive care it is of accepted value in the ventilation of patients with bronchopleural fistula and possibly in patients proving difficult to wean from a ventilator.

It is, as yet, of no proven advantage in the adult respiratory distress syndrome, despite having a number of theoretical advantages.

The main clinical problem is the monitoring of ventilation and by implication effective gas exchange. As yet this can only be determined intermittently, such as with arterial blood gas analysis, and remains a major problem with a sick unstable patient.

REFERENCES

Borg U, Eriksson I, Sjostrand U 1980 High frequency positive pressure ventilation (HFPPV): a review based on its use during bronchoscopy and for laryngoscopy and microlaryngeal surgery under general anaesthesia. Anesthesia and Analgesia 59: 594–603

Briscoe W A, Forster R E, Comroe J H 1954 Alveolar ventilation at very low tidal volumes. Journal of Applied Physiology 7: 27–30

Crawford M, Rehder K 1985 High frequency small volume ventilation in anaesthetised humans. Anesthesiology 69: 298–304

Drazen J M, Kamm R D, Slutsky A S 1984 High frequency ventilation. Physiological Review 64: 505–543

Gavriely N, Solway S, Loring S H, Butler J P, Slutsky A S, Drazen J M 1985 Pressure flow relationships of endotracheal tubes during high frequency ventilation. Journal of Applied Physiology 59: 3–11

Goldstein D H, Slutsky A S, Ingram R H, Westerman P, Venergas J, Drazen J M 1981 CO_2 elimination by high frequency ventilation (4 to 10 Hz) in normal subjects. American Review of Respiratory Diseases 123: 251–255

Haselton F R, Scherer P W 1980 Bronchial bifurcations and respiratory mass transport. Science 208: 69

Lehr J 1980 Circulating currents during high frequency ventilation. Federation Proceedings 39: 576

Rossing T H, Slutsky A S, Lehr J, Drinker P, Kamm R D 1981 Tidal volume and frequency dependance of carbon dioxide elimination by high frequency ventilaion. New England Journal of Medicine 305: 1375–1397

Slutsky A S, Lehr J, Shapiro A H, Ingram R H, Drazen J M 1980 Effective pulmonary ventilation with small volume oscillations at high frequency. Science 209: 609–611

6

S. A. Smith, W. A. Littler

Drugs used in the treatment of hypertension

INTRODUCTION

Data from life insurance statistics clearly demonstrate that patients with high casual blood pressure readings have a reduced life expectancy because of their increased susceptibility to cardiac and cerebrovascular disease. There is ample evidence in moderate and severe hypertension, and increasing evidence in mild hypertension, that reducing the blood pressure will minimize the risk of developing some of these complications. Physicians therefore find themselves obliged to reduce high levels of blood pressure by the chronic prescription of antihypertensive drugs. However, many important questions about the treatment of hypertension remain unanswered. What precise level of blood pressure requires treatment? Is it the systolic, diastolic or mean pressure that is most important? What are the long term metabolic effects of antihypertensive drugs? What is the aetiology of essential hypertension and are the complications caused by, or just associated with the level of pressure? A full discussion of these problems is outside the scope of this review, but the potential prescriber must bear them in mind when he initiates a lifelong course of treatment for an asymptomatic patient.

Many groups of drugs have antihypertensive activity. In this chapter we will confine ourselves to oral preparations that are prescribed specifically for long term treatment of hypertension. The list of drugs discussed is not intended to be comprehensive. We will provide an overview of the different classes of drugs which are currently available and say something about their use both as monotherapy and in combination.

Currently available antihypertensive drugs can be classified according to their mode of action into seven main categories, as follows:
Diuretics
Beta adrenoceptor antagonists
Alpha adrenoceptor antagonists
Calcium channel blocking agents
Angiotensin converting enzyme inhibitors
Direct acting vasodilators
Centrally acting agents

Diuretics

Diuretics have been used in the treatment of hypertension for almost 30 years. The first agent convincingly shown to lower blood pressure was the benzothiadiazine (thiazide), chlorthiazide, but it appears that all classes including loop and potassium sparing diuretics have some antihypertensive activity. Their mechanism of action, however, remains controversial and may differ for different types. It has been known for many years that salt restriction can be an effective method of lowering blood pressure in some individuals, and this group of patients is likely to respond well to diuretic therapy. The fall in pressure is related to a fall in body weight (due to loss of salt and water) and increasing the dose above that which causes maximum weight loss does not increase the hypotensive effect. However, natriuresis alone is not the sole mechanism.

Diuretics, particularly the thiazides, also act on peripheral blood vessels reducing vascular resistance and catecholamine responsiveness. There is little temporal relationship between the changes seen in plasma volume and changes in blood pressure; diuretic potency does not correlate well with antihypertensive effectiveness.

Thiazides are the most effective antihypertensive diuretics but even so their potency is not great. They can be used alone only in mild hypertension though they may be useful in combination with other drugs for more severe forms. Their action is on the distal part of the ascending limb of the loop of Henle promoting loss of potassium as well as sodium and water. They are ineffective in advanced renal failure.

The more powerful loop diuretics such as frusemide and bumetanide paradoxically are less potent antihypertensives. They act on the proximal part of the ascending limb of the loop of Henle increasing urine volume and promoting excretion of sodium, potassium and calcium (as opposed to thiazides which reduce urinary calcium). They have virtually no antihypertensive activity in many patients but are effective in conditions such as chronic renal failure and malignant hypertension when sodium retention contributes towards the raised blood pressure. They also potentiate the antihypertensive activity of angiotensin converting enzyme inhibitors (see below).

Potassium retaining diuretics include amiloride and triamterene which act on the distal convoluted tubule and spironolactone which is an aldosterone antagonist. They are relatively weak antihypertensives and are generally only used in combination with loop or thiazide diuretics to offset increased potassium losses. The importance of diuretic induced potassium depletion is controversial but in general it is more effective to add a potassium sparing diuretic than to give potassium supplementation. As a general rule monotherapy with these agents should be avoided, except in proven hyperaldosteronism when spironolactone is specifically indicated.

Diuretics are commonly prescribed in hypertension because they are cheap, experience with them is great and they are unlikely to cause side effects in the short term. However, longer term complications are common and potentially serious (Table 6.1). In particular, electrolyte imbalance may cause fatal arrhythmias and reduction of the high density to low density lipoprotien ratio may accelerate atherosclerosis. There has been some debate about whether these risks could outweigh the benefits in mild hypertension. Many of the adverse effects can be minimized by using low doses, and this policy makes sense as they have a flat dose response curve. MacGregor et al (1983) have shown that 12.5 mg per day of hydrochlorthiazide has the same antihypertensive potency as 50 mg per day.

The use of diuretics in hypertension is likely to decline as newer antihypertensives of other classes become available.

Table 6.1 Side effects of diuretic therapy

	Thiazide diuretics	Loop diuretics	Potassium sparing diuretics
Electrolytes	Hypokalaemia Hyponatraemia Hyperchloraemic alkalosis	Hyponatraemia Hypokalaemia Hypercaluria	Hyperkalaemia Hyponatraemia
Metabolic	Hyperuricaemia Glucose intolerance Hyperlipidaemia Pre-renal azotaemia	Hyperuricaemia Glucose intolerance Pre-renal azotaemia	
Others	Impotence Skin rashes Thrombocytopaenia	Ototoxicity Nephrotoxicity Myalgia (bumetanide)	Renal stones (triamterene) Gynaecomastia (spironolactone) Impotence Gastrointestinal disturbance

β Adrenergic antagonists (β blockers)

The sympathetic nervous system is important in short and long term regulation of blood pressure. End organ receptors for the system are broadly divided into two groups, α and β by their function and relative sensitivity to pressor amines. Drugs which block β receptors reduce blood pressure by a variety of mechanisms. They lower cardiac output by reducing myocardial contractility and heart rate, inhibit renin secretion, reset baroreceptors and reduce noradrenaline release from sympathetic neurones. They may also have a central effect on blood pressure regulation.

Since Pritchard & Gillam (1964) first demonstrated the antihypertensive effect of propranolol over 20 years ago more than 10 different β blockers have appeared on the market in most western countries, although only three, atenolol, propranolol and metoprolol are available in North America.

This proliferation of agents with a similar mode of action has led — often for commercial reasons — to extensive debate about the relative merits of other pharmacological properties which differ from drug to drug (Table 6.2). These properties include:

Cardioselectivity
Intrinsic sympathomimetic activity
Membrane stabilising activity and
Lipid solubility

Cardioselectivity. Cardioselective β blockers antagonize the mainly cardiac β_1 receptors more than pulmonary β_2 receptors. In theory this should reduce their adverse effects on peripheral vascular tone, glucose homeostasis and bronchial smooth muscle. However in practice these advantages are difficult to detect. Certainly even the most cardioselective β blockers can produce dangerous deterioration of pulmonary function in asthmatics.

Intrinsic sympathomimetic activity (ISA). The term intrinsic sympathomimetic activity (ISA) refers to the partial agonist effect possessed by some of these drugs. It has been claimed that this may offset side effects due to the lowered cardiac output and heart rate, and the increased peripheral resistance. It has not been convincingly

Table 6.2 Pharmacological properties of some β blockers

	Cardioselectivity	ISA	Membrane stabilizing activity	Lipid solubility
Acebutolol	–	+	+	+
Atenolol	+	–	–	–
Metoprolol	+	–	–	+
Nadolol	–	–	–	±
Oxprenolol	–	+	+	+
Pindolol	–	++	+	+
Propranolol	–	–	+	++
Sotalol	–	–	–	–
Timolol	–	–	+	+

shown that ISA is of clinical importance and in practice excessive ISA may reduce the antihypertensive effectiveness.

Membrane stabilising activity. Some β blockers possess a membrane stabilizing or 'quinidine like' activity which should in theory enhance their antiarrhythmic properties. However, the doses required to achieve this action are many times greater than those which give full β blockade. This pharmacological characteristic of some β blockers can be considered clinically irrelevant.

Lipid solubility. The importance of lipid solubility is better established. Highly lipid soluble drugs such as propranolol pass easily into the central nervous system and are rapidly eliminated by biotransformation in the liver. They are more likely to produce central adverse effects such as vivid dreams and should be avoided in liver failure. Lipid insoluble drugs such as atenolol are excreted unchanged by the kidneys and should be used in reduced dosage when renal failure is present.

In general there is little to choose between one β blocker and the next.

Side effects are common and may occasionally be catastrophic. Many are predictable and related to β blocking activity. These include excessive hypotension and bradycardia, decompensation of cardiac failure, bronchospasm and cold hands and feet. Other less predictable problems include vivid dreams, fatigue, sleep disturbance and impotence. In diabetes they mask the tachycardia and sweating of acute hypoglycaemia and inhibit glucose mobilization, thus increasing the risk of severe neuroglycopaenia.

Several large trials have shown that long term β blockade can improve survival following acute myocardial infarction (Singh & Vencatesh 1984). It is tempting to speculate that this cardioprotective action may also apply in hypertensive patients with ischaemic heart disease, but this hypothesis has not yet been confirmed in clinical trials.

Sudden withdrawal of β blockers in patients with ischaemic heart disease may be associated with an increase in angina, arrhythmias and sudden death (Nattel et al 1979). These drugs, like thiazide diuretics, will reduce the high density to low density lipoprotein ratio. This could theoretically increase the rate of atheroma formation, but the clinical significance of this effect is uncertain.

β-Blocking agents are potent drugs and remain in the first line of treatment for all grades of hypertension despite their many side effects.

α Adrenoceptor antagonists (α blockers)

In the context of blood pressure control α adrenergic receptors increase peripheral vascular tone and inhibit renin release. Over the last 10 years it has become apparent that there are two types of receptors termed α_1 and α_2 with different anatomical distribution and functions. The α_1 receptors are post-synaptic mediators of vasoconstriction while the pre-synaptic α_2 receptors inhibit noradrenaline release from nerve endings forming the basis of a negative feedback loop. Drugs which block α_1 receptors reduce peripheral resistance promoting a fall in blood pressure. They are particularly useful in combination with β blockers whose central cardiac β_1 hypotensive action tends to be opposed by peripheral vasoconstriction due to β_2 blockade. The most important drugs of this class are prazosin, indoramin and the combined α and β blocker labetalol. Phenoxybenzamine, a much older drug, is now rarely used because of its tendency to produce tachycardia, drowsiness and ejaculatory failure.

Prazosin is a quinazoline derivative that specifically antagonises α_1 receptors. It has a half life of about 4 hours and has to be given in divided doses. The tachycardia normally seen with peripheral vasodilation does not occur, though the reasons for this are not entirely clear (Graham & Pettinger 1979). The drug causes venous as well as arterial dilatation. The resulting decrease in venous return inhibits the expected reflex rise in cardiac output and further potentiates its hypotensive effect.

A proportion of patients get profound postural hypotension with the first dose but this becomes less obvious with continued treatment. In practice, this problem can be circumvented by starting with a small dose (0.5 mg) given immediately before the patient goes to bed. The dose can then gradually be increased over several weeks until therapeutic levels are reached. Fluid retention may occur at higher doses but this generally responds to diuretic therapy. Other problems include drowsiness, nasal congestion, blurred vision and impotence, though these are uncommon. Although not a very potent antihypertensive in its own right, prazosin remains a valuable adjunct to conventional therapy with β blockers and diuretics.

Indoramin is very similar to prazosin in action and side effects although they are not structurally related. It has potent selective α_1 blocking actions and is effective when given twice daily. It has a local anaesthetic type membrane stabilizing action which gives it class 1 antiarrhythmic properties.

Labetalol has combined α and β blocking properties, though the β effect is between three and seven times more potent than the α effect. Its action and side effects are identical to those that would be produced by a combination of prazosin and propranolol. The potential advantage of having both actions in one drug is to a certain extent minimized by the fact that it needs to be given in divided doses, often of more than one tablet. For practical purposes it can be regarded as a nonselective β blocking agent and it has typical β blocker side effects in asthma, heart failure and peripheral vascular disease. The usual α side effect of postural hypotension only occurs if high doses (in excess of 1500 mg/d) are used.

The α adrenergic blockers, though theoretically attractive, have a limited application in hypertension. The main problems are their side effects and lack of potency. Nevertheless, there is a place, particularly for prazosin, in selected resistant cases.

Calcium slow channel blocking agents (calcium antagonists)

Calcium antagonists have only recently been widely recognized as useful antihypertensive drugs. This heterogenous group of drugs act by blocking uptake of calcium into vascular and cardiac smooth muscle cells during the slow phase of depolarization. This lowers intracellular calcium concentration reducing contractility and automaticity. Their mechanism of action is not fully understood but it is certainly more complicated than simple blockade of slow calcium channels as was once thought (Braunwald 1982) and it appears to vary from drug to drug. Nevertheless, the final result is reduction of vascular smooth muscle tone and thus peripheral vascular resistance. The two most important calcium antagonists currently available for treating hypertension are *nifedipine* and *verapamil*, although two newer agents, felodipine and nicardipine will probably soon appear.

These drugs vary in their effect on vascular, myocardial and conducting tissue, though all exhibit a hypotensive effect which is mainly related to their vasodilating potency (Table 6.3).

Nifedipine is the calcium antagonist most widely used for hypertension. The standard preparation is rapidly and completely absorbed but has a half life of only 5–6 hours, necessitating thrice daily doses. A slow release preparation (Adalat retard) which can be given twice per 24 h is now available. It affects peripheral blood vessels much more than myocardial and conducting tissue and it can quite safely and effectively be combined with β blockers without the risk of bradycardia or excessive depression of cardiac output.

The main side effects, which comprise headache, flushing, palpitations and peripheral oedema, are related to the vasodilation and so are dose dependent (and relatively common). Occasionally, idiosyncratic hepatotoxicity can occur, and fatigue, depression and nausea, though unusual, can be troublesome.

Nifedipine is also a potent antianginal and is particularly useful for treating hypertensive patients with ischaemic heart disease. It has been shown to be effective when used alone (Bayley et al 1982) and in combination with β blockers, diuretics and methyl dopa (Guazzi et al 1980), but it may cause dangerous hypotension when combined with prazosin (Jee & Opie 1983).

The use of this drug is increasing and it may soon be competing with β blockers and diuretics for a place amongst the first line agents.

Verapamil is much less firmly established as an antihypertensive agent but still has a place when other agents have failed or are contraindicated. The oral preparation is rapidly absorbed but an extensive first pass metabolism allows only 10%–20% of the

Table 6.3 Calcium antagonists used for treating hypertension

Effect	Nifedipine	Verapamil	Felodipine	Nicardipine
Peripheral vasodilatation	++	+	+++	++
Negative inotropism	+	++	+	±
Conduction disturbance	0	+++	0	0
Reflex tachycardia	±	0	++	0
Hypotension	++	+	+++	++
Compatible with blocker	Yes	No	Yes	Yes

drug to reach the circulation leading to considerable variability in blood levels. Its chief metabolite, norverapamil, is pharmacologically active with about one tenth the potency of its parent. This may accumulate with time and cause further unpredictability of effect. The half life is short (2–4 h) and divided dosing is required, though a sustained release preparation is currently undergoing clinical trials and should soon be available (Schutz et al 1982).

The major problems with verapamil in hypertension are its negative inotropism which can precipitate cardiac failure, and its depressant effect on the AV node, causing heart block. It should not be used in patients with myocardial deficiency or conduction disturbances and only used with caution in patients concurrently receiving β blockers or digoxin. Constipation due to inhibition of gut motility occurs in 30% of patients and rashes, joint pains and hepatotoxicity have been described. Its action on conducting tissues however may make it a particularly useful drug for treating hypertension in patients with episodic supraventricular arrhythmias.

Felodipine and nicardipine are not yet commercially available but show considerable promise in clinical trials. They both act predominantly on vascular smooth muscle with minimal myocardial and conduction depressant effects.

Buhler (1983) maintains that calcium antagonists are more effective in elderly patients, particularly those with low plasma renin activity, but this view is by no means universally accepted. There is no doubt that interest in these drugs is increasing and they may well assume as much importance in the 1980s as thiazides and β blockers did in the 1970s.

Angiotensin converting enzyme inhibitors

The renin angiotensin system plays an important role in blood pressure homeostasis and salt and water balance (Fig. 6.1). Renin is produced by the kidney response, amongst other things, to a decrease in renal arterial pressure, and it acts upon circulating globulin, angiotensinogen, to produce angiotensin I. This is then converted to the octapeptide angiotensin II (AII) by angiotensin converting enzyme (ACE). AII is a powerful vasoconstrictor and also stimulates aldosterone release from the adrenal cortex. In normal individuals AII levels are sufficient to exert a significant pressor effect. In hypertension the significance of AII will depend upon the plasma renin activity (PRA) which is determined by renal perfusion and salt water balance. Very high renin levels are found in patients with compromised renal perfusion due to renal artery stenosis, and some renal parenchymal disease (renovascular hypertension). ACE is also responsible for breaking down the naturally occurring vasodilator bradykinin, though the significance of this in hypertension is not clear. Currently, only two oral ACE inhibitors, *captopril* and *enalapril* are available.

Captopril has been shown to be a potent antihypertensive agent in man. It has a short half life and needs to be given 3 times/24 h. The antihypertensive effect is mediated by vasodilatation due to the virtual abolition of circulating AII. The magnitude of the hypotensive effect is related to pre-treatment PRA and thus AII levels. Diuretic drugs which tend to increase PRA will potentiate its action whereas β blockers which inhibit PRA do not work well in combination (MacGregor 1982).

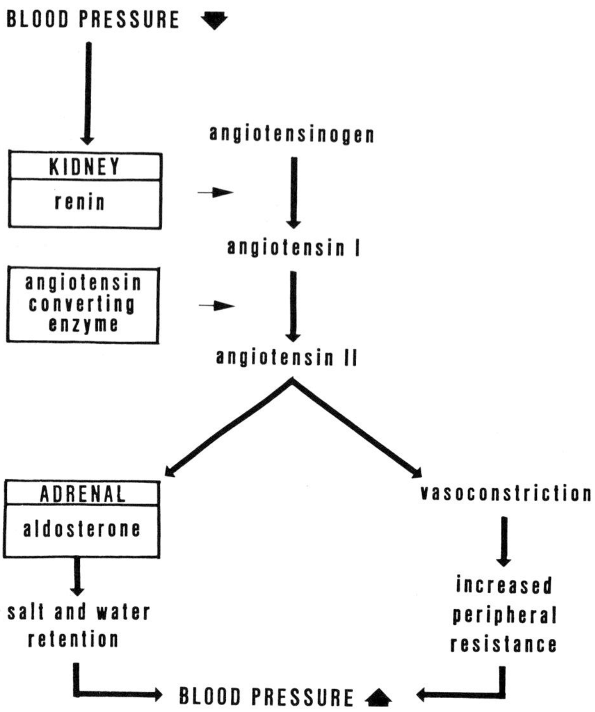

Fig. 6.1 Simplified diagram of the renin/angiotensin system.

Experience with captopril and calcium antagonists together is limited, but our initial impression of this combination is favourable.

Patients with renovascular hypertension are particularly suitable for ACE inhibitors but caution must be applied as captopril can impair renal function by deranging autoregulation of intrarenal blood flow. Acute renal failure has been caused in patients with bilateral disease or renal artery stenosis in a solitary kidney (Hricik et al 1983). Rather surprisingly, captopril has been shown to be of benefit in some cases of low renin hypertension, and even in anephric patients with limited endogenous sources of renin (Man in't Veld et al 1980).

Side effects are common and similar to those of penicillamine. They include rashes, arthralgia, fevers, leucopoenia, disturbance of taste and proteinuria. Their incidence can be greatly reduced by restricting the maximum daily dose to 150 mg. Many authors now regard the dose of 450 mg originally recommended by the manufacturers as being too high and well into the flat part of the dose response curve (Domby 1983).

A dramatic fall in blood pressure may occur on initial dosing. This is more likely to occur in patients rendered sodium deficient by previous diuretic therapy, but there is no good way of predicting exactly who will develop this problem (Hodsman et al 1983). Consequently, it is sensible to ensure that the first dose is given under medical supervision in a setting where resuscitation facilities (i.v. saline) are available. Potassium retention can occasionally occur and the serum electrolytes should be regularly monitored as should the white cell count and urine protein excretion. In view of these problems it is unlikely that captopril will find a large place in the treatment of hypertension outside hospital.

Enalapril, a newer drug, may have some advantages over captopril. It has a longer half life and so can be given only once or twice per 24 h, and it does not possess the sulphydryl group which is responsible for many of the side effects which have limited the usefulness of captopril. It does however have the same adverse effect on renal haemodynamics in renal artery stenosis and causes first dose hypotension which may be more severe and prolonged than with captopril.

ACE inhibition provides a new and pathophysiologically satisfying way of treating hypertension. Considerable research is going on in this branch of pharmacology and new drugs with fewer side effects will become available. ACE inhibitors will certainly play an increasing part in future antihypertensive prescribing.

Direct acting vasodilators

These structurally unrelated drugs are arbitrarily grouped together here because they all cause vasodilatation by direct action on vascular smooth muscle, reducing peripheral resistance and hence blood pressure. They achieve this by a variety of mechanisms which are often poorly understood. Their haemodynamic effects however are similar. The main contenders in this class are hydralazine, minoxidil and diazoxide, though the latter has lost popularity over the last 10 years because of side effects. The newer drug endralazine has been extensively studied recently but is not yet commercially available.

These drugs act predominantly on the arterial system with minimal effect on veins. If used alone they cause a reflex tachycardia and an increase in cardiac output which antagonizes their antihypertensive effect. They also cause salt and water retention by stimulating the renin angiotensin system and increasing intracapillary pressure.

Hydralazine has been used for over 30 years. It is rapidly absorbed from the gut, but has a half life of only 3 hours and divided dosing is necessary. Metabolism occurs in the liver by N-acetylation. This is of clinical significance as about 50% of the population are 'slow' acetylators and tend to accumulate the drug. A patient's acetylator status is determined genetically and can be measured by laboratory tests.

In some cases hydralazine produces a hypersensitivity syndrome which resembles systemic lupus erythematosis with skin rashes, arthralgia, fever, leucopaenia and lymphadenopathy. Antinuclear antibodies are usually found but the DNA binding test is characteristically negative. The syndrome will regress slowly after stopping the drug. It was once thought to be avoidable if the patient's acetylator status is checked and the total daily dose kept below 200 mg but Cameron & Ramsay (1984) have disputed this. Other side effects are related to vasodilatation and include flushing, tachycardia, headache, nasal congestion and postural hypotension.

Minoxidil is the most potent orally active vasodilator currently available and is often found to be effective when other treatment has failed. It is given 2 or 3 times per 24 h up to a maximum of 50 mg/24 h, although often as little as 2.5 mg bd will be effective. Unfortunately side effects are common. Reflex tachycardia and fluid retention are usually severe, making concomitant therapy with a β blocker and a diuretic mandatory, Glomerular filtration fraction is reduced, so considerable caution must be employed when using this drug in the presence of renal impairment. Pericardial and pleural effusions can occur, particularly in uraemic patients, and occasionally cardiac tamponade is produced.

A major problem with minoxidil is its ability to stimulate growth of body hair. Hypertrichosis is almost always found and can be severe. It may not be such a great problem in men who occasionally welcome the rugged appearance and reversal of male pattern baldness, though some baulk at the prospect of having to shave their foreheads! It is difficult to use this drug in women, even with the use of depilatory creams.

Diazoxide is structurally related to thiazide diuretics and shares some of their side effects. It has a greater adverse effect on glucose tolerance and most patients will require an oral hypoglycaemic agent to control blood sugar levels. It also produces hyperuricaemia and has theoretical adverse effects on lipid metabolism. Unfortunately it does not have the thiazide diuretic action and in fact will cause fluid retention secondary to vasodilatation. Largely because of these problems, diazoxide does not have a major part to play in the long-term management of hypertension, but it remains a very potent agent which can be employed in difficult hypertension.

Centrally acting agents

These drugs have been used for many years and are declining in popularity. They will not be discussed in detail here. The two most important are *methyl dopa,* which inhibits noradrenaline synthesis, and *clonidine,* which is a central α_2 stimulant that reduces sympathetic outflow. Methyl dopa was one of the drugs used in a large recently published trial of treatment of high blood pressure in the elderly (Amery et al 1985). The results suggest a significant reduction in cardiovascular mortality with active treatment. This may be a specific property of the drug or the effect of pressure reduction. We do not believe that the evidence from this trial alone is sufficient to justify a major revival of this drug.

These drugs have many side effects which include sedation, haemolytic anaemia, jaundice and impotence for methyl dopa, and sedation, dry mouth and rebound hypertension on withdrawal for clonidine.

GENERAL PRINCIPLES

Long term treatment of sustained hypertension

Current practice has evolved from a stepwise approach to therapy, starting with a β adrenergic blocking agent and/or a diuretic, and progressing to so-called 'third-line' drugs in resistant cases, or where first line drugs are contraindicated. This method may need to be modified in future as new calcium antagonists and angiotensin converting enzyme inhibitors become available. However, for the moment, the stepped therapy method remains a widely accepted and useful approach to planning antihypertensive treatment.

Most of the third line agents work, to a greater or lesser degree, by reducing peripheral vascular resistance, though often together with a variety of other actions. Some, such as minoxidil and hydralazine, will cause a reflex tachycardia and are best used only in combination with a β adrenergic blocking agent. Others, such as nifedipine and captopril, do not cause a tachycardia and can be used safely in patients when β blockers are contraindicated. The use of verapamil with β blockade can produce conduction disturbances and myocardial depression (Hutchinson et al 1984).

Unfortunately, choosing a third line drug to complement an antihypertensive regime remains as much an art as a science. The theoretically appealing approach of trying to correct underlying haemodynamic and endocrine abnormalities has proved difficult to achieve, and has not yet been demonstrated to be of benefit. Simply reducing the blood pressure is far more important than the manner in which the reduction is achieved.

When selecting a drug it is important to consider the patient as a whole. His age, ethnic origin, intelligence, occupation and the presence of other pathology could all influence the choice. Older patients often do not tolerate β blockers and potent vasodilators, but respond well to calcium antagonists and diuretics. Afrocaribbeans often have low renin hypertension which responds better to diuretics (and perhaps calcium antagonists) than to β blockers and captopril. Drugs which cause drowsiness or mental slowing should be avoided in those with occupations demanding high levels of mental or physical performance. The opportunity to use drugs which will also treat concurrent pathology should not be missed. Calcium antagonists are appropriate for patients with angina or tachyarrhythmias and diuretics for those with heart failure.

In general it is wise to adhere to a combination of drugs which has proved effective and to avoid those likely to be antagonistic. A summary of desirable and undesirable combinations is given in Fig. 6.2.

Once antihypertensive drugs are commenced, they will usually need to be

	Diuretics	Beta Blockers	Nifedipine	Verapamil	Captopril	Prazosin	Indoramin	Labetolol	Hydralazine	Minoxidil	Diazoxide	Methyl Dopa
Nifedipine	P	P										
Verapamil	P	D	N									
Captopril	R	P	P	P								
Prazosin	P	P	P	P	P							
Indoramin	P	P	P	P	P	N						
Labetolol	P	N	P	D	P	N	N					
Hydralazine	P	R	N	R	P	P	P	R				
Minoxidil	M	M	P	R	P	?	?	R	N			
Diazoxide	P	R	P	R	P	?	?	R	N	N		
Methyl Dopa	P	P	P	P	P	P	P	P	P	P	P	
Clonidine	P	N	P	P	P	P	P	P	P	P	P	N

Fig. 6.2 Possible combinations of antihypertensive drugs. M = mandatory, R = recommended, P = possible, N = not recommended D = dangerous, ? = unknown.

continued for life. In this context, even apparently very minor side effects will, with the passage of time, increase in their importance to the patient and the impact that they have on his quality of life. Adequate therapy should not only control his blood pressure, but leave him feeling as healthy as possible. Clinicians should be receptive to patients' complaints and be prepared to change offending drugs even if it seems that control may not be quite as good. The 'you will have to grin and bear it' approach eventually leads to poor compliance and increases the number of clinic defaulters. Thus, it is an advantage for the doctor to have a wide range of drugs in his therapeutic armamentarium. However, familiarity with a drug, its side effects, its interactions and its metabolism is also desirable, and we would encourage clinicians to familiarize themselves with a small range of agents which they use routinely, venturing outside this range only when circumstances dictate.

Patients with severe hypertension often require a considerable number of tablets. The chance of getting good compliance will diminish as the number of tablets and daily dosing times increase. In these patients particularly, the use of combination and sustained action preparations is desirable, despite their relative lack of flexibility and increased cost.

Short term treatment of hypertensive emergencies

As a rule high blood pressure should be gradually reduced over a period of weeks or months by careful titration of appropriate oral antihypertensive agents. This is important as cerebral blood flow can only be kept constant by autoregulation within a range of about 50 mmHg around the prevailing mean pressure. Rapid reduction of pressure will not allow the autoregulatory mechanisms to reset and may cause acute cerebral ischaemia or infarction (Graham 1975). Very rarely a sudden large increase in pressure may break through autoregulation at the upper end of this range and cause symptoms such as headache, confusion, seizures and coma (hypertensive encephalopathy). In this situation rapid reduction of blood pressure is essential, although it should only be brought down to the middle of the autoregulatory range for that patient, rather than to normotensive levels. Even more rarely, acute reduction of pressure is required to prevent progression of life threatening complications. A list of conditions which may require emergency antihypertensive therapy is given in Table 6.4.

When blood pressure reduction is required within minutes, parenteral therapy is necessary. Many drugs have been used for this purpose over the years (Table 6.5) and all have their advocates. We favour labetalol, sodium nitroprusside, diazoxide and hydralazine.

Labetalol is very effective but must be given cautiously as its onset of action may be delayed by as much as 20 minutes following an intravenous bolus. It has been (incorrectly) advocated for use in patients with a phaeochromocytoma because of its combined α and β adrenergic blocking effects. In these patients β blockade alone can paradoxically increase blood pressure by blocking the vasodilating peripheral vascular β_2 receptors while allowing unopposed a mediated vasoconstriction. Labetalol in fact has much more potent β blocking than α blocking activity and has the same problems as the pure β blockers. The α blocker phentolamine is much safer choice in this condition.

Table 6.4 Conditions in which emergency antihypertensive therapy may be required

Reason for emergency antihypertensive therapy	Associated disease process	Timescale for pressure reduction
Hypertensive encephalopathy	Malignant hypertension Acute glomerulonephritis Eclampsia Phaeochromocytoma Clonidine withdrawal Food interaction with MAO inhibitors	Minutes to hours
Prevention of life threatening complications	Acute aortic dissection	Minutes
	Intracerebral or subarachnoid haemorrhage	Minutes to hours
	Bleeding post cardiovascular surgery Eclampsia	
	Malignant hypertension Acute left ventricular failure	Hours

Nitroprusside and trimetaphan have the advantage of a rapid onset and short duration of action. They are given by continuous infusion and the desired level of blood pressure can be easily achieved by adjusting the infusion rate. Unwanted hypotension is treated simply by temporarily discontinuing the infusion. Nitroprusside solution reacts with light and it is necessary to cover the administration set with aluminium foil. Trimetaphan is a ganglion blocker and its hypotensive action may be augmented by head up tilting.

Diazoxide and hydralazine reduce blood pressure by reducing peripheral vascular resistance. They cause a reflex increase in heart rate and cardiac output which increases cardiac oxygen consumption and so are less desirable in patients with reduced coronary reserve or acute left ventricular failure.

Table 6.5 Drugs which may be used parenterally in a hypertension emergency

Drug	Route of administration	Dose (mg)	Onset of action	Duration	Comments
Diazoxide	i.v.	100–600	3–5 min	4–18 h	Increase cardiac oxygen consumption
Hydralazine	i.v., i.m.	10–30	3–6 min	3–8 h	Tachycardia
Labetalol	i.v., i.m., infusion	10–50	5–20 min	3–4 h	Not for phaeochromocytoma
Sodium nitroprusside	Infusion	0.03–0.5/mm	1–5 min	5–10 min	Unstable solution
Trimetaphan	Infusion	1–15	1–5 min	5–10 min	Helped by head up tilt; easy to control
Clonidine	i.v.	0.15–0.3	15–30 min	3–4 h	May cause an initial increase in pressure; sedative
Phentolamine	i.m.	10–20	15–30 min	5–6 h	Good for phaeochromocytoma; may cause severe hypotension

Parenteral therapy should only be used on the rare occasions that rapid reduction of blood pressure is imperative. In less urgent situations a nifedipine capsule crushed between the teeth is effective in about 30 minutes. The capsules contain a solution of nifedipine which is rapidly absorbed through the buccal mucosa. Treatment can be continued with slow release nifedipine tablets.

FUTURE DEVELOPMENTS

Many new compounds are currently undergoing clinical evaluation although only a small proportion will ever become available for general use. A few drugs with entirely novel modes of action are also being developed. One example of this is the serotonin antagonist ketanserin which has been found to lower blood pressure (Wenting et al 1982).

The range of antihypertensive agents currently available is large and this is bound to generate some confusion. As research into the pathophysiology of blood pressure and new drugs continues, the day is approaching when scientific and side effect free therapy will be possible. In the meantime we should try to remember that a patient's quality of life may be more important to him than the statistical risks of less than perfect control, and we should never forget that the people who sell us these drugs may have more than just our patient's health in mind.

REFERENCES

Amery A, Birkenhager W et al 1985 Mortality and morbidity results from the European Working Party on high blood pressure in the elderly trial. Lancet i: 1349–1354

Bayley S, Dobbs R J, Robinson B F 1982 Nifedipine in the treatment of hypertension: report of a double blind controlled trial. British Journal of Clinical Pharmacology 14: 509–512

Braunwald E 1982 Mechanism of action of calcium channel blocking agents. New England Journal of Medicine 307: 1618–1627

Buhler F R 1983 Age and cardiovascular response adaptation. Determinants of an antihypertensive treatment concept primarily based on beta-blockers and calcium entry blockers. Hypertension 5: 94–100

Cameron H A, Ramsey L E 1984 The lupus syndrome induced by hydralazine: a common complication with low dose treatment. British Medical Journal 289: 410–412

Dombey S 1983 Optimal dose of captopril. Lancet i: 355

Graham D I 1975 Ischeamic brain damage of cerebral perfusion type after treatment of severe hypertension. British Medical Journal iv: 739

Graham R M, Pettinger W A 1979 Prazosin, New England Journal of Medicine 300: 232–236

Guazzi M D, Fiorentine C, Olivari M T, Bastorelli A, Necchi G, Polese A 1980 Short- and long-term efficacy of a Ca-antagonistic agent (nifedipine) combined with methyldopa in the treatment of severe hypertension. Circulation 61: 913–919

Hodsman G P, Isles C G, Murray G D, Usherwood T P, Webb D J, Robertson J I S 1983 Factors related to the first dose hypotensive effect of captopril: prediction and treatment. British Medical Journal 286: 832–835

Hricik D G, Browning P J, Kopelman R, Goorno W E, Madias M E, Dzau V J 1983 Captopril induced functional renal insufficiency in patients with bilateral renal artery stenosis or renal artery stenosis in a solitary kidney. New England Journal of Medicine 308: 373–376

Hutchinson S J, Lorimer A R, Lakhdar A, McAlpin S G 1984 Beta blockers and verapamil: a cautionary tale. British Medical Journal 289: 659–660

Jee L D, Opie L H 1983 Acute hypotensive response to nifedipine added to prazosin in treatment of hypertension. British Medical Journal 287: 1514

MacGregor G A, Markandu N D, Banks R A, Roulston J E, Jones J C 1982 Captopril in essential hypertension; contrasting effects of adding hydrochlorthiazide or propranolol. British Medical Journal 284: 693–696

MacGregor G A, Banks R A, Markandu N D, Bayliss J, Roulston J 1983 Lack of effect of beta-blocker on flat dose response to thiazide in hypertension: efficacy of low dose thiazide combined with beta-blocker. British Medical Journal 286: 1535–1538
Man in't Veld A J, Schicht I M, Derkx F H M, de Bruyn J H B, Schalekamp M A D H 1980 Effects of an angiotensin-converting enzyme inhibitor (captopril) on blood pressure in anephric subjects. British Medical Journal 280: 288–290
Nattel S, Rangno R E, Van Loon G 1979 Mechanism of propranolol withdrawal phenomena. Circulation 59: 1158–1164
Pritchard B N C, Gillam P M S 1963 Use of propranolol (inderal) in treatment of hypertension. British Medical Journal 2: 725–727
Schutz et al 1982 Serum concentration and antihypertensive effect of slow release verapamil. Journal of Cardiovascular Pharmacology 3: 346–349
Singh B N, Venkatesh N 1984 Prevention of myocardial reinfarction and sudden death in survivors of acute myocardial infarction: role of prophylactic beta-adrenoceptor blockade. American Heart Journal 107: 189–200
Wenting G J, Man in't Veld A J, Woittiez A J 1982 Haemodynamic effects of ketanserin, a 5-hydroxytryptamine (serotonin) receptor antagonist, in essential hypertension. Clinical Science 63: 435s–438s.

Hypotensive anaesthesia

INTRODUCTION

The use of deliberate hypotension in anaesthesia is still a contentious issue. The advocates of the technique consider it to be without special problems, whereas others feel that its use should be restricted to making the impossible operation possible.

Awareness of blood pressure change during anaesthesia is surprisingly recent and its recording has become established practice only in the professional lifetime of practising anaesthetists. The concept of flow and perfusion is even more recent. Although initial reports on the use of deliberate hypotension appeared in the early 1950s, these were mainly clinical observations. It was almost 15 years later that significant scientific observations were made into the physiological changes produced by this technique.

PHYSIOLOGY

Measured blood pressure is a function of cardiac output and peripheral vascular resistance. Other factors —particularly viscosity — affect flow. Frequent references are made to Poiseuille's law and Reynolds number but they are of little relevance to clinical practice. Poiseuille stated that the pressure in a conduit was in inverse ratio to the fourth power of its radius. It relates to a homogenous fluid, with laminar flow in a non-distensible conduit. Reynolds number relates the velocity, viscosity and density of a fluid to the diameter of the conduit. A figure below 2000 indicates laminar (efficient) flow, and greater than 2000 turbulent (poor) flow.

The viscosity of blood is stated as four times that of water. However, this varies at different sites within the circulation (it falls in small vessels) and with different packed cell volumes (PCV). A rise in the PCV of 50% doubles the viscosity, while a fall of 25% halves it. Therefore, haemodilution by removing 1 litre of blood and replacing with a balanced salt solution materially improves perfusion.

Peripheral vascular resistance (PVR)

The major component of PVR occurs in the arterioles. Arterioles are classified as first to fourth order depending on their branching and size (200 μm down to 10 μm of the precapillary arteriole). Control tends to be neural in the larger arterioles and humoral in the smaller. The neural effect varies at different sites, but local metabolites act at the humoral sites. Catecholamines, vasopressin and angiotensin II are amongst the humoral pressors, while histamine, 5HT, bradykinin and prostaglandins have the reverse effect. Although cholinergic, vasodilator fibres have been described in skeletal muscle, the vast majority of neural control is via the sympathetic system. At rest, sympathetic impulses are about one per second, but under stress this multiplies 10-fold. Intense sympathetic activity increases the critical closing pressure (the pressure at which a vessel closes to redirect flow to essential circulation) to about 60 mmHg. Any agent which inhibits sympathetic discharge or its effects will, necessarily, reduce the closing pressure, usually to about 15 mmHg. Thus deliberate hypotension will maintain perfusion. Baroreceptors in the aortic arch and carotid sinus detect pressure changes and, via the vasomotor centre, affect sympathetic and vagal tone. The effects are seen mainly in the PVR and capacitance vessels and, to a lesser extent, in the cardiac output. Chemoreceptors in similar sites relate mainly to respiratory control, though hypoxia does cause a reflex increase in cardiac output and PVR. The role of peripheral chemoreceptors is uncertain, but hypoxia or hypotension may activate them and may be the mechanism by which respiratory effort — seen with very low blood pressure — is mediated. Anaesthesia itself inhibits both baroreceptor and chemoreceptor response.

Capacitance

75% of the blood volume is contained within the veins, the remainder in arteries and capillaries. The veins are rich in smooth muscle and are controlled in a manner similar to the arteries. They are able to contract around a diminishing blood volume to maintain cardiac return and output. Indeed, a blood loss of 500 ml reduces the central venous pressure by only 1 mmHg.

Cardiac output

The output of the heart produces the pressure head in the vasculature, and with a constant PVR the blood pressure will change accordingly. Venous return is the major factor determining cardiac output, with chronotropic and inotropic states playing a lesser role. Within specific limits, increased sympathetic tone will increase cardiac output. However, any abnormally high or low rate will result in a reduced cardiac output as a result of opposite changes in stroke volume.

Posture

Posture significantly affects pressures in both arteries and veins. In the arteries, for every 1 cm elevation above the site of measurement, the blood pressure will fall approximately 1 mmHg. Below the level of measurement, the converse is true. Similar changes are seen in venous pressure, but of a lesser magnitude in the elevated parts of the body. This orthostatic effect is magnified in association with general anaesthesia. In the head up position, the reduced muscle tone in the legs deprives the veins of external compression, and combined with reduced sympathetic tone, the veins dilate allowing more than 250 ml of blood to pool in the legs.

Ventilation

Intermittent positive pressure ventilation (IPPV) produces an initial rise in blood pressure as the increased intrathoracic pressure is transmitted directly to the arteries. However, the blood pressure then falls as venous return to the heart is reduced. Positive end expiratory pressure (PEEP) enhances the hypotension.

Auto regulatory blood flow

Blood flow varies in different tissue for different reasons, e.g. in skeletal muscle it is almost independent of sympathetic activity, but very responsive to vasodilator metabolites, whilst cutaneous blood is under mainly sympathetic control.

Coronary blood flow

Like systemic flow, coronary blood flow is a function of perfusion pressure and coronary vascular resistance. Coronary perfusion pressure is relatively high as both coronary arteries arise from the ascending aorta. At rest, 75% of flow in the coronary arteries occurs during diastole. Consequently a raised ventricular end diastolic pressure will effectively reduce the coronary perfusion pressure. During stress, the flow pattern is reversed, with most of the flow occurring during systole.

Coronary vascular resistance is determined by the lumen of the vessel and the muscle tone of the myocardium through which the vessel passes. Dynamic changes in the lumen occur mainly by changes in sympathetic tone, but metabolites — particularly carbon dioxide — play a major role. Static changes (e.g. atheroma) are more predictable in their effect. Stenosis, less than 70% of a vessel, produces little fall in flow unless under stress, but in excess of 90%, collateral vessels are required to maintain flow. The major coronary arteries are on the external surface of the heart, and must pass through the myocardium to supply the endocardium. It is the endocardium which is the first to suffer the effects of hypoperfusion. Myocardial hypertrophy per se reduces endocardial perfusion as does tachycardia — often seen as a baroreceptor response to hypotension.

The rate pressure product (heart rate × systolic blood pressure) is regarded as a useful indicator of ischaemia and, during anaesthesia, it should be kept below 12 000. It is not of great value during hypotensive anaesthesia.

Cerebral blood flow

Autoregulation of cerebral blood flow (CBF) is marked. There is relatively poor sympathetic innervation, but the vasodilator response to metabolites — especially carbon dioxide — is impressive. CBF is constant, with a mean arterial pressure above 60 mmHg. Below 50 mmHg, the CBF falls in direct proportion to the blood pressure, as autoregulation has failed and carbon dioxide now has no effect. In the untreated hypertensive, the pressure limits for maintaining CBF are higher, but with treatment they return to normal. In the presence of raised intracranial or venous pressure, a higher blood pressure is needed to maintain perfusion pressure and CBF. IPPV and PEEP have little effect on the cerebral venous pressure in the upright person, but in the supine position, the raised intrathoracic pressure is transmitted directly to the cerebral veins.

Blood flow to the parts of the brain furthest from the blood supply is relatively poor and more likely to be affected by a rise in intracranial pressure. These 'boundary areas' include the sulci of the cortex, hippocampus and basal ganglia. Consequently, survival following hypoperfusion states results in personality change and memory loss.

A sudden fall in the blood pressure has a greater effect on CBF as there is a lag in autoregulation. However, if the hypotension is drug induced, as opposed to haemorrhagic, the vasodilator effect of the drug (especially sodium nitroprusside) to some extent preserves the CBF and cortical oxygenation.

If hypotension is profound and prolonged, cerebral oedema occurs. Although this may not produce permanent damage, when perfusion is restored, recovery may occur in an erratic manner. The protective role of barbiturates in reducing cerebral oxidative metabolism has few advocates when induced hypotensive anaesthesia is used.

Renal blood flow

Like the brain, the kidneys have a marked metabolic autoregulatory system. Unlike the brain, it can be overridden by powerful sympathetic control. There is little change in perfusion and filtration above a mean arterial pressure of 70 mmHg, but below 60 mmHg, filtration stops and perfusion is dramatically reduced. Severe and prolonged hypotension results in acute tubular necrosis. Most volatile anaesthetic agents reduce renal blood flow independent of any hypotension they may produce.

Hypotension activates the renin-angiotensin axis. Renin is released from the juxtaglomerular apparatus and this activates angiotensin I. Although angiotensin I is not very vasoactive, passage through the lungs converts it to angiotensin II — a highly vasopressor substance. This sequence is seen particularly following hypotension with sodium nitroprusside.

Pulmonary function

It is well established that arterial oxygenation falls during general anaesthesia, as a result of reduced alveolar ventilation and an imbalance in the ventilation–perfusion ratio ($\dot{V}/\dot{Q}$) in dependent parts of the lungs. This fall in oxygenation is increased during induced hypotension. The change in $\dot{V}/\dot{Q}$ ratio is particularly marked during spontaneous ventilation and may well be affected by the action of drugs on the bronchial musculature. IPPV and PEEP improve the $\dot{V}/\dot{Q}$ ratio, but at the expense of obstructing pulmonary capillary flow and cardiac output. Drug induced, as opposed to haemorrhagic, hypotension obtunds the hypoxic pulmonary vasoconstrictor response — an homeostatic response to improve the $\dot{V}/\dot{Q}$ ratio. In a spontaneously breathing patient, the $P\text{CO}_2$ rises while the pO_2 falls. The $\dot{V}/\dot{Q}$ ratio improves with IPPV but at the expense of cardiac output.

Patients lying supine do not show as great a change in blood gases as those in a head up tilt. IPPV does not improve the gas picture as much as would be expected, but it does reduce cardiac output, which is said to improve the bloodless field. The raised

$P\text{CO}_2$ seen in spontaneous ventilation does maintain cardiac output and cerebral blood flow but may increase bleeding.

INDICATIONS AND COMPLICATIONS

All indications and contraindications must be relative rather than absolute. By far the most common indication for the use of induced hypotension is to improve the surgical field. Less blood obscuring the field allows for greater surgical accuracy in identifying vital structures and pathological tissue. During microsurgery, a minute quantity of blood may totally obscure the surgical field. A relatively bloodless field can substantially reduce operating times, but this should never be a prime consideration.

Reduced blood loss during surgery leads to a reduced requirement for blood transfusion — an expensive and potential dangerous fluid. In a Jehovah's Witness, it is a major factor to consider.

Reduced blood loss is usually associated with less peri-and post-operative oedema — crucial in skin flaps and pedicles or in other areas of compromised blood supply. Within limits, perfusion is improved despite reduction in systemic blood pressure.

The use of deliberate hypotension during anaesthesia must relate not only to the experience of the anaesthetist, but the familiarity of the surgeon with the technique. The ultimate decision is that of the anaesthetist.

Patients with pre-existing cardiovascular disease must be considered carefully. The hypertensive patient will probably have reset his autoregulation at a higher level than normal. In these patients hypotension must be regarded as a fall in the systolic pressure of 33%. Treated hypertensives should continue their treatment, but their medication will be potentiated by anaesthesia, and per-operative hypotensive agents. Drugs blocking α adrenergic receptors may well have bound permanently to the receptor. Existing myocardial ischaemia is often improved by hypotension — provided any infarct occurred more than 6 months pre-operatively. Intra-operative myocardial ischaemia can be identified by careful monitoring (vide infra) and if the fall in blood pressure is corrected immediately, there is no evidence that permanent damage ensues (Rollason & Hough 1969). Thompson (1978) and her colleagues, in a wider study, found no biochemical changes as a result of hypotension. Cerebral disease, whether vascular or from other pathology, tolerates hypotension well as cerebral blood flow (down to a mean pressure of 50 mmHg) is more dependent on changes in carbon dioxide than blood pressure. However, patients with established infarcts should not be hypotensed for fear of extending the infarct in areas of critical flow. Eckenhoff et al (1964) and Rollason et al (1971) could not detect changes by psychometric testing following hypotensive anaesthesia, even in the elderly.

Consideration must be given to the changes in blood gases in patients with respiratory disease and the effects of hypotensive agents on bronchical structures, particularly in asthmatics. Asthmatics should not be given ganglion blockers and; there is usually some hyperinflation and they do not readily tolerate the valsalva manoeuvre associated with IPPV. Poor renal and hepatic function may be aggravated by hypotension in these organs.

Ganglion blockade enhances the effect of insulin in diabetic patients. Those insulin dependent are further at risk, as they have abnormally responsive cerebral blood flow and may be unable to compensate for hypotension (Dandona et al 1978).

Anaesthesia itself can produce problems in pregnant women. Induced hypotension should be avoided, as the effects of the technique on the blood flow in the uterus and fetus are uncertain. Initial enthusiasm for induced hypotension in the early 1950s rapidly waned as a result of the apparent increase in morbidity and mortality. Hampton & Little (1953) quoted a mortality of approximately 1:500, three times that of normotensive anaesthesia, and with a comparable rise in morbidity. Although figures produced at this time are open to criticism, the use of controlled hypotension would have become historical interest but for the enthusiasm of anaesthetists such as Enderby and later Eckenhoff, to whom must go credit for their scientific application. More recent estimates of mortality and morbidity (Enderby 1980) show that with improved selection and technique, morbidity and mortality compares favourably with normotensive anaesthesia.

MONITORING

The mercury manometer or its aneroid equivalent has been the time honoured method of measuring blood pressure during anaesthesia, but it is slow and cumbersome. The oscillotonometer is a better instrument and, suitably modified, it can be left inflated and can act as a continuous monitor of pulse and trends in the systolic pressure. Most automatic blood pressure recorders work on the oscillotonometric principle, but they have a slow cycle time. Most read low — a safety factor. Intra-arterial cannulation — usually of the radial artery — gives a direct and accurate reading of the blood pressure. Although considered to have complications, the incidence of permanent sequelae is minimal. It is a low risk, high benefit, method of patient monitoring (Slogoff et al 1983). Allens test to predict occlusive problems is probably of little value (Wilkins 1985). A 20G Teflon cannula is preferred. Intra-arterial cannulation also offers the facility for blood gas measurement. Hypoxia produced by hypotension can be accurately compensated for and $P\text{CO}_2$ measurement is particularly useful to monitor cerebral blood flow. In the absence of blood gas estimation, an end tidal CO_2 meter is of value.

The electrocardiogram is a good indicator of cardiac rhythm. During anaesthesia the selection of lead II is often standard. However, this is a poor indicator of myocardial ischaemia, for which lead V5 should be selected. A modified V5 may be produced by placing RA on the right side of the chest, LA in the position of V5 with the reference electrode in any convenient position.

The cerebral function monitor (CFM) is an integrated electroencephalogram with both amplitude and frequency modified. Two electrodes are placed parietally. It indicates global rather than focal hypoperfusion or hypoxia and the record will remain normal while the systolic blood pressure is above 60 mmHg, and the fall in blood pressure is not greater than 10 mmHg/min. The CFM tells of hypoxic events, but some time after they have occurred and consequently it is of little value in clinical practice.

Changes in blood volume in an hypotensed patient have a greater physiological effect than in a normotensive patient. A blood loss as small as 100 ml may have a significant hypotensive effect, while the infusion of a similar amount of fluid have the reverse effect. It is important to estimate blood loss accurately and have a reliable intravenous infusion.

It is easy to concentrate on instruments and their readings. But this should not replace observation of the patient.

TECHNIQUES

Hypotension has been defined as a fall of 33% in the systolic blood pressure. In practice the systolic blood pressure is reduced to 60–80 mmHg. During normal sleep, the systolic pressure may not be much greater than 80 mmHg. There has been debate as to whether a reduced cardiac output, rather than hypotension, is the greater factor in producing a relatively ischaemic surgical field. Hypotension is probably the major factor (Sivarajam et al 1980). The use of high spinal analgesia to create intra-operative hypotension — though hardly controlled — was reported by Koster as early as 1928. Griffiths & Gilles used the technique more widely and reported their results in 1948. Three years later Bromage advocated the use of epidural anaesthesia for hypotension (Bromage 1951). Total sympathetic blockade has now no part in hypotensive anaesthesia, but more limited blockade, using spinal or epidural analgesia, has an important role in producing an ischaemic surgical field.

Haemorrhagic hypotension —arteriotomy following by autotransfusion — as practiced by Gardner in 1946, was associated with many problems and gained little acceptance. However haemodilution, with or without hypotension, is now practised. The viscosity of blood is reduced and tissue perfusion improved at the expense of a slight rise in cardiac output. Fahmy and colleagues (1980) report a marked reduction in the need for donor blood transfusion using this technique. The development of drugs able to block the autonomic ganglia (Paton & Zaimis 1948) heralded the hesitant beginning of hypotensive anaesthesia as we know it today, and became the basis of 'pharmacological blockade' (vide infra). Of the early ganglion blocking drugs, pentolinium and trimetaphan are the only ones which remain in use. Both have a competitive blocking action on the autonomic ganglion, similar to that of D-tubocurarine.

Pentolinium

Pentolinium is presented as 10 mg in 2 ml ampoules. The dose required is variously reported as between 0.05 mg/kg and 0.3 mg/kg. Fit, young patients require higher doses, as do patients breathing spontaneously. Posture and volatile anaesthetic agents have a marked synergism on the hypotensive effect. An accurate initial dose is important, as it is usually the only effective dose, subsequent doses having a lesser effect. When used during cardiopulmonary bypass, only 0.5 mg may be required to achieve hypotension. There is a great individual response to pentolinium, the maximal effect occurring within 30 minutes and lasting between 1 and 4 hours. However, many of its effects may last much longer — e.g. cycloplegia up to 12 hours. The drug is not metabolized and is excreted unchanged in the urine.

Trimetaphan

Trimetaphan was first used clinically in the early 1950s (Magill et al 1953). The hypotensive effect of ganglion blockade is potentiated by a direct vasodilator action and histamine release. An ampoule of 250 mg in 5 ml is normally diluted to 0.1% solution and administered by continuous infusion. Hypotension occurs in approximately 3 minutes and last 15 minutes. Tachyphalaxis is marked, but the total dose should never exceed 1 g. As a sole hypotensive agent, it has been superseded by sodium nitroprusside, but is returning in popularity in a combination of trimetaphan/sodium nitroprusside. Its metabolic pathway has never been established, but one-third appears unchanged in the urine.

β Adrenergic blockade

β Adrenergic blockade with propanolol has been used to control the tachycardia produced by hypotensive anaesthesia for 20 years (Hellewell & Potts 1966). Its use is firmly established, although there are now more cardioselective blockers such as practolol and atenolol. The effects of these drugs on cardiac output is an important factor in achieving a bloodless surgical field.

β Adrenergic stimulation is usually seen during hypotension with the directly acting vasodilators, sodium nitroprusside and trinitroglycerine. This activates the renin–angiotensin axis, making per-operative control of blood pressure difficult and post-operative hypertension frequent. β Blockade inhibits the renin–angiotensin reaction (Khambatta et al 1981), but renin activation is not seen as a result of ganglion blockade.

Labetolol

Labetolol, an α and β adrenergic blocker, is marketed to treat hypertensive patients with associated angina. Its use in anaesthesia was first reported by Scott and colleagues in 1976. Its hypotensive effect occurs mainly by lowering the peripheral resistance and, to a lesser extent, reducing the cardiac output. Given in 5 mg increments, to a maximum of 25 mg in 10 minutes, its effects are rapidly apparent. The hypotension is potentiated by volatile anaesthetic agents and head up tilt. As with most other hypotensive agents, moderation is needed in the elderly, in whom bradycardia, extending well into the post-operative period, may be marked. Although this can be effectively treated with atropine, profound hypotension may be difficult to reverse because of the α blockade.

Direct acting vasodilators

It was a quarter of a century after its initial clinical use that sodium nitroprusside (SNP) was first used in anaesthesia (Moraca et al 1962). It is now probably the most common agent used to reduce the blood pressure during anaesthesia. It is presented as a powder, 50 mg, which must be reconstituted immediately prior to use and is normally diluted in 500 ml, 5% dextrose for use as a continuous infusion. SNP is rapidly decomposed by light to aquapentaferrocyanate, a substance which releases free cyanide. Protected from light, a solution should be discarded 4 hours after preparation.

In the body, toxic cyanide ions are converted into non-toxic cyanmethaemoglobin and thiocyanate. Although excess cyanide ions can be absorbed by the administration of sodium thiocyanate, it is better to reduce the risk of cyanide poisoning by restricting the dose of SNP. The recommended maximum safe dose is accepted as 1.5 mg/kg over a short period and 0.5 mg/kg per hour for prolonged administration. The rate of infusion should not exceed 10 μg/kg per minute. Patients with B_{12} deficiency should not be given SNP as they have defective cyanide metabolism. The effect of SNP is directly on the vascular smooth muscle, the exact mode being of continuing speculation, but effects are more marked in arterial muscle than venous muscle. Onset of hypotension occurs within 1 minute and normal blood pressure is restored within 4 minutes of ceasing the infusion. Moderate tachycardia, a baroceptor response, is usual. The effects on myocardial perfusion and oxygen demand are confusing, but both are probably reduced, making it useful to control ischaemic hypertension during coronary artery surgery.

Cerebral perfusion is increased, causing an initial rise in the intracranial pressure. For this reason it has been suggested that an infusion of SNP does not begin until the dura has been opened. SNP is the drug of choice for hypotension during neurosurgery, as its effects are solely vascular and readily reversible. MacRae (1981) has described the combined infusion of trimetaphan/SNP (10:1). Hypotension is good with greatly reduced doses of individual drugs, thereby reducing their individual toxicities.

Trinitroglycerin (TNG), like SNP, has a direct action on blood vessel musculature, but unlike SNP its effects are mainly venous. It is presented as 1 mg/ml in 10 ml ampoules, which is diluted to 100 ml for infusion. It is usually used to reduce cardiac pre-load and dilate the coronary vasculature and to this end, it is an excellent hypotensive agent during cardiac surgery. Its role as an hypotensive agent in patients without ischaemic heart disease is less certain. It will produce hypotension in normal patients, but the dose required is often very high. In combination with SNP, good hypotension is achieved and this use may be indicated for hypotensive anaesthesia in patients with proven myocardial ischaemia.

Volatile agents

Halothane potentiates most hypotensive drugs, though its use as a sole hypotensive agent is limited. Autonomic depression does occur, together with a reduced cardiac output and reduced peripheral vascular resistance. Alone it produces adequate hypotension, particularly in the elderly, but a concentration of 3% with intermittent positive pressure ventilation may be necessary. Enflurane produces similar effects but it is unlikely that isoflurane will contribute much to hypotensive anaesthesia, as with this drug cardiac output is maintained.

Pharmacological blockade (Enderby 1974)

This is a concept which explains hypotension produced by several factors:
Ganglion blockade (pentolinium, trimetaphan).

Beta blockade (propanolol, practolol, atenolol).
Volatile agents (halothane, enflurane).
Posture (25% head up tilt).
IPPV ± PEEP.

It is a safe technique employed and recorded during many thousands of general anaesthetics by anaesthetists trained and experienced in the technique. However, for the anaesthetist called upon to provide hypotensive anaesthesia less frequently, it is probably not the method of choice. Instead they should consider a technique involving IPPV with a volatile agent and posture which produce satisfactory results, supplemented by SNP or labetolol. There can be no dogma relating to spontaneous respiration or intermittent ventilation, but oxygen enriched mixtures are mandatory.

Deliberate hypotension in anaesthesia is a safe procedure which can materially benefit surgery. With careful selection of patients and administration of the technique, there should be no greater incidence of complications than with normotensive anaesthesia.

REFERENCES

Bromage P R 1951 Anaesthesia 6: 26

Dandona P, James A M, Newbury M L, Beckett A G 1979 Instability of cerebral blood flow in insulin dependent diabetics. Lancet ii: 1203–1205

Eckenhoff J E, Compton J R, Larson A, Davies R M 1964 Assessment of cerebral effects of deliberate hypotension by psychological measurements. Lancet ii: 711–714

Enderby G E H 1974 Pharmacological blockade. Postgraduate Medical Journal 50: 572–575

Fahmy N R, Chandler H P, Patel D G, Lappas D G 1980 Haemodynamics and oxygen availability during acute haemodilution in conscious man. Anesthesiology 53: 584

Gardner W J 1946 The control of bleeding during operation by induced hypotension. Journal of the American Medical Association 132: 572–574

Griffiths H W C, Gilles J 1948 Thoracolumbar splanchnicectomy and sympathectomy: anaesthetic procedure. Anaesthesia 3: 134–136

Hampton L J, Little D M 1953 Results of a questionnaire concerning controlled hypotension in anaesthesia Lancet : 1299–1300

Hellewell J, Potts M 1966 Propanolol during controlled hypotension. British Journal of Anaesthesia 38: 794–801

Khambatta H J, Stone J G, Khan E 1981 Propanolol alters renin release during nitroprusside induced hypotension and prevents hypertension on discontinuation of nitroprusside. Anesthesia and Analgesia (current researches) 60: 569–573

Koster H 1928 Spinal anaesthesia with special reference to its use in surgery of the head, neck and thorax. American Journal of Surgery 5: 554

Magill I W, Scurr C F, Wyman J B 1953 Controlled hypotension by a thiophanium derivative. Lancet i: 219–220

Moraca P P, Elmers M B, Hale D E, Wasmuth C E, Pontasse E F 1962 Clinical evaluation of sodium nitroprusside as an hypotensive agent Anesthesiology. 23: 193

Paton W D M, Ziamis E J 1948 Curare like action of polymethylene bis-quaternary ammonium salts. Nature 161: 718–719

Rollason W N, Hough J M 1969 A re-examination of some electrocardiographic studies during hypotensive anaesthesia. British Journal of Anaesthesia 41: 985–986

Sivarajan M, Amory D W, Everett G B, Buffington C 1980 Blood pressure not cardiac output determines blood loss during induced hypotension. Anesthesia and Analgesia (current researches) 59: 203–206

Slogoff S, Keats A S, Arlund C 1983 On the safety of radial artery cannulation. Anesthesiology 59: 42–47

Thompson G E, Miller R D, Stevens W C, Murray W R 1978 Hypotensive anaesthesia for total hip arthroplasty. A study of blood loss and organ function (brain, heart, liver and kidney). Anesthesiology 48: 91–96

Wilkins R G 1985 Radial artery cannulation and ischaemic damage: a review. Anaesthesia 40: 896–899

Further reading

Enderby G E H (ed) 1985 Hypotensive anaesthesia. Churchill Livingstone, Edinburgh

D. W. Davies, A. J. Camm

A classification of antiarrhythmic drugs and common cardiac arrhythmias

INTRODUCTION

A large number of antiarrhythmic drugs are currently available to practising doctors, with even more waiting in the wings at the stage of clinical research. None is a panacea and all may aggravate or provoke rather than relieve arrhythmias (proarrhythmic effect). Careful consideration is therefore necessary before prescription of any of these agents. The most important factor in choosing an antiarrhythmic drug is the arrhythmia to be treated. In this chapter, we will therefore briefly outline the arrhythmias commonly encountered in terms of their presentation, electrocardiographic features, underlying mechanism and their clinical significance before proceeding to discuss the drugs used in their management in Chapter 9. The references for both chapters are listed at the end of Chapter 9.

Many drugs have lapsed into relative disuse because of the advent of a more effective or less toxic agent while other new agents do not offer any advantage over existing, tried and trusted drugs. Such new drugs are unlikely to replace these successful older drugs and so we will concentrate on those drugs commonly used and the new drugs likely to become future favourites. For the sake of convenience, we will employ the *Vaughan-Williams classification* of antiarrhythmic drugs (Table 8.1). This classification is based on the cellular electrophysiological effects of antiarrhythmic drugs whereby they are divided in to four main classes, I–IV. This is not always clinically relevant because, although the classification usually allows prediction of sites of action and inaction, there is often considerable variation in terms of clinical effect even between drugs in the same group.

The class I antiarrhythmic drugs

The class I antiarrhythmic drugs are subclassified as Ia, Ib and Ic drugs according to their different effects upon the action potential (Table 8.1). The predominant effect of all class I drugs is to reduce the rate of maximal depolarization of myocardial cells and Purkinje tissue. The resting transmembrane potential is little affected whereas the threshold for depolarization is raised, conduction velocity depressed and refractory periods prolonged. The spontaneous diastolic deplorization which identifies pacemaker cells is also inhibited, this effect being seen more readily, i.e. at lower drug concentrations, than the effects on threshold and conduction. This combination of properties makes arrhythmias which are due both to foci of increased

Table 8.1 The Vaughan-Williams classification

Class	Effects	Examples
Ia	Membrane stabilization Prolonged action potential duration	Quinidine Procainamide Disopyramide
Ib	Membrane stabilization Shortened action potential duration	Lignocaine Mexiletine Tocainide
Ic	Membrane stabilization Varied action potential duration	Flecainide Propafenone
II	β-Blockade	Propranolol Metoprolol Acebutolol
III	Action potential prolongation	Amiodarone Bretylium
IV	Calcium antagonism	Verapamil Diltiazem Tiapamil

automaticity and to reentry susceptible to class I agents. The subdivision of the group is based upon their differing effects on the subsequent duration of the action potential, i.e. the time taken for repolarization. Drugs of class la prolong this, class Ib agents shorten it and flecainide acetate (the first representative of class Ic) prolongs repolarization of atrial and ventricular myocardium while shortening that of the His-Purkinje system. These different properties might explain some of the differences in their antiarrhythmic effects. Those which prolong the action potential duration are effective against atrial flutter and fibrillation (reentry atrial arrhythmias influenced by tissue refractoriness) whereas those of class Ib are not, their activity being restricted to ventricular arrhythmias. Because of their effects upon the His-Purkinje system, all class I drugs are relatively contraindicated in patients with conduction abnormalities. The efficacy of class I drugs depends upon the potassium concentration. Hypokalaemia renders them less effective (and is itself proarrhythmic) whereas hyperkalaemia accentuates their effects. With the possible exceptions of mexiletine, tocainide (Ib) and propafenone (Ic), all are at least moderately negatively inotropic and left ventricular function should be considered before prescription of class I agents.

The class II antiarrhythmic effect

The class II antiarrhythmic effect is β-blockade. Thus arrhythmias influenced by sympathetic tone are affected. These include those related to ischaemia and the long QT syndromes although the most profound electrophysiological effect of β-blockade is seen at the AV node where refractoriness is increased and conduction velocity decreased. The antiarrhythmic uses of the drugs are therefore mainly to reduce conduction of atrial arrhythmias via the AV node (and thereby the ventricular response rate) or more rarely to prevent or terminate junctional reentry arrhythmias which use the AV node as at least one limb of the reentry circuit. The major cellular electrophysiological effect is to depress phase 4 depolarization, although at relatively high concentrations some have independent class I effects. Chronic β-blockade (> 3 weeks) results in slight but statistically significant QT prolongation.

The class III antiarrhythmic effect

The class III antiarrhythmic effect is related purely to prolongation of action potential duration. The major example of the group is amiodarone (Singh & Vaughan-Williams 1970) which also exhibits a mild non-competitive antisympathetic effect (Charlier 1970). The effect is widespread throughout the heart, this being mirrored by the diversity of the arrhythmias treatable by amiodarone.

The class IV antiarrhythmic drugs

The class IV antiarrhythmic drugs are a heterogenous group sharing the property of slow-channel (calcium dependent) blockade. Accordingly, they are collectively known as calcium antagonists. The slow channel is particularly important in the formation and propagation of impulses at the sinus and AV nodes. The major antiarrhythmic effects of slow channel blocking drugs are seen at the AV node; they are often used in the same context as β-blockers. Not all possess antiarrhythmic effects. Nifedipine is a member of the group which does not have an antiarrhythmic property at clinical concentrations, exerting its effect predominantly upon vascular smooth muscle.

ARRHYTHMIAS

Only the drug treatment of *tachy*arrhythmias will be considered because, with the exception of acute emergencies, drugs have no place in the modern management of bradyarrhythmias. Cardiac arrhythmias may usefully be described according to their site of origin: atrial, AV junctional and ventricular (Table 8.2).

Atrial arrhythmias

Atrial arrhythmias share a number of features in terms of both presenting symptoms, electrocardiographic appearance and therapy. They usually present as paroxysmal palpitations although all (particularly atrial fibrillation) may become incessant or permanent. As with all arrhythmias however, they are often asymptomatic and non-specific symptoms such as fatigue, dyspnoea or dizziness are common. Symptoms depend to a large extent on the rate of the atrial arrhythmia, its conduction to the ventricles and ventricular function. Most are facilitated by increased sympathetic tone, caffeine and alcohol. Electrocardiographically, they usually appear as narrow QRS complex tachycardias unless there is bundle branch block or ventricular pre-excitation via an accessory AV pathway as in the Wolff-Parkinson-White syndrome. The ventricular rate is dependent on both the rate of the atrial arrhythmia and the degree of AV block. In all cases, therapy may be aimed at either

Table 8.2 Common cardiac arrhythmias

Arrhythmia	Causes	℞ aim	Drugs	Disadvantages
Atrial				
Tachycardia	—	Prevention ↓Vr	Ia, Ic, III II, IV, dig	Ia may ↑Vr No prevention
Flutter	CAD, MVD	Prevention ↓Vr	Ia, III II, IV, dig	Ia may ↑Vr No prevention
Fibrillation	CAD, MVD, Ca, τT4	Prevention ↓Vr	Ia, Ic, III II, IV, dig	Ia may ↑Vr No prevention
Junctional				
AVNRT	DAH	Prevention	All but Ib	Potentially proarrhythmic
AVRT	AP	Prevention	All but Ib	Potentially proarrhythmic
Ventricular				
Ectopics	None, CAD, CM, MVP	Prevention	I, II, III	Potentially proarrhythmic
Tachycardia	CAD, CM, None	Prevention	I, II, III	Potentially proarrhythmic

Abbreviations: AP = accessory pathway; AVNRT = atrioventricular nodal reentry tachycardia; AVRT = atrioventricular reentry tachycardia; Ca = bronchial carcinoma; CAD = coronary artery disease; CM = cardiomyopathy; DAH = dual atrio-His conduction; dig = digoxin; MVP = mitral valve prolapse; ℞ = treatment; τT4 = thyrotoxicosis; Vr = ventricular response rate; (↑) = increase; (↓) = decrease.

prevention of paroxysms (with class I, II or III drugs) or reduction of ventricular rate (and thereby the severity of associated symptoms and haemodynamic disturbance) in the event of sustained arrhythmia (with digoxin or class II or IV drugs).

Atrial ectopic beats

Atrial ectopic beats commonly occur in normal people but increase with atrial disease and occur frequently in the sick sinus syndrome. They are mostly asymptomatic and usually require no treatment. The exceptions are those which are symptomatic or initiate other arrhythmias.

Atrial tachycardia

Atrial tachycardia is a relatively uncommon but sometimes distressing clinical problem. As a rule, there is no underlying heart disease to be found but cardiomyopathy is an occasional association. The relationship between the abnormal P waves and the QRS complexes may be fixed or variable (Wenckebach phenomenon) and is determined by AV nodal conduction properties. Both the diagnosis and choice of preventative therapy can often only be made following electrophysiological study.

Atrial flutter and fibrillation

Atrial flutter and fibrillation often coexist in the same patient, atrial flutter sometimes being a transitory stage between atrial fibrillation and sinus rhythm. Atrial flutter represents a single intra-atrial macroreentry circuit whereas atrial fibrillation is the result of multiple, discrete and independent microreentry circuits. Chronically, they both usually reflect atrial disease, most commonly in association with coronary artery disease, mitral valve disease, bronchial carcinoma, the sick sinus ('brady-tachy') syndrome, or more rarely with cardiomyopathies, mitral valve prolapse or atrial tumours. The 'lone fibrillators' do not suffer from identifiable pathology and in acute toxic illnesses such as pneumonia or hyperthyroidism, both arrhythmias may occur transiently without cardiac disorder, only to disappear once the toxicity is treated. Both may complicate pericarditis. Symptomatic paroxysmal palpitations are typically described as irregular and a common occasional presenting complication of atrial fibrillation is thromboembolism especially in the presence of mitral stenosis. The development of atrial fibrillation under any circumstance is associated with an adverse prognosis.

Junctional arrhythmias

Junctional arrhythmias are of three types, two of which are reentrant in nature. The exception is the rare *ectopic junctional or His bundle tachycardia.* This arrhythmia is almost always seen in children either after surgical correction of congenital heart disease or spontaneously within the first 6 months of life. The diagnosis is made from the surface ECG which reveals a narrow complex tachycardia with dissociated P waves. It is virtually unresponsive to drug therapy with the exception of the experience of Bucknall and co-workers (Bucknall et al 1985) who were able to control the arrhythmia with either disopyramide, mexilitine or amiodarone, alone or in combination, in four out of five patients. Apart from their experience, the prognosis is generally regarded as poor.

The reentrant junctional tachycardias

The reentrant junctional tachycardias occur as the result of there being at least two routes for conduction between atria and ventricles. Normally, both pathways conduct anterogradely in response to sinus rhythm. However, the refractory properties of the two pathways differ so that a premature (usually atrial) ectopic depolarization may find one of them still refractory. Conduction will proceed along the other, 'second' pathway and is then able to return to the atria via the now recovered 'first' pathway. A reentry circuit is thereby created for a depolarization wavefront which, in the case of intra-AV nodal reentry tachycardia, is contained within the AV node and in the case of atrioventricular reentry tachycardia consists of the AV node, ventricular myocardium, an extra-AV nodal accessory pathway and atrial myocardium. Typically, symptoms are of paroxysmal regular palpitations of sudden onset and termination. Associated symptoms depend on the rate and duration of tachycardia and include dizziness, chest pain and dyspnoea. Electrocardiographically they appear as regular, usually narrow QRS complex, tachycardia. In the case of atrioventricular reentry tachycardia, the retrograde P wave may sometimes be seen in the ST segment but this can be difficult to detect with certainty especially with very rapid tachycardia. In typical intranodal tachycardia, QRS complexes and P waves occur simultaneously and so the P wave is obscured.

It can be seen that choice of therapy will be considerably helped by knowledge of which type of reentry circuit is operating. For intra AV nodal reentry, digoxin and drugs of classes II or IV might be expected to be particularly useful whereas with atrioventricular reentry, drugs of classes Ia, Ic and III would be preferable because of their depressant effects on the other parts of the circuit, especially the accessory pathway. Rapid anterograde conduction to the ventricles of atrial tachyarrhythmias such as atrial fibrillation is a potentially dangerous complication of such pathways which might therefore be avoided by the use of such agents. Because reentry arrhythmias are likely to be initiated by atrial (or ventricular) ectopic beats, suppression of these by drugs of classes Ia, Ic and III might also reduce the incidence of both types of junctional reentry tachycardia. It must be remembered that the propensity to reentry in an individual patient depends, not only on the number of ectopic beats occurring, but also upon the relative properties of the two pathways. By altering these with a drug, it is possible to paradoxically facilitate the onset and perpetuation of reentry.

Ventricular tachyarrhythmias

The significance of ventricular tachyarrhythmias depends on underlying heart disease. Ventricular tachycardia does not much affect prognosis in individuals with otherwise normal hearts whereas, in the presence of underlying heart disease, lesser grades of arrhythmia such as frequent ventricular ectopic beats are associated with an increased risk of sudden death. Different ventricular arrhythmias carry different prognostic weight, especially in the context of acute myocardial infarction and the Lown classification was designed accordingly so that therapy could be aimed at the higher risk patients identified by the higher grades of their arrhythmias (Table 8.3). However, the applicability of this classification to patients without recent myocardial infarction is limited. Treatment of ventricular arrhythmias can be achieved with drugs of classes I, II and III and, in the rare fascicular ventricular tachycardia, with class IV (Ward et al 1984) drugs. Electrocardiographic diagnosis of ventricular tachycardia traditionally causes problems. These problems appear to be related to difficulty in distinguishing ventricular tachycardia from aberrantly conducted supraventricular tachycardia. Points which are specific for ventricular tachycardia are: dissociated P waves, fusion beats which are narrower than the tachycardia complexes, R wave only in V_1, initial R taller than R' of an RSR' deflection in V_1, Rs deflection in V_1, QS deflection in V_6 and QRS width > 140 ms. A feature which is

Table 3 The Lown classification of ventricular arrhythmias

Grade	Arrhythmia
0	None
1	Occasional, isolated, unimorphological VPB
2	Frequent (> 1/min or 30/h), isolated, unimorphological VPB
3	Multimorphological VPB
4	Repetitive VPB (a) couplets (b) salvoes
5	Early VPB (R-on-T)

VPB = ventricular premature beats

highly suggestive of, but not totally specific for, ventricular tachycardia is a frontal plane axis of < -30 (left axis deviation) of a wide complex tachycardia.

Torsade de pointes is an unusual arrhythmia which resembles non-sustained ventricular fibrillation. It is typically seen in situations associated with a long QT interval such as the congenital syndromes of Romano and Ward, and Jervell and Lange-Nielsen, bradycardia or phenothiazine toxicity. For the congenital variety, the treatment varies from atrial pacing with β-blockade to left stellectomy to correct a supposed autonomic imbalance. Treatment for the aquired forms is in many ways opposite to that of the congenital forms since the aim is to shorten the QT interval. The treatment of choice is therefore isoprenaline which is contraindicated for the congenital syndromes.

Acknowledgement

The authors are supported by the British Heart Foundation.

REFERENCES

See end of chapter 9.

9 *D. W. Davies, A. J. Camm*

Individual antiarrhythmic drugs

QUINIDINE

Quinidine is a cinchona derivative, being the dextroisomer of quinine. It is usually prescribed as the sulphate or gluconate forms and may be given both orally and parenterally although intramuscular injection is painful and intravenous injection is dangerous. The gluconate form is absorbed rather more slowly after oral dosage with peak blood levels occurring at 3–4 hours compared with 1.5–2 hours for the sulphate. The relatively short half life of 6–10 hours, increasing with age, has led to the use of slow release preparations (e.g. Kinidin Durules) which may be taken twice a day. The therapeutic range lies between 2 and 5 μg/ml (plasma concentration) and a high incidence of toxic side effects is encountered at levels above 7 μg/ml. The majority of the drug undergoes hepatic oxidative metabolism with only 10–20% being excreted unchanged in the urine. Because the drug is basic, this may be increased by acidification of the urine. The metabolites are incompletely investigated but do possess antiarrhythmic activity. Quinidine is useful against atrial and ventricular arrhythmias as well as those junctional reentry tachycardias utilizing an accessory AV pathway. The drug also possesses some α-blocking properties.

Quinidine has a low toxic/therapeutic ratio and this has led to its decreased use. Approximately one-third of patients have to discontinue therapy because of unwanted side effects. These include gastrointestinal disturbance, thrombocytopenia, haemolytic anaemia and arrhythmogenic effects, either aggravation or development

Table 9.1 Pharmacokinetics and dynamics of antiarrhythmic drugs

Drug	Administration route	Therapeutic level	Plasma half life	Elimination route
Quinidine	oral	2–5 μg/ml	6–7 hours	Hepatic
Procainamide	oral/i.v.	4–10 μg/ml	3–5 hours	Renal/hepatic
Disopyramide	oral/i.v.	2–4 μg/ml	4–10 hours	Renal/hepatic
Lignocaine	i.v.	1–5 μg/ml	1–3 hours	Hepatic
Mexiletine	oral/i.v.	1–2 μg/ml	9–12 hours	Hepatic
Tocainide	oral/i.v.	3–10 μg/ml	10–15 hours	Renal/hepatic
Flecainide	oral/i.v.	160–980 ng/ml	12–27 hours	Hepatic/renal
Propafenone	oral/i.v.	Variable	3–6 hours	Hepatic
Amiodarone	oral/i.v.	1.5–3 mg/l	7–40 days	Hepatic/renal
Verapamil	oral/i.v.	50–250 ng/ml	5–10 hours	Hepatic/renal
Diltiazem	oral/i.v.	100–200 ng/ml	4–6 hours	Hepatic/renal
Digoxin	oral/i.v.	2–2.5 ng/ml	33–38 hours	Renal

of conduction abnormalities, or provocation of ventricular arrhythmias. It interacts with other drugs, in particular with digoxin, the serum levels of which approximately double when quinidine is added at a therapeutic dose. The dose of digoxin should therefore be halved. Quinidine potentiates the neuromuscular blocking effects and ventilatory depression of succinylcholine, decamethonium and tubocurarine (Miller et al 1967). By depressing clotting factor synthesis, quinidine potentiates the effect of coumarin anticoagulants. As with any drug extensively metabolised in the liver, its levels are significantly influenced by those drugs which induce hepatic enzymes such as phenytoin and rifampicin.

PROCAINAMIDE

Procainamide was developed after the antiarrhythmic effects of the local anaesthetic procaine were noticed 30 years ago. It is available both for oral and parenteral use. As with quinidine it needs to be given frequently because of its short half life of 6–10 hours. This is dependent upon whether the patient is a fast or a slow acetylator. However, its major metabolite, N-acetylprocainamide (NAPA) has significant electrophysiological effects which are similar to the effects of procainamide except for the absence of effect on the His-Purkinje system. A sustained release preparation is available. The therapeutic plasma concentration lies between 4 and 10 μg/ml, toxic side effects being uncommon with levels below 12 μg/ml but common above 16 μg/ml. Procainamide is eliminated by both renal and hepatic routes with approximately 75–95% appearing in the urine, 30–60% as the unchanged drug. Its spectrum of antiarrhythmic activity is identical to quinidine and so are its electrocardiographic side effects. Other common unwanted side effects include gastrointestinal disturbance and a drug-induced lupus syndrome. It is contra-indicated in patients with myasthenia gravis for fear of aggravation. There are relatively few drugs which interact with procainamide although, being weakly basic, its renal elimination will be increased by urinary acidification.

DISOPYRAMIDE

Disopyramide's antiarrhythmic effects were first described in 1962 and are essentially the same as those of quinidine and procainamide. It is active both parenterally and orally, the majority of the drug being excreted unchanged in the urine. At therapeutic levels (2–4 μg/ml), about 40% of the drug is protein bound. It follows first order kinetics for a two compartment model, the unbound drug level being proportional to the dose. Plasma half life is in the order of 7 hours but increases with renal impairment and after myocardial infarction. A sustained release preparation is available allowing twice daily dosage.

Although disopyramide's antiarrhythmic effects are similar to those of quinidine and procainamide, its unwanted side effects, although numerous, are not so serious. It has therefore become the most widely used drug in this group in the UK. The major unwanted effects are anticholinergic, due mostly to its N-monodealkylated metabolite. Dry mouth is the commonest of these but the drug should be avoided in patients with narrow angle glaucoma and used with great care in those with symptoms of prostatism.

LIGNOCAINE

Lignocaine has been used as an antiarrhythmic agent since 1950. Because of an extensive first pass hepatic metabolism to inactive metabolites, it is only active when given parenterally. This limits its use to the treatment of non-recurrent ventricular arrhythmias such as those seen in the acute stages of myocardial infarction. The half life following intravenous bolus is about 1.5 hours so that a continuous infusion is required after the initial bolus, the infusion being titrated against the clinical effect. The usual infusion rate is between 1 and 4 mg per hour. Toxic side effects, especially central nervous effects, occur at whole blood levels in excess of 5–6 μg/ml, therapeutic levels needing to be in excess of 1–2 μg/ml. It is certainly active against reentrant ventricular arrhythmias but its ability to suppress automatic foci is controversial. The most important unwanted effects are related to the central nervous system. These range from drowziness to psychotic reactions and grand mal seizures. They are dose related. Predictable electrocardiographic side effects such as the development or aggravation of conduction disorders occur as well as sinus bradycardia, sinus arrest and sinoatrial block. It is a negatively inotropic drug which requires careful monitoring when used in patients with impaired left ventricular function. In terms of drug interactions, there are relatively few which are unexpected. One is the reduction in lignocaine clearance seen in people also receiving propranolol; sympathomimetic agents have the opposite effect. Halothane decreases lignocaine metabolism, perhaps by reducing hepatic blood flow or possibly by affecting hepatic enzymes. Therapeutic serum lignocaine concentrations reduce the anaesthetic requirements for halothane and nitrous oxide (Himes et al 1977).

MEXILETINE

Mexiletine, a relatively new drug, was synthesized and studied in the early 1970s and has similar local anaesthetic and antiarrhythmic effects to lignocaine. It differs from lignocaine in having a high degree of bioavailability after oral administration followed by a long half life of about 9 hours when taken via this route. It is extensively metabolized in the liver both by oxidation and reduction, the metabolites being unlikely to have significant antiarrhythmic properties since these decline with the mexiletine level. Under 10% of the drug appears unchanged in the urine, a figure which could also be increased by urinary acidification since mexiletine is weakly basic. Therapeutic plasma levels lie between 0.75 and 2.0 μg/l, above which side effects are seen with increasing frequency. The drug is negatively inotropic but this effect is not marked at clinical antiarrhythmic doses. However, the effects in patients with pre-existing heart failure are not known. Like lignocaine it is only active on ventricular arrhythmias with perhaps a particular effect on torsade de pointes (Krikler & Curry 1976). Its unwanted side effects, both intra- and extra-cardiac, are also similar although the commonest side effect is nausea and vomiting. There is little evidence of significant interaction with other drugs other than those which induce its hepatic metabolism.

TOCAINIDE

Tocainide is the result of an attempt to find a drug similar to lignocaine but which would be active when taken orally. Elimination half life after oral dosage is between 10 and 15 hours and is little affected by myocardial infarction. Elimination of the drug is shared between renal excretion of the unchanged drug and glucuronidation in the liver. Therapeutic levels are above 3 μg/l with toxic effects being increasingly encountered above 10 μg/l. As with mexiletine, negative inotropism is a property but the effect at a clinical dosage is minimal. It is active primarily against ventricular arrhythmias but has been shown to terminate junctional reentry tachycardia (Waleffe et al 1979). It has also been used to treat paramyotonia congenita (Dengler & Rudel 1979) and tinnitus although this can paradoxically also be a side effect of tocainide therapy. Not surprisingly, in patients with pre-existing conduction abnormalities, these were aggravated when tocainide was given in combination with the β-blocker metoprolol with three patients developing asystole (Ikram 1980). Hepatic enzyme induction does not appear to significantly affect its metabolism (Elvin et al 1980).

ENCAINIDE

Encainide is an interesting antiarrhythmic drug whose antiarrhythmic effects after oral dosage differ from those after intravenous use because of the significant antiarrhythmic effects of two metabolites produced after oral administration. Its propensity to provoke malignant ventricular arrhythmias will probably severely limit its future use.

FLECAINIDE

First reported 10 years ago, flecainide is a potent antiarrhythmic agent with a wide spectrum of activity. It is active after both intravenous and oral administration with a half life after a single dose (via either route) of about 13 hours, this ranging from 12 to 27 hours after repeated oral doses. It can therefore be taken twice a day with peak plasma levels being seen at 2–4 hours after a single oral dose. Approximately 60% is metabolized by the liver (one of the products having weak antiarrhythmic activity) the rest being excreted unchanged, mostly in the urine but a small amount appearing in the faeces. The clinical effects of flecainide within the heart are widespread: PA (right atrial conduction time), AH (AV nodal conduction time), HV (His-Purkinje conduction time) and QRS duration are all prolonged. Although the QT is also prolonged, this prolongation is composed solely of increased QRS duration, the JT being unaffected. Atrial and ventricular refractory periods are slightly prolonged, but the most marked prolongation of refractoriness in response to flecainide is seen with anomalous AV pathways both intra- and extra-AV nodal with the effect being most marked in the retrograde direction. In terms of arrhythmias, all are susceptible to flecainide therapy, the least sensitive being atrial flutter.

Of its unwanted effects, a strong negative inotropic effect is the most commonly encountered and is therefore an important limiting factor especially in patients with impaired left ventricular function. Proarrhythmic effects include the aggravation/ production of conduction abnormalities, and a nearly 5% incidence of serious ventricular arrhythmias is reported (Nathan & Hellestrand 1984). The risks of these effects are greater in patients with coronary artery disease, myocardial infarction, pre-existing ventricular tachycardia or congestive cardiac failure. Pacing thresholds are elevated by the drug to a far greater extent than observed with other drugs. Extracardiac effects are predominantly central nervous with dizziness and visual disturbance being the commonest. Little is known of drug interactions but there is an increase in both rate of absorption and peak levels of digoxin in patients given flecainide although steady state levels are little affected.

PROPAFENONE

Propafenone, although being predominantly a class Ic agent, also possesses class II, III and weak class IV activities (Dukes & Vaughan Williams 1984). It slows conduction and prolongs the refractory periods of atrial, junctional (including accessory) and ventricular tissue. After a single dose, its half life is about 3.5 hours increasing to 6 hours with multiple doses but appears to have considerable and unpredictable individual variation. Elimination is by hepatic metabolism. The drug is of limited use in the conversion or prophylaxis of atrial flutter or fibrillation although its effects upon accessory AV conduction are sufficient for it to be effective in the termination and prevention of reentry arrhythmias using such pathways (Rudolph et al 1979). Ventricular premature beats and sustained tachycardia are also susceptible to the drug (Salerno et al 1984, Shen et al 1984). The significant side effects are related to its negative inotropism, the production of conduction abnormalities and proarrhythmic effects. The unwanted effects encountered most commonly are gastrointestinal disturbance and dizziness.

THE β-BLOCKERS

The β-blockers: this group contains more drugs than any of the other groups, reflecting the diverse uses of β-blockade. The electrophysiological effects of β-blockers are principally the result of sympathetic blockade. Thereby, they depress excitability and conduction, especially of the sinus and AV nodes, and by reducing ischaemic episodes, perhaps decrease automaticity and inhibit reentry at ventricular level. Although all these drugs appear as racemic mixtures for clinical use, virtually all the β-blocking effect is within the L-isomer. Many has class I 'local anaesthetic' properties but these are not seen at therapeutic levels. They are subdivided according to properties such as cardioselectivity and intrinsic sympathomimetic activity but these do not effect their antiarrhythmic effects. Sotalol, however, is interesting among the β-blockers because of its additional class III effect (predominantly in the D-isomer). All β-blockers prolong the QT interval when used chronically. However, this is a small effect compared with that observed with sotalol, with which the effect is most marked after an intravenous bolus. Specific β-blockers and their special properties are well described elsewhere (Silverman & Frishman 1983) and so they will not be discussed further here.

AMIODARONE

Amiodarone is the most important representative of those drugs possessing class III effect. It is unique amongst antiarrhythmic drugs in many ways. It was introduced as an antianginal drug, the mode of action being vasodilatation, its antiarrhythmic effect being discovered later (Charlier et al 1968, Marcus et al 1981, Ward et al 1980). It has a major advantage in that it is not negatively inotropic and therefore may even be haemodynamically beneficial to patients with impaired left ventricular function through its vasodilatory effect. Amiodarone has an extremely long half life of 7–40 days (Holt et al 1983). This probably reflects the high lipid solubility of the drug, its volume of distribution being estimated at about 5000 litres. The sole metabolite is des-ethyl amiodarone, the antiarrhythmic effects of which are unknown. Its concentration, however, always exceeds that of the parent compound except in fat. Elimination is by biliary and gastrointestinal excretion, little of either the drug or its metabolite appearing in the urine. The extremely long half life is both a disadvantage and an advantage. The problems associated with this are that antiarrhythmic effects may not be seen for several days because of its wide distribution and the electrophysiological confirmation of effect is therefore difficult. In fact, conventional assessment by electrophysiological study may not be possible for this drug. Furthermore, discontinuation of the drug is followed by a long and variable period during which the extent of amiodarone's remaining effects are uncertain and the patient therefore extremely difficult to assess. The advantage of the long half life is seen with chronic therapy, which can be with once daily dosage, and in those patients with life threatening arrhythmias where short term cessation of therapy (inadvertent, diarrhoea) will not have catastrophic results. In order to shorten the delay to onset of antiarrhythmic efficacy, loading by means of high dose intravenous infusion has recently been used. Any advantage that this may have over oral loading is uncertain as is the nature of action of the drug when used intravenously.

The spectrum of oral amiodarone's antiarrhythmic effects is wide. It has been used successfully in the prophylactic treatment of all forms of atrial, junctional and ventricular arrhythmias. However, because of the problems associated with its use, this has tended to be restricted to arrhythmias refractory to more conventional drugs and to those patients with life threatening arrhythmias in the presence of poor left ventricular function. Apart from the difficulties associated with the drug's pharmacokinetics, unwanted effects are another discouragement to its use. Although many are dose related, it is their serious nature and the difficulty associated with their reversal (because of the long drug elimination time) which present the problems. The commonest is photosensitivity of varying severity but which may necessitate withdrawal of the drug in extreme cases. In some, this may be followed by an asymptomatic and permanent bluish discolouration of exposed areas associated with deposition of lipofuschin. Next commonest are side effects on the neurological system varying from insomnia and nightmares to axonal degeneration producing peripheral neuropathy which may also leave permanent sequelae unless the drug is stopped promptly. Corneal microcrystal deposition is seen in every patient but seldom causes a problem. Occasionally, 'gritty' eye occurs or the crystals are deposited in the visual field; short term discontinuation of the drug is usually enough to relieve the latter problem as the crystals are reabsorbed. Hyperthyroidism is increasingly recognized among patients on long term amiodarone although hypothyroidism is also seen. Rarely, severe alveolitis with associated radiological shadowing is encountered, usually with high doses. However, subclinical deterioration in lung function is seen more often, the changes being in diffusing capacity. The problem resolves with steroid therapy and withdrawal of treatment which is only necessary for the clinically overt syndrome. Gastrointestinal effects are uncommon with nausea, vomiting and constipation occasionally encountered, especially during the loading period. A chemical hepatocellular hepatitis is seen in about 15% of patients but resolves spontaneously even with continued therapy at the same dose in the majority of cases.

In terms of drug interactions, because of its protein and tissue binding, other drugs such as digoxin and anticoagulants are displaced although alternative explanations for the increased plasma concentrations of the drugs exist. With digoxin, there may be interference with its excretion and warfarin's metabolism may be impaired by hepatic microsomal enzyme inhibition. Amiodarone has an additive effect with beta blockers, verapamil and diltiazem in depressing sinus and AV nodal function.

BRETYLIUM

Bretylium is an adrenergic neurone blocker with a class III antiarrhythmic effect. Its use is restricted to refractory ventricular arrhythmias, especially fibrillation. It is given intravenously because of poor and unpredictable absorption after oral administration. The adrenergic neurone blocking effects are probably not relevant to its antiarrhythmic effects which are seen in denervated and catecholamine depleted hearts as well as those where the blockade has been reversed by using tricyclic antidepressant drugs. Also, the antifibrillatory effects of bretylium are not shared by guanethidine (Bacaner 1968) despite the shared adrenergic neurone blocking effects. It has an advantage that, being a vasodilator, it can be used readily in patients with poor left ventricular function.

Drug interactions such as the increased efficacy of supportive pressor amines can be predicted from knowledge of the adrenergic neurone blocking properties of bretylium.

SOTALOL

Initially introduced as a non-selective β-blocker without sympathomimetic nor membrane stabilizing activity, Sotalol has subsequently been demonstrated to possess class III antiarrhythmic properties seen especially after intravenous bolus administration although also detectable after chronic oral use to a degree more than might be expected from pure β-blockade. However, the clinical advantage of this additional property is uncertain, there being no demonstrable increase in antiarrhythmic effect compared with β-blockade alone. The drug is a racemic mixture of the L and D-isomers. It appears that most of the β-blocking effect is contributed by L-sotalol and so D-sotalol is currently being investigated as a class III antiarrhythmic drug (although it is also a weak β-blocker).

VERAPAMIL

Verapamil is a synthetic papaverine derivative and is used for its antiarrhythmic, antianginal and antihypertensive properties. Of the calcium antagonist group, it is the most widely used for an antiarrhythmic effect. It reduces the amplitude of transmembrane action potentials in the SA and AV nodes and prolongs AV nodal refractoriness. Although active both orally and parenterally, there is extensive first pass metabolism so that, to overcome this, the oral dose used is about 10 times the intravenous dose. After either oral or intravenous administration there is an initial distribution phase (α) of about 20–30 minutes followed by a more gradual elimination (β) phase with a half life of 3–7 hours. Following an intravenous bolus, the onset of effect is within 2 minutes, peaking at 10 minutes. After oral administration, effects appear at 2 hours and peak at 5 hours. Less than 5% of the drug appears unchanged in the urine. With the solitary exception of fascicular tachycardia (Ward et al 1984), verapamil is inactive on ventricular arrhythmias. The effect upon supraventricular arrhythmias depends on the role of the AV node in the arrhythmia. When it merely transmits an atrial tachyarrhythmia to the ventricles, the effect will be to decrease the ventricular response rate as in atrial tachycardia, flutter and fibrillation whereas, when the AV node is an essential part of the tachycardia substrate as in junctional reentry tachycardia, then the arrhythmia will usually be terminated.

In that it interferes with calcium mediated myocardial excitation–contraction coupling, verapamil has a negatively inotropic effect. This has to be balanced against the beneficial effects of vasodilatation but overall, care is required in patients with impaired left ventricular function. Other unwanted cardiac effects include sinus bradycardia, sinus arrest, AV block, ventricular arrhythmias and ventricular asystole. Extracardiac side effects include headaches, flushing and constipation. Verapamil interacts with other drugs, principally digoxin and β-blockers. The former interaction is synergistic whereas the combination of β-blockade and verapamil aggravates the negatively inotropic properties of both drugs and can lead to asystole (Krikler & Spurrell 1972). The usual interactions with protein bound drugs such as warfarin occur and verapamil when used in conjunction with class I agents may cause profound myocardial depression. Although reentry tachycardias in association with the Wolff-Parkinson-White syndrome may be terminated by verapamil, conduction of atrial tachyarrhythmias via an accessory pathway may be accelerated. A number of verapamil derivatives, such as Tiapamil, have been developed and are structurally and functionally similar to the parent compound.

DILTIAZEM

Apart from verapamil, diltiazem is the only calcium antagonist used frequently for its antiarrhythmic effect. This is similar to verapamil although it differs in being a less effective peripheral vasodilator and is less negatively inotropic. Also, as a result of less hypotensive effect, there is less reflex sympathetic response. However, the pharmacokinetics and pharmacodynamics of the two drugs are very similar. Diltiazem has fewer side effects, thanks mainly to the relative absence of negative inotropism although constipation is also uncommon.

DIGOXIN

The antiarrhythmic effects of digoxin in man are restricted to the AV node. There is no overall effect upon sinus cycle length nor atrial refractory period. Ventricular refractoriness is reduced and there is evidence that accessory pathway refractoriness is also reduced (Wellens & Durrer 1973). Both these effects may be proarrhythmic whereas the effects on the AV node are to prolong its conduction time and refractory period. Thereby, digoxin may be useful in controlling the ventricular response rate to an atrial tachyarrhythmia such as atrial fibrillation (its main use) or in terminating or preventing an arrhythmia for which the AV node is essential such as AV nodal reentry tachycardia. Its uses are therefore similar to those of verapamil but its side effect profile is different. It has been used in the past for a positive intropic effect. Whilst the importance of this effect is controversial, it is certainly not negatively inotropic like verapamil and so the same precautions about its use in patients with poor left ventricular function are not necesary. However, its proarrhythmic effects should be remembered in such patients. Any arrhythmia can be provoked by digoxin and the proarrhythmic effects are usually dose related. Heart block is particularly common as are ventricular ectopics. Hypokalaemia potentiates the effects of digoxin and may therefore be responsible for toxic effects being seen at therapeutic levels. Serum levels are of little benefit in making the diagnosis of digoxin toxicity which should therefore be made from clinical criteria such as arrhythmias and symptoms which include nausea, anorexia and central nervous effects. Subjective visual disturbances are common. These unwanted effects are particularly common amongst the elderly, especially those with renal impairment in whom renal excretion of the unchanged drug is reduced.

The drug is given orally once daily in view of its long half life with the usual dosage being between 0.125 and 0.5 mg daily. Loading is required, usually with an increased oral dose for the first 24 to 36 hours but this can be accelerated by intravenous use, care being taken to monitor for potential proarrhythmic effects. Treatment of intoxication consists of correcting electrolyte abnormalities where they exist and withdrawal of the drug. These measures usually suffice but where more urgent treament is required, class Ib agents may be used to treat ventricular arryythmias until the drug level subsides and temporary pacing may also be indicated for a similar period in patients with severe bradycardia as a result of digoxin induced heart block. More aggressive methods such as adsorptive haemoperfusion or the use of digoxin-specific antibodies are rarely required.

CONCLUSIONS

We have attempted to summarize the antiarrhythmic drugs in common use. Although the anticipated antiarrhythmic effects of many of them will overlap, there is considerable individual variation in the observed clinical antiarrhythmic effects, even of drugs with apparently identical spectra of basic and clinical electrophysiological effects. This implies that much remains to be learnt regarding the precise mechanism of the arrhythmias and the drugs' antiarrhythmic effects.

Acknowledgements

The authors are supported by the British Heart Foundation.

REFERENCES

Bacaner M B 1968 Quantitative comparison of bretylium with other antifibrillatory drugs. American Journal of Cardiology 21: 504–512

Bucknall C, Laudusans E, Tynan M J, Curry P V L 1985 Ventricular tachycardia masquerading as supraventricular tachycardia: management of His bundle tachycardia. British Heart Journal 53: 681 (Abstract)

Charlier R, Deltour G, Baudine A, Chaillet F 1968 Pharmacology of amiodarone, an antianginal drug with a new biological profile. Arzneimittel Forschung 18: 1408–1417

Charlier R 1970 Cardiac actions in the dog of a new antagonist of adrenergic excitation which does not produce competitive blockade of adrenoreceptors. British Journal of Pharmacology 39: 668–673

Dengler R, Rudel R 1979 Effects of tocainide on normal and myotonic mammalian skeletal muscle.Drug Research 29: 270–273

Dukes I D, Vaughan Williams E M 1984 The multiple modes of action of propafenone. European Heart Journal 5: 115–125

Elvin A T, Lalka D, Stoeckel K et al 1980 Tocainide kinetics and metabolism: effects of phenobarbital and substrates for glucuronyl transferase. Clinical Pharmacology and Therapeutics 28: 652–658

Himes R S, DiFazio C A, Burney R G 1977 Effects of lidocaine on the anaesthetic requirements for nitrous oxide and halothane. Anesthesiology 47: 437–440

Holt D W, Tucker G T, Jackson P R, Storey G C A 1983 Amiodarone pharmacokinetics. American Heart Journal 106: 840–847

Ikram H 1980 Hemodynamic and electrophysiologic interactions between antiarrhythmic drugs and beta-blockers, with special reference to tocainide. American Heart Journal 100: 1076–1080

Krikler D, Spurrell R 1972 Asystole after verapamil. British Medical Journal 2: 405 (Letter)

Krikler D M, Curry P V L 1976 Torsade de pointes, an atypical ventricular tachycardia. British Heart Journal 38: 117–120

Marcus F, Fontaine G H, Frank R, Grosgogeat Y 1981 Clinical pharmacology and therapeutic applications of the antiarrhythmic agent, amiodarone. American Heart Journal 101: 480–493

Miller R D, Way W L, Katzung B G 1967 The potentiation of neuromuscular blocking agents by quinidine. Anesthesiology 28: 1036–1041

Nathan A W, Hellestrand K J 1984 Flecainide acetate: a review. Clinical Progress in Pacing and Electrophysiology 2: 43–53

Rudolph W, Petri H, Kofk W, Hall D 1979 Effects of Propafenone on the accessory pathway in patients with WPW syndrome. American Journal of Cardiology 43: 430 (Abstract)

Salerno D M, Granrud G, Sharkey P et al 1984 A controlled trail of propafenone for treatment of frequent and repetitive ventricular premature complexes. American Journal of Cardiology 53: 77–83

Shen E N, Sung R J, Morady F et al 1984 Electrophysiologic and hemodynamic effects of intravenous propafenone in patients with recurrent ventricular tachycardia. Journal of the American College of Cardiology 3: 1291–1297

Singh B N, Vaughan-Williams E M 1970 The effect of amiodarone, a new anti-anginal drug on cardiac muscle. British Journal of Pharmacology 39: 657–667

Silverman R, Frishman W H 1983 Drug treament of cardiac arrhythmias: propranolol and other beta-blockers. In: Gould L A (ed) Drug treatment of cardiac arrhythmias. Futura Press, New York, ch 11

Waleffe A, Brunix P, Mary-Rabine L, Kulbertus H E 1979 Effects of tocainide studied with programmed electrical stimulation of the heart in patients with reentrant tachyarrhythmias. American Journal of Cardiology 43: 292–299

Ward D E, Camm A J, Spurrell R A J 1980 Clinical antiarrhythmic effects of amiodarone in patients with resistant paroxysmal tachycardias. British Heart Journal 44: 91–95

Ward D E, Nathan A W, Camm A J 1984 Fascicular tachycardia sensitive to calcium antagonists. European Heart Journal 5: 896–905

Wellens H J J, Durrer D 1973 Effect of digitalis on atrioventricular conduction in circus movement tachycardia in patients with Wolff-Parkinson-White syndrome. Circulation 47: 1229–1233

Young M D, Hadidian Z, Horn H R et al 1980 Treatment of ventricular arrhythmias with oral tocainide. American Heart Journal 100: 1041–1045

10 *G. Farnsworth*

Anaesthesia for cardiac surgery and post-operative care

During the last 10 years there has been a marked increase in the number of cardiac surgical operations performed in the UK. The UK cardiac surgical register shows that in 1977 there were 11 602 operations and by 1982 this had risen to 15 890. Adult valvular heart disease and congenital heart disease have remained constant at 4000–5000 and 3000–3500 per year respectively while those for ischaemic heart disease have increased from 3000 to 7000 cases per year (English et al 1984) (Table 10.1). This review is concerned with anaesthesia for adult cardiac surgery and does not include anaesthesia for congenital heart disease in paediatric patients.

The risks of cardiac surgery have fallen with the result that in 1982 in the UK, the mortality within 30 days of operation was 7.1%. Factors associated with increased risk include unstable angina, recent myocardial infarction, poor left ventricular function, age greater than 65 years, obesity, reoperation, heart failure and emergency surgery. A prospective study from the Montreal Heart Institute demonstrated a mortality of 0.4% in the absence of any of these factors rising to 3.1% if one is present and to 12.2% for more than one factor (Paiement et al 1983).

Newer surgical operations include ablation of arrhythmogenic areas in refractory arrhythmias, heart transplants, combined heart and lung transplants and implantation of a total artificial heart.

Table 10.1 Number (percentage mortality[a]) of all cardiac operations 1977–82 (Reproduced from English 1984 with kind permission of the British Medical Journal)

Year	Valvular heart disease	Ishaemic heart disease	Congenital valve disease	Adult miscellaneous acquired heart disease	Total
1977	4832 (8.9)	3040 (9.3)	3344 (10.1)	386 (22.8)	11 602 (9.8)
1978	4873 (9.5)	3345 (7.5)	3385 (11.1)	340 (22.1)	11 943 (9.8)
1979	4791 (9.2)	3688 (8.4)	3275 (10.5)	402 (19.2)	12 156 (9.6)
1980	4814 (7.0)	5011 (6.1)	3472 (11.0)	442 (15.4)	13 739 (7.9)
1981	4762 (6.9)	6123 (5.8)	3501 (8.9)	401 (19.7)	14 787 (7.3)
1982	4652 (6.7)	7403 (5.2)	3392 (9.9)	443 (21.7)	15 890 (7.1)
Total	28 724 (8.1)	28 610 (6.6)	20 369 (10.0)	2414 (19.9)	80 117 (8.5)

[a]Mortality (%) defined as death at or within 30 days after operation (English 1984).

PRE-OPERATIVE PREPARATION

Patients presenting for operation should be prepared with the adjunct of drugs to be in the best possible medical condition.

Valvular disease

Patients with valvular disease may have heart failure which is controlled by diuretics and digoxin. Those with mitral valve disease may be in atrial fibrillation and although digoxin has traditionally been used to slow the ventricular rate by blocking atrioventricular conduction, verapamil, a calcium antagonist may be used instead or in combination with digoxin.

Coronary artery disease

Patients with coronary artery disease are commonly treated with β adrenergic antagonists, calcium antagonists and vasodilators, i.e. triple-drug therapy.

β Adrenergic blocking drugs

Newer β blocking drugs may have a greater selectivity for the β_1 adrenergic receptors in cardiac muscle and have a lesser effect on the β_2 receptors in bronchial muscle and the peripheral circulation. Such cardioselective drugs are metoprolol and atenolol and these may be useful in patients with respiratory disease leaving the β_2 receptor unblocked. However, even the cardioselective β blockers may aggravate bronchospasm in some asthmatic patients. Absorption and metabolism of β blockers determine the onset of their action and the duration of clinical effect. Propranolol is lipid soluble, is almost completely absorbed from the gastrointestinal tract and is metabolized by the liver. Its elimination half life is 3.5–6 h and administration is 3–4 times per 24 h. Atenolol is water soluble, is completely absorbed from the gut and is eliminated unchanged by the kidney. Its elimination half life is 6–9 h and once per 24 h dosage is appropriate (Frishman 1981). All β blockers can be dangerous in patients with compromised ventricular function and can precipitate pulmonary oedema, hypotension and heart block.

Calcium antagonists

The calcium antagonists are a developing group of drugs which inhibit calcium ion flux in smooth muscle. Verapamil, nifedipine and diltiazem are used for their effects on cardiac and vascular muscle. They produce vasodilation, particularly of the arterial bed and the coronary arteries appear to be especially sensitive. In stable, effort induced angina, coronary vasospasm may add to the obstructive coronary artery disease and further reduce blood flow. Other factors involved in amelioration of anginal symptoms are given in Table 10.2. Headache from cerebral arteriolar dilatation and postural hypotension are among the side effects. Since verapamil and β blockers both have negative inotropic activity and depress atrioventricular conduction, the effects of verapamil and β blockers can be additive. If intravenous β

Table 10.2 Mechanisms of beneficial effect of Ca^{2+} channel blocking agents in stable angina (Reproduced from Braunwald 1982 with kind permission of the New England Journal of Medicine)

1 Increased myocardial oxygen supply
 A Coronary artery dilation
 B Improved subendocardial perfusion

2 Decreased myocardial oxygen demand
 A Decreased peripheral resistance
 B Decreased myocardial contractility (verapamil)
 C Decreased heart rate (verapamil)

Table 10.3 Side effects of anti-anginal drugs (Reproduced from Braunwald 1982 with kind permission of the New England Journal of Medicine)

Drug	Hypotension; flushing; headache	Left ventricular dysfunction	Decreased heart rate; atrioventricular block	Gastrointestinal symptoms	Broncho-constriction
β Blockers	0	++	+++	+	+++
Diltiazem	+	+	+	0	0
Nifedipine	+++	0	0	0	0
Verapamil	+	+	++	++	0
Nitrates	+++	0	0	0	0

Abbreviations: 0 = absent; + = mild; ++ = moderate; +++ = sometimes severe.

blocking drugs are given to patients taking verapamil, there is an increased risk of bradycardia and hypotension. (Table 10.3).

Nitrates

Nitrates, because of their vasodilating properties, are the third group of drugs used to stabilize patients with coronary artery disease. The vasodilation is mainly venous, producing a lower ventricular filling pressure and a reduction in myocardial wall tension and myocardial work. By lowering ventricular diastolic pressure they also permit an increased blood flow as this depends on the difference between aortic and ventricular diastolic pressures. Sublingual glyceryl trinitrate is particularly useful for acute events and more sustained action can be achieved with absorption through the skin. Other longer acting nitrates have been developed for oral use such as isosorbide dinitrate and pentaerythritol tetranitrate. Glyceryl trinitrate and isosorbide dinitrate can also be administered by intravenous infusion to patients with prolonged or severe rest pain.

Patients may find waiting for surgery to be stressful and it is therefore routine practice to continue all medical therapy up to and including the day of operation.

OPERATIVE MANAGEMENT

Monitoring

One of the major tasks of an anaesthetist is to maintain the patients' physiological functions during surgical events. Being forewarned is to be forearmed and it is

Table 10.4 Monitoring during cardiac anaesthesia

System monitored	Measurement
Cardiovascular	Electrocardiogram Blood pressure via arterial cannulae Central venous pressure Pulmonary artery pressure Left atrial pressure
Respiratory	Airway pressure Blood gases
Central nervous	Pupil size Cerebral function trace
Renal	Urine output Serum potassium Acid–base status

advantageous to have adequate monitoring established before anaesthesia and surgery commence. Parameters often monitored are shown in Table 10.4. In addition central temperature is usually measured by a nasopharyngeal probe. Some of the measurements such as pupil size cause minimal hazard to the patient but invasive cardiovascular monitoring carries the risk of infection, haemorrhage, thrombosis and embolism. The risks associated with monitoring have to be balanced against the protection they afford the patient.

Arterial lines

The radial artery is most used and a number of workers have looked at the incidence of complications, especially that of thrombosis. Bedford & Woolmer (1973) in a prospective study found that 40 of their 105 patients (38%) developed vessel occlusion. In a study in New Zealand the incidence was reduced to 3% when 20 g teflon canulae were used instead of 18 g polypropylene (Davis & Stewart 1980). However, workers in Texas with the largest prospective series yet reported comprizing 1699 patients, had an overall incidence of 25% abnormal flow and also failed to show that catheter size (18 g or 20 g) or material altered this figure (Slogoff et al 1983). These authors also queried the predictive value of an Allen's test for collateral ulnar flow. 411 patients were examined and 16 had an abnormal test ($>$ 15 s). None of the 16 patients had signs of ischaemia during cannulation and none had abnormal flow after decannulation.

Regular examination of the patients hand will identify ischaemic changes. If there is a persistent decrease in temperature or skin mottling, the catheter should be removed,

Central venous lines

As well as providing a measurement of right atrial pressure, these lines are used for administration of vasoactive and irritant drugs. The insertion of more than one line allows infusion of such drugs to proceed without interference from CVP measurements or bolus injections. A trilumen catheter has recently been introduced (Deseret Medical). Luer-lock connections help to reduce the risk of accidental disconnection and air embolism.

Pulmonary artery catheters

These are widely used in patients in North America having heart surgery but are inserted more selectively in the UK. Pulmonary artery wedge pressure is considered equivalent to left atrial pressure providing the catheter is free from clot and its tip is at or below the level of the left atrium. In the upper zones of the lung, alveolar pressure may occlude pulmonary vasculature, produce intermittent blood flow and a wedge pressure may not correspond to that of the left atrium. In conditions where the right and left filling pressures of the heart are different (e.g. mitral valve disease, poor left ventricular function) pulmonary artery catheters may provide additional information to that obtained from central venous pressure measurement. The main indication for use in cardiac surgical patients is an unstable patient with poor left ventricular function. Arrhythmias and premature beats can occur during catheter insertion. In a recent prospective study of 500 patients (Boyd et al 1983) this occured in 100 (20%). Serious complications occured in 23 patients (4.3%) including ventricular tachycardia (8), pulmonary heamorrhage (1), pulmonary infarction (7) and septicaemia(7).

Left atrial lines

These are placed by the surgeon at operation either directly into the left atrium or via the right atrium through the atrial septum. Embolism is a particular danger. The line should be clearly labelled, not used for infusion or injection of drugs and removed as soon as possible.

Choice of anaesthetic agent

Many techniques and anaesthetic drugs have been described for use in cardiac anaethesia. It would appear to be primarily important to maintain cardiovascular stability and the drugs an individual anaesthetist chooses to achieve this are of less importance. It has been shown that peri-operative ischaemia can influence the incidence of post-operative myocardial infarction after coronary artery bypass surgery (Slogoff & Keats 1985). Endotracheal intubation, the surgical stimulation of skin incision and sternal splitting accounted for half of these ischaemic episodes. Nine anaesthesiologists were involved in the study, one being associated with a significantly higher incidence of peri-operative ischaemia and post-operative myocardial infarction.

Anaesthetic drugs (recently introduced)

Isoflurane This inhalational agent causes a drop in blood pressure by a reduction of systemic vascular resistance. Vasodilation and a fall in blood pressure would seem very useful properties in patients with coronary artery disease but a clinical study by

Reiz et al (1983) revealed possible hazards. Isoflurane (1% end-tidal) was administered to patients with coronary artery disease having major vascular surgery of the aorta or iliac vessels. Ten of the 21 patients developed ECG changes with ST depression or T wave inversion. Coronary blood flow did not alter in these 10 patients but lactate extraction decreased markedly. It is postulated that a reduction in perfusion pressure may lead to regional ischaemia in the area supplied by the stenosed coronary arteries. Thus isoflurane should be used with care in patients with critical coronary stenoses.

Vecuronium Pancuronium has been used as a neuromuscular blocking agent in many cardiac procedures as blood pressure is maintained but the tachycardia is a disadvantage. This does not occur with the short acting monoquaternary steroid, vecuronium bromide.

Atracurium This interesting muscle relaxant undergoes degradation with increase in pH and temperature. If given to a cold patient, e.g. one cooled in cardiopulmonary bypass, additional incremental doses are unnecessary.

Management on bypass

One of the important tasks is to ensure adequate heparinization during cardiopulmonary bypass. Too little leads to the risk of emboli while the filters of the bypass system may become blocked; too much leads to difficulty in reversing the anticoagulation at the end of the procedure. The management of the anticoagulation has been greatly assisted by the use of the activated clotting time (ACT). 2–3 ml of blood are added to 12 mg of celite which reduces the whole blood clotting time to 90–130 s. Adequate heparinization is achieved by prolonging the ACT to at least three times baseline levels. Two groups of patients, those with recent subacute bacterial endocarditis and those on intra-aortic balloon pumps may require more than 3 mg/kg to do this (Kamath & Fozard 1980).

Perfusion of vital organs such as the brain, heart and kidneys may alter when the patient is no longer dependent on his own cardiac output but that produced by a machine. Patients with cerebrovascular disease are more susceptible to falls in blood pressure and reduced blood flow. In a retrospective survey of 3206 patients Bojar et al (1983) showed that of the 32 patients developing a major neurological deficit, six had carotid or vertebral stenoses. Monitoring pupil size is a simple way of assessing gross cerebral perfusion and more sophisticated methods involve the electroencephalogram (EEG). The EEG during ischaemia shows a decline in electrical activity. There is a decrease in faster waves with an increase in slower waves leading to electrical silence. The cerebral function monitor was designed to follow the electrical activity from a single pair of parietal electrodes. The position of the trace indicates the overall cerebral energy and the width of the trace shows the variation in wave form. The cerebral function analysing monitor is a further refinement giving a more detailed plot of the β, α, θ and δ waves (Maynard & Jenkinson 1984) (Fig. 10.1).

For some procedures involving the correction of complex cardiac defects in small infants or for aortic arch surgery in adults, complete cessation of the cerebral circulation may be required. What is considered to be a safe time of circulatory arrest at a given temperature? Treasure (1984) studied hypothermic circulatory arrest in a small mammal, the gerbil. There is no circle of Willis in these animals and carotid

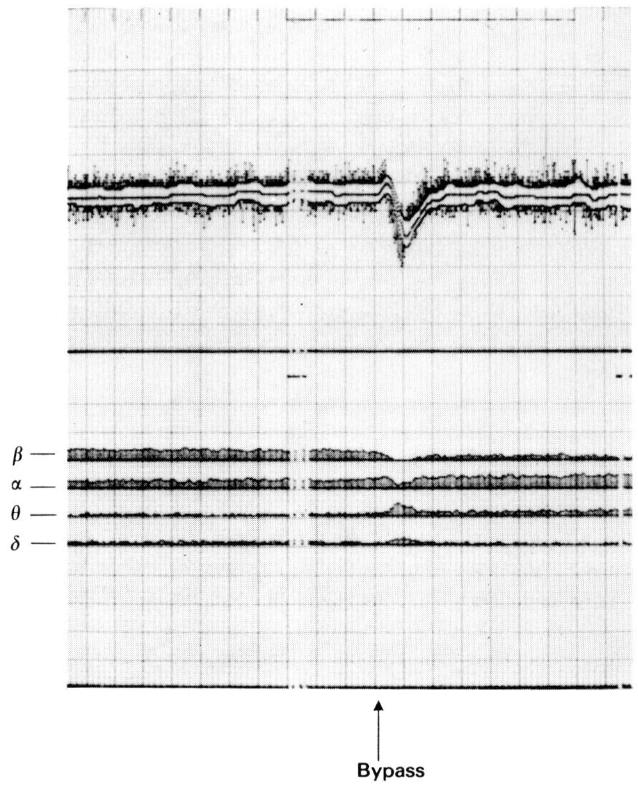

Fig. 10.1 Cerebral function analysing monitor trace recorded as patient went on to cardiopulmonary bypass. A fall in mean voltage is seen which recovers within 2 minutes. There is also a decrease in β and α wave activity with an increase in θ and δ wave activity.

occlusion leads to a cessation of cerebral blood flow. With brain temperatures of 20°C the gerbils had periods of cerebral ischaemia for times ranging from 0 to 180 minutes and were then examined metabolically, functionally and morphologically. Although one hour of circulatory arrest at temperatures below 20°C has been considered acceptable, Treasure convincingly suggested that this time should be revised to 20 minutes if the risk of irreversible brain damage is to be minimized.

Technical developments

Oxygenators

The most common type of oxygenator is a bubble oxygenator and damage to blood cell membranes can occur at the blood-gas interface. Membrane oxygenators are similar to the physiological arrangements in the lungs as the perfusion fluid and gases are separated by a polypropylene or silicone membrane. Membrane oxygenators cause less haemolysis, and higher platelet and white cell counts are obtained than when bubble oxygenators are used (Pierce 1980). Although they are more expensive and may take longer to set up, membrane oxygenators offer advantages for lengthy procedures. They can also be used for patients requiring long term support on partial cardiopulmonary bypass.

Biochemical measurements

Advancing technology allows for the rapid determination of pH, serum potassium and blood gases. Intravascular probes have been used to give continuous measurement of Po_2 but because probes are 5 French gauge, they are more suited to insertion into a central line than into a peripheral artery. An on-line oxygen electrode has been developed for use in the arterial or venous lines of the cardiopulmonary bypass to give a continuous reading of Po_2 (Claremont et al 1984).

POST-OPERATIVE CARE

Cardiovascular system

Following cardiac surgery the patient may develop life threatening complications and is therefore transferred to an intensive care ward for intensive monitoring. Monitoring is continued during the transfer using portable ECG and blood pressure equipment. Cardiovascular stability may require the use of ionotropes, vasodilators, dysrhythmic drugs, pacemakers and intra-aortic balloon pumps. Replacement of blood loss is important to maintain adequate filling pressures for the right and left atria. Autologous blood transfusion using a closed collecting system (commercially available from Sorensen Research Corporation) can reduce the requirement for banked blood (Johnson et al 1983).

Respiration

In the early post-operative period respiration is usually maintained by mechanical ventilators. The reasons for this are as follows.

1. The patient may have been in heart failure pre-operatively and still have residual pulmonary oedema.
2. High doses of opiates can markedly depress respiration.
3. Patients may be cool both centrally and peripherally and have greater oxygen demands when warming.
4. An increase in alveolar-arterial Po_2 difference is seen for at least 3 hours after operation (Sanchez de Leon et al 1982). A fall in colloid osmotic pressure occurs during bypass due to crystalloid fluid in the bypass priming fluid. This may cause interstitial pulmonary oedema and an increasing alveolar-arterial oxygen gradient. The time course for the restoration of colloid osmotic pressure and haematocrit parallels that of the restoration of the alveolar-arterial gradient.

More recently a number of workers have questioned the need to ventilate post-operatively patients with stable cardiovascular systems. Quasha et al (1980) studied patients following elective coronary artery bypass grafts. They compared a group of 18 patients who had spontaenous respiration and early extubation at a mean of 2 hours post-operatively with 20 patients who were ventilated overnight and extubated late at a mean of 18 hours. There was a significant reduction in the amount of analgesics and sedatives given to the early extubation group. There was a reduction in the amount of vasodilator drugs required to keep the systolic and diastolic pressures under 160 mmHg and 90 mmHg respectivelyalthough this did not reach statistical significance. One patient was reintubated when his PCO_2 reached 56 mmHg (kPa 7.46). Schuller et al (1984) have also reported on their practice of early extubation in children and had a low reintubation rate of 2.4%.

Humidification

For those who are ventilated, heating and humidification of the inspired gases has been provided by heated water reservoirs. Simpler hygroscopic condenser humidifiers are now available. Fully humidified expired gases at 37°C contain 44 mg water vapour per litre, which falls to 19.5 mg/l at 22°C in a heat and moisture exchanger. If a hygroscopic surface is added expired gases leave with only 9 mg water vapour per litre leaving 35 mg for humidification of inspired gas. A device such as the Servo-Humidifier (Siemans-Elema) is thus capable of providing inspired gases at a temperature of 5°C below body temperature and a relative humidity of 75% (Gedeon & Mebius 1979). The Pall Ultipor hydrophobic filter, designed as a bacterial filter, can also function as a humidifier. It compares well with other devices and has the added advantage of bacterial filtration (Bethune 1985).

Sedation

Regimes for sedation of patients on ventilators have come under scrutiny following the increased mortality in patients receiving etomidate infusions (Ledingham & Watt 1983). Etomidate infusions can no longer be recommended while althesin has been withdrawn from use (see also p. 219).

Combinations of analgesics and sedatives are often employed. A water soluble benzodiazepine, midazolam, has the advantage of being non-irritant to veins and has a short half life of 60–90 minutes (Dundee et al 1980) (see also p. 218).

REFERENCES

Bedford R F, Woolmer H 1973 Complications of percutaneous radial artery cannulation: an objective prospective study in man. Anesthesiology 38: 228–236

Bethune D W 1985 Hydrophobic versus hygroscopic heat and moisture exchangers. Anaesthesia 40: 210–211

Bojar R M, Hassan N, DeLaria G A, Sherry C, Goldin M D 1983 Neurological complications of coronary revascularisation. Annals of Thoracic Surgery 36: 427–432

Boyd K D, Thomas S J, Gold J, Boyd A D 1983 A prospective study of complications of pulmonary artery catheterisations in 500 consecutive patients. Chest 84: 245–249

Braunwald E 1982 Mechanism of action of calcium-channel blocking agents. New England Journal of Medicine 307: 1618–1627

Claremont D J, Pagdin T M, Walton N 1984 Continuous monitoring of blood $P\text{O}_2$ in extracorporeal systems. An in vitro evaluation of a re-usable oxygen electrode. Anaesthesia 39: 262–269

Davis F M, Stewart J M 1980 Radial artery canulation: a prospective study in patients undergoing cardiothoracic surgery. British Journal of Anaesthesia 52: 41–46

Dundee J W, Samuel I O, Toner W, Howard P J 1980 Midazolam: a water-soluble benzodiazepine. Studies in volunteers. Anaesthesia 35: 454–458

English T A H, Bailey A R, Dark J F, Williams W G 1984 The UK cardiac surgical register 1977–82. British Medical Journal 289: 1205–1208
Frishman W H 1981 β-Adrenoceptor antagonists: new drugs and new indications. New England Journal of Medicine 305: 500–506
Gedeon A, Mebius C 1979 The hygroscopic condenser humidifier. A new device for general use in anaesthesia and intensive care. Anaesthesia 34: 1043–1047
Johnson R G, Rosenkrantz B A, Preston R A, Hopkins C, Daggett W M 1983 The efficacy of postoperative autotransfusion in patients undergoing cardiac operations. Annals of Thoracic Surgery 36: 173–179
Kamath B S K, Fozard J R 1980 Control of heparinisation during cardiopulmonary bypass. Experience with the activated clotting time method. Anaesthesia 35: 250–256
Ledingham I M, Watt I 1983 Influence of sedation on mortality in critically ill multiple trauma patients. Lancet i: 1270
Maynard D E, Jenkinson J L 1984 The cerebral function analysing monitor. Initial clinical experience, application and further development. Anaesthesia 39: 678–690
Paiement B et al 1983 A simple classification of the risk in cardiac surgery. Canadian Anaesthetists Society Journal 30: 61–68
Pierce E C 1980 The membrane versus bubble oxygenator controversy. Annals of Thoracic Surgery 29: 497–499
Quasha A L, Loeber N, Feeley T W, Ullyot D J, Roizen M F 1980 Postoperative respiratory care: A controlled trial of early and late extubation following coronary-artery bypass grafting. Anesthesiology 52: 135–141
Reiz S, Balfors E, Sorenson M B, Ariola S, Friedman A, Truedsson H 1983 Isoflurane — a powerful coronary vasodilator in patients with coronary artery disease. Anesthesiology 59: 91–97
Sanchez De Leon R, Paterson J L, Sykes M K 1982 Changes in colloid osmotic pressure and plasma albumin concentration associated with extracorporeal circulation. British Journal of Anaesthesia 54: 465–473
Schuller J L, Bovill J G, Nijveld A, Patrick M R, Macelletti C 1984 Early extubation of the trachea after open heart surgery for congenital heart disease. A review of 3 years experience. British Journal of Anaesthesia 56: 1101
Slogoff S, Keats A S, Arlund C 1983 On the safety of radial artery cannulation. Anesthesiology 59: 42–47
Slogoff S, Keats A S 1985 Does perioperative myocardial ischemia lead to postoperative myocardial infarction? Anesthesiology 62: 107–114
Treasure T 1984 The safe duration of total circulatory arrest with profound hypothermia. Annals of the Royal College of Surgeons of England 66: 235–240

11

P. M. Bailey, C. S. Child

Endocrine response to surgery

INTRODUCTION

Trauma, whether accidental or surgical, induces a series of circulatory, endocrine, metabolic and immunological changes which are known as the stress response.

In 1942 Cuthbertson divided the stress response into an ebb phase and a flow phase (Cuthbertson 1942) and in 1953 Moore described four separate metabolic phases associated with surgery — an adrenergic/corticoid phase, a corticoid withdrawal phase, an anabolic phase and a fat gain phase (Moore 1953). The ebb or adrenergic/corticoid phase lasts between 1 and 5 days and consists of a series of emergency responses designed to ensure the immediate survival of the individual. Four catabolic hormones, catecholamines, cortisol, growth hormone and glucagon are involved while the actions of insulin are suppressed. This results in an increase in the production and delivery of readily utilizable fuel sources (glucose and free fatty acids) to organs vital for fight and flight, namely the heart, the brain and muscle. The ebb phase gives way to the flow phase (the corticoid withdrawal phase, Moore 1983) when catabolic activity decreases and the metabolic effects of insulin predominate.

The flow or anabolic phase usually starts 2–10 days after the initial trauma and during this time there is a positive nitrogen balance as the protein loss which occurred in the initial phases is replaced. Fat stores are also replaced during the fat gain phase. However the whole anabolic process may be protracted and last several months.

Metabolic changes may occur in the pre-operative phase in the patient who is unduly anxious or who has severe pain, but the main causative factor is surgical trauma resulting in afferent nerve stimulation and increased production of hormones. Anaesthesia per se has little overall effect in initiating the response although different techniques have been developed to limit the consequences thereof.

It has been suggested that attempts to suppress the metabolic response to surgery are unnecessary or even harmful. The view has been propounded that the traumatized animal survives because of the response but it is illogical to suggest that this situation is analogous to that seen following surgical trauma. By suppressing the stress response the loss of energy stores and tissues can be minimized. During the stress response extensive amounts of hormones are released and the management of this at operation appears to be turning towards preventing their release and instituting appropriate hormone therapy as necessary.

In addition Akiyoshi et al (1984) have shown that immunodepression occurs following major abdominal surgery while Mani et al (1984) found a similar effect occurred following cardiac surgery. Animal studies by Fujiwara (1984) referred to the role of surgical stress in suppressing the graft versus host reaction following trauma. All these findings suggest that modifying the endocrine response to trauma may be an important factor in improving immunocompetence following major surgical procedures, with the result that post-operative complications may be minimized so that an earlier return to normal health is possible.

This chapter reviews the hormonal and metabolic changes that occur in response to surgery and trauma, the mechanisms by which they are initiated and the methods available to clinical anaesthetists to modify the response.

HORMONAL RESPONSE TO SURGERY

Catecholamines

The adrenergic response to surgery provides the anaesthetist with an important guide to depth of anaesthesia and adequacy of analgesia. The response is initiated by emotion, pain, hypotension, hypoxia and exposure to cold, and it manifests itself as an increase in adrenergic nerve activity intra-operatively with an increase in the circulating levels of catecholamines post-operatively (Halter et al 1977, Nistrup Marsden et al 1978).

The effects of a large increase in adrenergic activity are widespread. There is an increase in peripheral vascular resistance, heart rate and cardiac contractility, resulting in a rise in blood pressure, cardiac output and myocardial oxygen consumption. There are a series of metabolic responses which are mainly attributed to the effects of adrenaline, which has eight times the metabolic effects of noradrenaline and which is secreted in larger quantities, especially in the immediate post-operative period. Glycogenolysis is stimulated in muscle by a β adrenergic effect, which is cyclic AMP dependent and results in a rise in plasma lactate. In the liver glycogenolysis is an α effect and is dependent on calcium ions. There are several factors which reduce glucose utilization: these include a reduction in glycogen formation by an inhibition of glycogen synthase activity, a reduction in insulin activity and an increase in the formation of alternative fuel sources, e.g. fat. In addition, α adrenergic stimulation suppresses the release of insulin from the β pancreatic cells (Allison 1971).

The lipolytic effects of catecholamines produce free fatty acids, glycerol and 3-hydroxybutyrate. This β adrenergic, cyclic AMP effect of noradrenaline is brought about by an increase in activity of the enzyme triglyceride lipase. Noradrenaline is also responsible for an increase in heat production in brown adipose tissue (Hall & Lucke 1982). Although this may be important to the neonates the significance to the adults has yet to be determined.

The release of other catabolic hormones, such as growth hormone and cortisol, may be affected by an increase in adrenergic activity. α Adrenergic stimulation promotes the release of growth hormone from the pituitary while α adrenergic blockade has the opposite effect (Ishibashi & Yamaji 1984). These effects are probably mediated by dopamine receptors. Release of corticotrophin releasing factor (CRF), and hence adrenocorticotropic hormone and cortisol, may also be affected by adrenergic activity (Rees et al 1970, Gignere et al 1981, Grossman & Besser 1982).

The methods of assaying hormones and technical difficulties may make studies on plasma catecholamine levels appear contradictory. Thus the precise role of catecholamines in the metabolic response to surgery is still unclear.

Adrenocorticotropic hormone and cortisol

Early investigations into cortisol and adrenocorticotropic hormone (ACTH) secretion relied on the presence of indirect indicators such as eosinophilia. It was not until 1953 that plasma cortisol could be measured directly in the plasma (Weichselbaum et al 1953), while it was not until 1962 that ACTH could be assayed (Cooper & Nelson 1962). However, inspite of these difficulties, Long (1946) recognized that afferent nerve stimulation produced an endocrine response, including the release of ACTH and cortisol. In 1953 Hume described the nervous pathways in an elegant series of experiments on dogs. In the same year Moore (1953) measured urinary excretion of 17 ketosteroids during the 'four phases of convalescence'. The steroid excretion rose intra-operatively and in the immediate post-operative period, and then fell 2–5 days post-operatively to subnormal levels, for a period of several weeks.

It has since been shown that the plasma cortisol levels may rise to five times normal or more during major surgery (Thomasson 1959) or severe trauma. Levels usually remain high for 1–3 days. Factors such as severity of trauma, pain, hypovolaemia, hypoxia, sepsis and emotional upset increase cortisol production. Afferent neuronal blockade, central depression of ACTH and pharmacological inhibition of cortisol manufacture by agents such as etomidate (Ledingham & Watt 1983, Fry & Griffiths 1984) will reduce the adrenocortical response. There is a loss of the normal negative feedback control of ACTH by cortisol.

High circulating levels of corticosteroids will have effects on the circulation, on metabolism and on immunological systems. Some of their effects are due to a selective increase in enzyme production brought about when the steroids bind to nuclear chromatin and increase RNA production.

Cortisol is 95% bound to transcortin and albumin and only the free, unbound form is active. Its half life is 80 minutes and it is excreted by the kidneys after conjugation in the liver. It is possible that part of the increase in circulating cortisol levels during surgery is due to a decrease in liver blood flow resulting in a decrease in conjugation and excretion with also a reduction in protein binding.

The circulatory effects of the corticosteroids result in a decrease in peripheral resistance, an increase in cardiac output and an improvement in tissue perfusion (Samblin et al 1965). Hepatic blood flow and glomerular filtration rate are also improved. Cortisol has a mild sodium and water retaining effect and is important in maintaining the correct cell membrane permeability to electrolytes.

Cortisol inhibits the actions of insulin. This results in hyperglycaemia as glucose utilization is reduced while gluconeogenesis in the liver results in increased production of glucose. Cortisol also increases lipolysis. The effects of cortisol on protein metabolism are controversial and it is unclear whether it increases catabolism (Simmons et al 1984), decreases anabolism, or both (Hoover-Plow & Clifford 1978). The increase in protein catabolism may only occur when circulating levels are very high (Munro 1979) and in the absence of ketosis (Williamson et al 1977). That is, it may not be of significance in starved patients. It has been suggested that cortisol may not be an important wound hormone leading to post-traumatic muscle wasting and nitrogen loss (Baracos et al 1983, Clowes 1983, Bessey 1984, Gelfand et al 1984).

High circulating levels of cortisol will also have immunological effects, depressing allergic and inflammatory responses by decreasing antibody formation, decreasing numbers of circulating lymphocytes and eosinophils, decreasing the mass of lymphatic tissue, and inhibiting the activity of granulocytes and monocytes. There is a selective depression of T lymphocytes relative to B lymphocytes. If the high level of cortisol persists there may be an increased susceptibility to infection, inhibition of fibroblasts with an increased risk of bruising and poor wound healing, increased erythropoeisis, osteoporosis, and mood and behaviour changes.

Growth hormone

The factors effecting the release of growth hormone from the pituitary include pain, trauma, emotional stress, α adrenergic stimulation, antidiuretic hormone, deep sleep, fasting, protein depletion, glucagon, arginine and insulin hypoglycaemia (Newsome 1975). Growth hormone (GH) is inhibited by somatostatin, produced by 'D' cells of the pancreas (it also inhibits release of insulin and glucagon), and hyperglycaemia. However, during surgical stimulation GH is released in large quantities despite the presence of hyperglycaemia. Its effects are to produce hyperglycaemia, lipolysis and protein synthesis. Its effects on protein metabolism are probably mediated by somatomedin, a peptide produced by the liver, which stimulates amino acid uptake and protein synthesis and hence promotes nitrogen retention. It is likely that GH reduces the loss of protein that would otherwise occur during surgery, for it has been found that infusions of GH and calories in patients with burns will result in a positive nitrogen balance (Wilmore et al 1974). GH produces a decrease in glucose utilization but this tendency is partially offset as it sensitizes the β islet cells to produce more insulin. As with ACTH, the normal control of growth hormone release is lost during stress. There may be an adrenergic mechanism in GH release during stress as α blockade can inhibit its release. (Imura et al 1971, Ishibashi & Yamaji 1984).

Glucagon

Glucagon is a polypeptide secreted from the α islet cells of the pancreas (Unger & Orci 1976). The difficulty in assaying glucagon has meant that little information about its role in the stress response is available. Its release is initiated by hypoglycaemia, starvation, exercise, stress, pancreozymin and gastroinhibitory peptide: glucagon release is inhibited by somatostatin, α stimulation and β blockade.

Its effects are to produce hyperglycaemia by stimulation of hepatic glycogenolysis and gluconeogenesis, to produce a rise in circulating free fatty acids by increasing lipolysis, and to increase protein breakdown. It also stimulates insulin release.

Insulin

Insulin is the main anabolic hormone involved in the stress response. Under non-stressful circumstances it is released from the β islet cells of the pancreas by an increase in blood glucose levels, by amino acids such as phenylalanine, anginine, leucine and histidine, by other hormones such as ACTH, growth hormone and glucagon, by β adrenergic stimulation, vagal stimulation, and by secretin and cholecystokinin. Its release is inhibited by somatostatin, α adrenergic stimulation, β adrenergic blockade, thiazide diuretics and phenytoin.

During surgery the circulating levels of insulin fall probably as a result of α adrenergic stimulation on insulin release (Allison 1971, Walsh et al 1982). This fall in circulating levels occurs despite the high blood glucose levels, suggesting there is resistance of the normal response to hyperglycamia. This is most marked during major surgery and severe trauma and results in a decrease in the body's glucose utilization. The cells are unresponsive to the effects of endogenous insulin in the non-diabetic patient (Buckingham et al 1976, Meyer et al 1979) and to endogenous insulin in diabetics (Meyer et al 1979). Those cells not solely dependent on glucose metabolism will therefore turn to alternative fuel sources such as free fatty acids.

In the hours following surgery the circulating levels of insulin begin to increase but its effects are still inhibited by cortisol, growth hormone, glucagon and adrenaline with hyperglycaemia persisting for 24–48 hours.

The actions of insulin are wide ranging. Its main effects are on carbohydrate metabolism increasing membrane transport, and hence the utilization of glucose. It also increases the storage of glucose in the form of fat or glycogen. It stimulates RNA and DNA synthesis and inhibits lipolysis.

Many of the metabolic effects of surgery are brought about by the actions of catabolic hormones during a time of inhibition of the main anabolic hormone, insulin. Indeed, many of the metabolic effects of surgery can be prevented by a per-operative infusion of insulin (Woolfson et al 1979).

There are certain problems with the interpretation of the measurements of peripheral levels of insulin because of the very rapid and variable liver metabolism of the hormone and it has been suggested that measurement of C-peptide, which is secreted molecule for molecule with insulin, may provide a better guide to the insulin secretion rate (Jaspan et al 1984).

Antidiuretic hormone

Antidiuretic hormone, or arginine vasopressin (ADH) is an octopeptide released from the neurosecretory cells of the supraoptic and paraventricular nuclei of the hypothalamus (Moran 1971). After combining with a polypeptide carrier, neurophysin, it migrates down the axons and is stored in the posterior pituitary. Its release from the posterior pituitary is controlled by osmoreceptors in the hypothalamic region, volume receptors in the left atrium, and baroreceptors in the carotid sinus and aortic arch. In low doses ADH increases the distal tubular reabsorbtion of water without solute. In intermediate doses it increases solute reabsorbtion, possibly through a reduction in glomerular filtration rate, while in high doses it produces vasoconstriction. It is one of the most potent endogenous vasoconstrictors in man. The half life of ADH is only 3 minutes and it undergoes rapid hepatic clearance. 10% is excreted unchanged in the urine. Normal circulating levels are 1–2 pg/ml. During surgical stress levels of up to 120 pg/ml have been reported. Anaesthesia per se has little effect on ADH secretion in comparison to surgery (Philbin & Coggins 1978).

The effects of artificial ventilation on ADH levels is still uncertain but IPPV and PEEP probably do not directly increase secretion (Kumar et al 1974), though there is a secondary increase due to a fall in cardiac index. Hypercarbia is a stimulus to ADH secretion (Philbin et al 1970).

Renin angiotensin aldosterone

Renin is a proteolytic enzyme released from the macula densa of the juxtaglomerullar apparatus (Miller 1981). It breaks an α 2 globulin in the plasma to produce angiotensin I, a decapeptide which releases catecholamines from the adrenal gland resulting in an increased blood pressure and also producing a sensation of thirst. Most angiotensin I is transformed into angiotensin II in the lungs by a converting enzyme. Angiotensin II is a vasoconstrictor with a positive inotropic effect on the heart; it also stimulates catecholamine release. It has a short half life, measured in seconds. It is metabolized in the plasma and the liver by angiotensinase to angiotensin III. Both angiotensin II and angiotensin III are potent releasers of aldosterone while angiotensin II will also stimulate ACTH release. The ACTH releases cortisol which also has a mild mineralocorticoid effect. Aldosterone will increase water and sodium retention in the kidney resulting in an increased potassium loss.

During major surgery there may be a three- to four-fold increase in plasma renin activity (PRA). The actual increase will depend on the blood loss and fluid administration during surgery (Bailey et al 1975). Renin is released by a variety of mechanisms. A fall in renal perfusion will be detected by renal baroreceptors. Hypovolaemia will result in increased renal nerve and adrenergic receptor activity with an increased level of circulating catecholamines. Decreased glomular filtration rate results in a rise in urinary sodium concentration. All these mechanisms result in increased renin secretion, conserving sodium and water in an attempt to maintain cardiac output. In addition, hormones such as ACTH, adrenal corticosteroids and oestrogens, and changes in posture as well as hypothermia will all increase PRA. Angiotensin II and ADH reduce PRA.

Other hormones

Plasma thyroxine remains unchanged during surgery whilst plasma triiodothyronine is decreased during and after surgery. Testosterone and prolactin are increased. The significance of these findings is not fully understood.

Wound hormones

Phagocytic cells can produce hormone like substances which have been given a variety of names such as leucocytic pyrogen, endogenous pyrogen, leukocytic andogenous mediator, neutrophil releasing factor, lymphocyte activating factor and, most recently, Interleukin I (ILI) (Dinarello 1984).

These substances are involved in the production of post-traumatic fever, the production and release of neutrophils from the bone marrow, hepatic production of acute phase reactants such as C-reactive protein, fibrinogen, ceruloplasmin and antitrypsin, and also in the hepatic uptake of amino acids. They are also capable of proteolysis (Clowes 1983), possibly by increasing prostaglandin E_2 synthesis in muscle (Baracos et al 1983).

The extent to which ILI is involved in the metabolic response to surgery has yet to be decided. If wound hormones do play a large part then it is obvious that afferent blockade alone will not completely obtund the stress response.

METABOLIC RESPONSE TO SURGERY

Carbohydrate metabolism

Following surgery the blood glucose levels rise from their normal level of 3.5–5 mmol/l to as much as 8–10 mmol/l. The blood sugar may remain elevated for more than 24 hours if trauma is severe. Under resting conditions in the adult, the liver can produce about 10 g of glucose per hour, of which 6 g/h will be utilized by the brain while both white cells and red blood cells will each use 2 g/h. The glucose is manufactured from lactate and pyruvate, which is released from muscle (following the breakdown of muscle glycogen), from amino acids (from muscle protein breakdown), from liver glycogen stores, and from glycerol and free fatty acids (from adipose tissue breakdown).

During surgery the break down of liver glycogen increases, though liver glycogen stores may be low following pre-operative fasting. This is an α adrenergic, calcium ion dependent effect which is enhanced by glucagon and cortisol. In muscle β adrenergic cyclic AMP dependent mechanisms cause glycogen breakdown with the production of lactate and pyruvate, which are metabolized to glucose in the liver. Protein breakdown is increased with the production of more amino acids for gluconeogenesis and lipolysis while glyceroland free fatty acid production is also increased. Gluconeogenesis is encouraged by cortisol, growth hormone and thyroxine. Glucose utilization is reduced due to the low level of insulin and the inhibition of the effects of insulin by catecholamines, glucagon, growth hormone and cortisol (Stanley 1981a–c).

Protein metabolism

Following surgery there is a period of negative nitrogen balance which lasts for 2–10 days, depending on the severity of the surgery and on the presence of complications such as sepsis. The loss of nitrogen may vary from 5–20 g/d, following uncomplicated surgery in patients on no nutritional support, to 50 g/d in hypercatabolic states after burns or multiple injuries. Each 50 g of nitrogen represents a loss of 1.25 kg of muscle mass.

There are many causes of protein loss including hypothermia. Prevention of heat loss in the elderly during surgery prevents most of the peri-operative nitrogen losses (Carli et al 1982). Cortisol levels which are elevated two to three times that of normal during surgical stress may effect the breakdown of myofibrillar protein (Thomas et al 1979). The increased secretion of glucagon, growth hormone and catecholamines and reduced insulin activity all promote catabolism.

However, infusions of the four catabolic hormones, adrenaline, growth hormone, cortisol and glucagon, resulted in blood glucose changes similar to those seen during surgery, but the effects on protein metabolism were less impressive (Bessey et al 1984, Gelfand et al 1984). It was concluded that the catabolic hormones contributed to, but were not the sole mediators of, the muscle wasting seen after surgery.

There has been a recent resurgence of interest in wound hormone. Interleukin I is a polypeptide which is released from activated monocytes and macrophages after tissue damage (Dinarello 1984). It is known to increase protein breakdown in muscle without affecting synthesis and it is possible that it plays a role in post-operative nitrogen loss (Baracos et al 1983, Clowes et al 1983).

The breakdown of muscle protein in the peri-operative period is of value because this source of amino acids can be used to provide glucose by gluconeogenesis in the liver and to provide new proteins for antibody production, wound healing and acute phase reactant synthesis. In addition, the branched chain amino acids can be used within the muscle as a direct source of energy.

Fat metabolism

Lipid metabolism shows great individual variation and is affected by fasting and by surgery (Stanley 1981a,b). Lipolysis is caused by all the catabolic hormones — cortisol, glucagon, growth hormone and especially the catecholamines. The increase in lipolysis is due to increased activity of triglyceride lipase caused by a cyclic AMP dependent mechanism. Free fatty acids are released into the circulation and are converted to ketone bodies in the liver. Both free fatty acids and ketone bodies are used by muscle as fuel sources and ketone bodies are used by the brain and renal cortex as a fuel source during prolonged fasting. The brain's glucose requirements during starvation may fall from 120 g/d to 35 g/d as the brain begins to utilize ketone bodies. Insulin is released in response to high circulating levels of ketone bodies and it will also inhibit further lipolysis.

The changes in lipid metabolism during the surgical period will depend on the individual's fat content and individual metabolic profile, the severity of trauma, the level of anxiety and the duration of fasting. Fasting alone may raise free fatty acid and ketone body levels in the plasma more than surgery (Foster et al 1979).

CAUSES OF THE STRESS RESPONSE

The most important initiator of the stress response to surgery or trauma is stimulation of afferent somatic and autonomic nerves at the wound site. The relative importance of somatic, parasympathetic and sympathetic afferent pathways has still to be determined although complete blockade of all afferent pathways is necessary for obtunding the stress response (Engquvist et al 1977).

Physiological factors such as hypothermia (Carli et al 1982), hypoxia, hypercarbia, infection and hypotension all play a part in initiating the stress response, as will psychological factors such as fear and anxiety. Clowes et al (1983) and Baracos (1983) have recently scrutinized the part played by wound hormones and bacterial forms.

Advantages and disadvantages of the stress response

The immediate benefits of the stress response are to maintain blood flow to vital organs and to increase the delivery of readily utilizable fuel sourses to those organs. The supply of fuel is then maintained by the continuing process of catabolism until the patient has recovered sufficiently to resume normal food intake. However, afferent nerve stimulation activates the response in an indiscriminant manner producing an excess of hormones which may be life saving in some patients, but can be disadvantageous in others. Oxygen consumption is increased and there is a relative hypoxia in non vital organs such as the lung, kidney and intestines. An increase in blood pressure, heart rate and hence cardiac work may be detrimental to patients with coronary artery disease while the high level of adrenergic activity may increase the risk of life threatening arrhythmias. Acidosis may inhibit myocardial function. Muscle protein breakdown produces negative nitrogen balance which, if severe, may delay wound healing. There may be an increased risk of infection due to depression of the immune response by corticosteroids while stress can play a part in initiating disorders such as malignant hyperpyrexia. There is also an increase in the blood coagulability which can lead to the production of microemboli and deep vein thrombosis (Ellis & Humphrey 1982).

ANAESTHETIC MANAGEMENT OF THE ENDOCRINE RESPONSE

There has been a widespread increase in interest in developing anaesthetic techniques which are believed to suppress the endocrine response to surgical trauma.

Psychological preparation

It has long been said that the pre-operative visit by the anaesthetist is as effective in relieving stress as premedication. Anxious patients have higher circulating catecholamine (Hjenidahl & Eliasion 1979). Recent studies have shown that acute and chronic psychogenic stress in animals are important factors in initiating the stress response (Armanio et al 1984). The effect of pre-surgical psychological counselling and preparation is currently being studied (Salmon 1986; personal communication).

High dose opioid anaesthesia

Morphine and nalorphine have been shown to suppress the cortisol response to surgery (McDonald 1959) and this has led to other studies of the use of large doses of intravenous morphine to modify the stress response (George et al 1974). The advent of more potent short acting analgesic agents has led to the use of fentanyl, alfentanil and sufentanyl.

Unfortunately the dose of intravenous opioids necessary to suppress the endocrine response was such that there was still profound respiratory depression at the end of operation, long after cessation of surgical stimulation. The use of high dose morphine implied that it could only be used in patients who were due to be ventilated post-operatively (e.g. after cardiac surgery). The technique was not suitable for patients who were expected to be returned to a normal surgical ward (Brandt et al 1978). Fentanyl, with a shorter plasma half life seemed more promising in inhibiting hypothalamic-pituitary stimulation but post-operative respiratory depression has also occurred. This has led to interest in even shorter acting drugs such as alfentanil and sufentanyl (Bovill et al 1983, Moller et al 1985).

It has been demonstrated that, as with morphine, the dose of fentanyl necessary to suppress the endocrine response is largely dependent upon the degree of surgical stimulation suffered by the patient. Thus a dose of 10 μg/kg body weight was sufficient to modify the rise in cortisol and hyperglycaemia seen during abdominal surgery (Haxholdt et al 1981) but that 50 μg/kg body weight was necessary during upper abdominal surgery and its modifying action lasted for only half as long (Cooper et al 1981). A similar effect could be seen in patients undergoing cardiac surgery using fentanyl in doses in excess of 50 μg/kg. Despite the use of high doses cardiopulmonary bypass, with the use of cold perfusate, and the attendant haemodynamic changes and surgical stimulation overcame the inhibitory effects of the opioid (Sebel et al 1981, Walsh et al 1981).

Maller (1985) has continued the study into the post-operative period after using alfentanil at a loading dose of 150 μg/kg body weight, followed by an infusion of 3 μg/kg/min in patients undergoing abdominal surgery. This dose suppressed the endocrine response during the surgical procedure but the effect had worn off after 2–3 hours into the post-operative period when the opioid levels had fallen. By this time the patients had returned to their wards and were receiving routine intramuscular opioid injections on demand for analgesia.

Bent et al (1984) have examined the effect of giving a known suppressive dose of fentanyl to patients in whom the endocrine response has already been established. Their patients received fentanyl 30 μg/kg body weight during pelvic surgery after 1 hour of surgery using inhalational anaesthesia alone. This resulted in a fall in blood lactate levels possibly due to a decrease in plasma catecholamines but the levels of cortisol and glucose which were already raised were unaffected, demonstrating the inability of high dose opioids to alter the established endocrine response. Hay et al (1985) confirmed this by demonstrating the inability of meptazinol or morphine to alter the established endocrine response when given at the end of surgery.

It has been suggested that endogenous opioids play an important role in the endocrine response, and that during high dose opioid anaesthesia there may be a negative feedback mechanism. Hall et al (1983) examined the role of endogenous opioids by using an infusion of naloxone, a potent opiate antagonist, in patients undergoing pelvic surgery with inhalational anaesthesia. He found no significant alteration in the levels of insulin, cortisol or growth hormone and concluded that endogenous opioids played only a minor role in the endocrine response.

Thus, in clinical practice it has become apparent over the last few years that high dose opioid anaesthesia is effective in suppressing the endocrine response only if it is initiated before surgical stimulation, and that it may be overcome if the stimulus is sufficiently strong. Suppression will only last for as long as adequate opioid levels are maintained. This implies that patients have to be ventilated in the post-operative period.

Afferent neuronal blockade

In clinical practice afferent neuronal blockade may be achieved either by local anaesthetics or by opioids given extradurally or intrathecally. The fact that afferent blockade may modify the endocrine response has been known for some years since animal studies showed that denervation of a limb prior to trauma to that limb prevented the rise in cortisol levels (Wise et al 1972). Recent advances have been achieved by employing a variety of different drugs and techniques to achieve this.

Bromage et al (1971) showed that, following epidural blockade with local anaesthetics for upper abdominal surgery, there was a suppression of the glucose response but plasma cortisol levels still rose with surgery despite adequate analgesia.

Engquvist et al (1977) confirmed this by demonstrating that for pelvic surgery a very extensive epidural blockade from T_4 to S_5 was required for complete suppression of the endocrine response: surgery in the upper abdomen, or incomplete blockade still caused a rise in cortisol levels.

Traynor et al (1982) combined thoracic epidural analgesia with the use of a vagal blockade at operation in patients undergoing upper abdominal surgery and although the hyperglycaemic response was suppressed there was still a rise in plasma cortisol levels. This was confirmed by Tsugi et al (1983) who used combined extradural analgesia with vagal blockade for gastrectomy, but in both these studies vagal blockade was performed after the onset of surgical stimulation. Epidural blockade and intravenous opioids are ineffectual in modifying the endocrine response if administered after surgical stimulation (Moller et al 1982). Tsuji (1983), however, noted that epidural blockade combined with splanchnic nerve blockade successfully suppressed the rise in cortisol levels.

Intrathecal local anaesthetics also suppressed the endocrine response but is only effective during the duration of the blockade (Moller et al 1984). Lush et al (1972) confirmed this finding with extradural local anaesthesia. In clinical practice this has led to epidural blockade being more widely used as the block may be maintained for longer into the post-operative period via an indwelling catheter, with the use of an infusion pump. In this way it is hoped that a more prolonged suppression of the endocrine response can be extended into the post-operative period. Kehlet et al (1980) and Rem et al (1980) have both shown that following epidural anaesthesia there is less immunodepression and nitrogen balance is maintained.

The use of opioids to provide analgesia when given extradurally and intrathecally has become more widespread since it was first described by Yaksh (1976). The apparent advantage for the patient over local anaesthetics is prolonged analgesia without the risk of sympathetic or motor blockade. After intrathecal diamorphine the average time for post-operative analgesia has been up to 16 hours (Child & Kaufman 1985) with 33% of the patients requiring no supplementary analgesia in the first 24 hours.

Christensen et al (1982) and Jorgensen et al (1982) showed that extradural morphine (4 mg) suppressed the adrenocortical and hyperglycaemic responses to surgery post-operatively but had little effect intra-operatively and that in fact a local anaesthetic, bupivacaine, produced greater suppression. This failure could be due to the need to use a higher dose when given extradurally as suggested by Bromage et al (1980), especially when a poorly lipid soluble drug such as morphine is used, which will only slowly cross the dura to its site of action on the opioid receptors of the dorsal columns of the spinal cord.

Child & Kaufman (1985) have shown that suppression of the endocrine response can be achieved intra-operatively by the use of intrathecal diamorphine which presents a high dose of opiate directly to the receptors before surgery starts. However, sympathetic and proprioceptive afferents are not effected by opioids (Kitihata & Collins 1981) and this may be the reason for incomplete suppression seen with spinal opiates. Again to reinforce the concept of multiple pathways transmitting afferent nociceptive responses, Piv et al (1983) have demonstrated in animals pathways, dependant upon γ-amino-butyric acid transmitter, which are unaffected by opioids but may be blocked by midazolam given intrathecally.

Efferent neuronal blockade

The interruption of the efferent limb of the sympathetic reflex, by α and β blockade has been studied to examine the role of the sympathetic system in initiating the endocrine response to surgery.

Giguene et al (1980) showed that α_1 blockade in rats reduced the release of ACTH from the pituitary, and α blockade by phentolamine reversed the insulin suppression that occurred during surgical stimulation (Walsh et al 1982). Labetalol, a combined α and β blocker was shown to reduce cortisol levels probably via an α mediated pituitary action (Child 1984).

β Blockade with propranolol 0.15 mg/kg in patients undergoing pelvic surgery was shown to have little effect on the hyperglycaemic response although insulin levels were decreased at 60 and 90 minutes into the operation as its β stimulated release was blocked (Cooper et al 1980). However, Lowidsen et al (1983) showed that β blockade prolonged hypoglycaemia by increasing tissue uptake of glucose directly and not by decreasing the hormones inhibiting insulin (epinephnine and growth hormone). These results show that adrenaline induced hepatic glycogenolysis is a major cause of the hyperglycaemia seen intra-operatively.

Hormone manipulation

Most of the anaesthetic techniques for modifying the endocrine response to surgery have concentrated on blocking the pathways transmitting stimuli which inhibit or stimulate the various hormones involved in the response. Recent work has studied manipulating the hormone levels directly.

The idea of being able to modify cortisol levels directly arose after it was discovered that patients being ventilated in certain intensive care units had lower cortisol levels than in groups previously treated and the only change in their overall management had been the introduction of the anaesthetic agent etomidate for their long term sedation (Fellows et al 1983).

Since then the exact nature of this suppression of cortisol has been elucidated, and it is apparent that adrenocortical function is altered by the inhibition of 11 β hydroxylation and 17 α hydroxylation. This is seen transiently after a bolus dose of etomidate (de Jong 1984) while a more prolonged suppression can be obtained with an etomidate infusion (Moore et al 1985) when aldosterone suppression is also seen.

It is unclear as yet whether this has any beneficial long term effect on the catabolic phase of negative nitrogen balance normally associated with raised cortisol levels. No patients showed any cardiovascular instability during this infusion despite low recorded cortisol levels of <100 mol/l.

Insulin appears to be the most important short term anabolic hormone effected during the stress response, and while many anaesthetic techniques have been used to prevent this inhibition, insulin levels can readily be maintained by intra-operative infusion. Hall et al (1983) have studied this by instituting a low dose insulin infusion regime on patients undergoing pelvic surgery. They showed that by increasing plasma levels, blood glucose fell during the surgical period, probably as a result of increased peripheral glucose uptake. The inhibition of substrate mobilization was continued with the reduction in fat metabolism, as plasma non-esterified fatty acids and later 3-hydroxybutyrate levels fell.

General patient care

Irrespective of the anaesthetic technique, the overall management of the patient has been shown to have some influence on the endocrine response. Mullin & Kilpatrick (1981) showed that good nutritional support both pre-operatively and post-operatively in surgical patients resulted in better immunocompetence with an increase in circulating lymphocytes, while there is evidence that adequate nutritional support post-operatively reduces the catabolic phase and decreases overall nitrogen losses. Many patients would benefit from a period of pre-operative feeding rather than undergoing surgery at the earliest convenient moment.

Although it is accepted practice to nurse neonates at an optimal temperature to minimize heat loss and reduce calorie demands, adult surgical patients have not been shown to benefit in the long term from being maintained in a thermoneutral environment during the post-operative period. Carli et al (1982) have shown that the prevention of intra-operative heat loss, however, has resulted in a decreased nitrogen loss post-operatively in elderly patients undergoing abdominal surgery. This may reflect the role of heat loss as an initiating factor in the stress response and the importance of preventing initiation rather than attempting to alter the established endocrine response.

CONCLUSIONS

Debate continues as to whether the endocrine response or its suppression is beneficial. However, the controversy has led to the introduction of many new drugs and techniques and has stimulated detailed research projects, one of which has served to improve patient care and wellbeing (see Update section).

REFERENCES

Akiyoshi T 1984 Immunodepression after surgery: impaired production of interleukin 2. Japanese Journal of Surgery 14: 384–386

Allison S P 1971 Changes in insulin secretion during open heart surgery. British Journal of Anaesthesia 43: 138–142

Armanio A 1984 The effect of acute and chronic psychogenic stress on corticoradrenal and pituitary-thyroid hormones in male rats. Hormone Research 20: 241–245
Bailey D R, Miller E D, Kaplan A J, Rogers P W 1975 The renin-angiotensin-aldosterone system during cardiac surgery with morphine-nitrous oxide anaesthesia. Anesthesiology 42: 538–541
Baracos V, Rodemann H P, Dinarello C A, Goldberg A 1983 Stimulation of muscle protein degradation and prostaglandin E_2 release by leukocytic pyrogen: a mechanism for the increased degradation of muscle proteins during fever. New England Journal of Medicine 308: 553–558
Bent J M, Paterson J L, Mashiter K, Hall G M 1984 Effects of high dose fentanyl anaesthesia on the established metabolic and endocrine responses to surgery. Anaesthesia 39: 19–24
Bessey P Q, Watters J W, Aoki T T, Wilmore P W 1984 Combined hormonal infusion simulates the metabolic response to injury. Annals of Surgery 200: 264–267
Bovill J G, Sebel P S, Tiolet J W, Tauber J L, Philbin D M 1983 The influence of sufentanil on endocrine and metabolic responses to cardiac surgery. Anesthesia and Analgesia 62: 391–395
Brandt M R, Harshin J, Prange Hausen A, Hummer L, Nistup Modsen S, Lugg I, Hellet H 1978 Influence of morphine anaesthesia on the endocrine-metabolic response to open heart surgery. Acta Anaesthetica Scandanavica 22: 400–405
Bromage P R, Camporesi E, Chestnut D 1980 Epidural narcotics for postoperative analgesia. Anaesthesia and Analgesia 59: 473–476
Bromage P R, Shibata H R, Willoughby H W 1971 The influence of prolonged epidural blockade on blood sugar and cortisol responses to operations upon the upper part of the abdomen and thorax. Surgery Gynecology and Obstetrics 132: 1051–1054
Buckingham J M, Palumbo P J, Woods J E 1976 Plasma insulin and glucose levels after renal transplantation. Urology 83: 210–212
Carli F, Clark M M, Woollen J W 1982 Investigation of the relationship between heat loss and nitrogen excretion in elderly patients undergoing major abdominal surgery under general anaesthesia. British Journal of Anaesthesia 54: 1023–1025
Child C S 1984 The effect of labetolol on the cardiovascular, hyperglycaemic and adrenocortical responses to surgery. Anaesthesia 39: 1192–1196
Child C S, Kaufman L 1985 Effect of intrathecal diamorphine on the adrenocortical hyperglycaemic and cardiovascular responses to major colonic surgery. British Journal of Anaesthesia 57: 389–393
Christensen P, Brandt M R, Pen J, Kellet H 1982 Influence of extradural morphine on the adrenocortical and hyperglycaemic response to surgery. British Journal of Anaesthesia 54: 23–27
Clarke R S J 1970 The hyperglycaemic response to different types of surgery. British Journal of Anaesthesia 42: 45–48
Clowes G H A Jr, George B C, Villee C A Jr, Saravis C A 1983 Muscle proteolysis induced by a circulating peptide in patients with sepsis or trauma. New England Journal of Medicine; 308: 545–459
Cooper C E, Nelson D H 1962 ACTH levels in plasma in pre-operative and surgically stressed patients. Journal of Clinical Investigation 41: 1599–1603
Cooper G M, Paterson J L, Mashiter K, Hall G M 1980 Beta adrenergic blockade and the metabolic response to surgery. British Journal of Anaesthesia 52: 1231–1236
Cooper G M, Paterson J L, Ward I D, Hall G M 1981 Fentanyl and the metabolic response to gastric surgery. Anaesthesia 36: 667–671
Cuthbertson D P 1942 Post-shock metabolism. Lancet 1: 433
Dinarello C A 1984 Interleukin-1. Reviews of Infectious Diseases 6: 51–55
Engquvist A, Brandt M R, Fernandes A, Kellet H 1977 The blocking effect of epidural analgesia on the adrenocortical and hyperglycaemic responses to surgery. Acta Anaesthesia Scandanavica 21: 330–335
Ellis F R, Humphrey D E 1982 Clinical aspect of endocrine and metabolic changes relating to anaesthesia and surgery. In: Watkins J, Salo M (Eds) Trauma, Stress and Immunity in Anaesthesia and Surgery. Butterworth Scientific, Guidford
Fellows I W, Bastaw M D, Byrne A J, Allison S P 1983 Adrenocorticol suppression in multiple injured patients: a complication of etomidate infusion. British Medical Journal 287: 1835–1837
Foster K J, Alberti K G M M, Binder C et al 1979 Lipid metabolites and nitrogen balance after abdominal surgery in man. British Journal of Surgery 66: 242–247
Fry D E, Griffiths H 1984 The inhibition by etomidate of the 11 beta hydroylation of cortisol. Clinical Endocrinology 20: 625–628
Fugiwara R 1984 Suppressive influence of surgical stress on the graft versus host reaction in mice. Acta Medica Okayama 38: 439–446
Gelfand R A, Matthews D E, Bier D M, Sherwin R S 1984 Role of counter regulatory hormones in the catabolic response to stress. Journal of Clinical Investigation 74: 2238–2240
George J M, Peier C E, Lavese R R, Rawer J M 1974 Morphine anaesthesia blocks cortisol and

growth hormone response to surgical stress in humans. Journal Clinical Endocrinology and Metabolism 38: 736–739
Gignere V, Cate J, Labine F 1981 Characteristics of the alpha adrenergic stimulation of adrenocorticotrophin secretion in rat anterior pituitary cells. Endocrinology 109: 757–762
Grossman A, Besser G M 1982 Opiates control ACTH through nonadrenergic mechanism. Clinical Endocrinology 17: 287–290
Hall G M, Adrian T E, Bloom S R, Mashiter K 1983 The effects of naloxone on the circulating metabolites, gluco-regulatory hormones and gut peptides during pelvic surgery. Clinical Physiology 3: 49–58
Hall G M, Lucke J N 1982 Editorial. Brown fat — a thermogenic tissue of anaesthetic importance? British Journal of Anaesthesia 54: 907
Hall G M, Walsh E S, Paterson J L, Mashiter K 1982 Low dose insulin infusion and substrate mobilisation during surgery. British Journal of Anaesthesia 54: 517–521
Halter J B, Pflug A E, Porte D 1977 Mechanism of plasma catecholamine increases during sugical stress in man. Journal of Clinical Endocrinology and Metabolism 45: 936–939
Haxholdt O, Kehlet H, Dyrberg V 1981 The effect of fentanyl on the cortisol and hypoglycaemic response to abdominal surgery. Acta Anaesthetica Scandanavica 25: 434–436
Hoover-Plow J L, Clifford A J 1978 The effect of surgical trauma on protein turnover in rats. Biochemical Journal 176: 137–140
Hjeindahl P, Eliasson K 1978 Sympatho-adrenal and cardiovascular response to mental stress and orthostatic provocation in latent hypertension. Clinical Science 57: 293–296
Hume D M 1953 The neuroendocrine response to injury — the present status of the problem. Annal of Surgery 138: 548
Imura H, Kato Y, Ikeda M, Morimoto M, Yanvata M 1971 The effect of adrenergic blocking or stimulating agents on plasma growth hormone, immunoreactive insulin and blood free fatty acid levels in man. Journal of Clinical Investigation 50: 1069
Ishibashi M, Yamaji I 1984 Direct effects of catecholamines, thyrotropin releasing hormone and somatostatin on growth hormone and PRL secretion from adenomatous and non-adenomatous human pituitary cells in culture. Journal of Clinical Investigation 73: 66
Jaspan J B, Cohen D M, Karrison T, Tager H S, Rubenstein A H 1984 C-peptide and insulin secretion. Relationship between peripheral concentrations of C-peptide and insulin and their secretion rates in the dog. Journal of Clinical Investigation 74: 1821
De Jong F H, Mallias C 1984 Etomidate suppresses adrenocortical function by the inhibition of 11 beta hydroxylation. Journal of Clinical Endocrinology and Metabolism 59: 1143
Jorgensen B C, Andersen H B, Engquvist A 1982 Influence of epidural morphine on post-operative pain, endocrine-metabolic and renal responses to surgery. A controlled study. Acta Anaesthesica Scandanavica 26: 63
Kay N H, Allen M C, Bullingham R E S et al 1985 The influence of meptazinol on the metabolic and hormonal responses following major surgery; a comparison with morphine. Anaesthesia 40: 223–228
Kehlet H, Brandt M R, Pen J 1980 The role of neurogenic stimuli in mediating the endocrine-metabolic response to surgery. Journal of Parenteral and Enteral Nutrition 4: 152–156
Kitihata L M, Collins J G 1981 Spinal action of narcotic analgesics. Anesthesiology 54: 153
Kumar A, Pontopprdan H, Baraty R A, Laver M B 1974 Inappropriate response to increased plasma ADH during mechanical ventilation in acute respiratory failure. Anesthesiology 40: 215
Ledingham I M, Watt I 1983 Influence of sedation on mortality in critically ill multiple trauma patients. Lancet 1: 1270
Long C N H 1946 Relations of cholesterol and ascorbic acid to secretion of the adrenal corten. Recent Progress in Hormonal Research 1: 99
Lowidsen U, Christensen N, Lyngsoe J 1983 Effects of non-selective and beta selective blockade on glucose metabolism and hormone responses during insulin induced hypoglycaemia in normal man. Journl of Clinal Endocrinology and Metabolism 56: 876
Lush D, Thorpe J N, Richardson D J, Bowen D J 1972 The effect of epidural anaesthesia on the adrenocortical response to surgery. British Journal of Anaesthesia 44: 1169
McDonald R K, Evans F T, Weise V K, Patrick R W 1959 The effect of morphine and nalorphine on plasma hydrocortisone levels in man. Journal of Pharmacology and Experimental Therapy 125: 241–245
Mani F 1984 Depression of host defence mechanisms following cardiac surgery. Japanese Journal of Surgery 14: 377–383
Meyer E J, Lorenzi M, Bohannon N V 1979 Diabetic management by insulin infusion during major surgery. American Journal of Surgery 137: 323
Miller E D 1981 The role of the renin-angiotensin-aldosterone system in circulatory control and in hypertension. British Journal of Anaesthesia 53: 711

Moller I W, Rem J, Brandt M R, Kehlet H 1982 The effect of post-traumatic epidural analgesia on the cortisol and hyperglycaemic response to surgery. Acta Anaesthesica Scandanavica 26: 56–58

Moller I W, Hjouts E, Krantz T, Wardell E, Kehlet H 1984 The modifying effect of spinal anaesthesia on intra and postoperative advenocortical and hyperglycoenic responses to surgery. Acta Anaesthesica Scandinavica 28: 266–270

Moller I W, Krantz T, Wardell E, Kehlet H 1985 The effect of alfentanyl anaesthesia on the adrenocortical and hyperglycaemic response to abdominal surgery. British Journal of Anaesthesia 57: 591–594

Moore R W, Allen M C, Wood P J, Rees L S, Sear J W 1985 Perioperative endocrine effects of etomidate. Anaesthesia 40: 124–31

Moore F D 1953 Bodily changes in surgical convalescence I. The normal sequelae — observations and interpretations. Annals of Surgery 137: 289

Moran W H 1971 CPPB and vasopression secretion: editorial views. Anesthesiology 34: 501

Mullin T J, Kilpatrick J R 1981 The effect of nutritional support on immune competency in patients suffering from trauma, sepsis or malignant disease. Surgery 90: 610–615

Munro H N 1979 Editorial. Hormone and the metabolic response to injury. New England Journal of Medicine 300: 41

Newsome H H 1975 Editorial. Growth hormone in surgical stress. Surgery 77: 475

Nistrup Masden S, Fog-Moller F, Christiansen C, Vester-Andersen T, Engquvist A 1978 Cyclic AMP, adrenaline and noradrenaline in plasma during surgery. British Journal of Surgery 65: 191

Philbin D M, Baratz R A, Patterson R W 1970 The effect of carbon dioxide on plasma antidiuretic hormone levels during intermittent positive pressure breathing. Anesthesiology 33: 345

Philbin D M, Coggins C H 1978 Plasma antidiuretic hormone levels in cardiac surgical patients during morphine and halothane anaesthesia. Anesthesiology 49: 95

Piv D, Whitwam J G, Lok L 1983 Depression of nociceptive sympathetic reflexes by the intrathecal administration of midazolam. British Journal of Anaesthesia 55: 541

Rees L, Butler P W P, Gosling L, Besser G M 1970 Adrenergic blockade and the corticosteroid and growth hormone responses to methylamphetamine. Nature 22: 565

Rem J, Brandt M R, Kehlet H 1980 Prevention of postoperative lymphopenia and granulocytosis by epidural analgesia. Lancet 1: 283

Sambhi M P, Weil M H, Udhoji U N 1965 Acute pharmacodynamic effects of glucocorticoids. Cardia output and related haemodynamic changes in normal subjects and patients inshock. Circulation 31: 523

Sebel P S, Bovill J G, Shellenkus A P M, Hawker C D 1981 The hormonal responses to high dose fentanyl anaesthesia. A study in patients undergoing cardiac surgery. British Journal of Anaesthesia 53: 941–948

Simmons P S, Miles J M, Gerich J E, Haymond M W 1984 Increased proteolysis — an effect of increases in plasma cortisol within the physiological range. Journal of Clinical Investigation 73: 412

Stanley J C 1981a The glucose-fatty acid cycle. British Journal of Anaesthesia 53: 123

Stanley J C 1981b The glucose-fatty acid ketone body cycle. British Journal of Anaesthesia 53: 131

Stanley J C 1981c The regulation of glucose production. British Journal of Anaesthesia 53: 137

Thomasson B 1959 Studies on the content of 17 hydroxyortico steriods and its diurnal rhythm in the plasma of surgical patients. Scandinavian Journal of Clinicaland Laboratory Investigation 11: Supplement 42

Tomas F M, Munro H N, Young V R 1979 Effect of glucocorticoid administration on the rate of muscle protein breakdown in vivo in rats, as measured by urinary excretion of N-methylhistidine Biochemic Journal 178: 139

Traynor C, Paterson J L, Ward I D, Morgan M, Hall G M 1982 Effects of extradural analgesia and vagal blockade on the metabolic and endocrine responses to upper abdominal surgery. British Journal of Anaesthesia 54: 319–323

Tsugi H, Asoh T, Takenchi Y, Shirosaka C 1983 Attenuation of adrenocortical response to upper abdominal surgery with epidural blockade. British Journal of Surgery 70: 122–124

Tsugi H, Shirosaka C, Asoh T, Takenchi Y 1983 Influences of splanchnic nerve blockade on endocrine-metabolic responses to upper abdominal surgery. British Journal of Surgery 70: 437–479

Unger R H, Orci L 1976 Physiology and pathophysiology of glucagon. Physiological Reviews 56: 778

Walsh E S, Patterson J L, O'Riordon J B A, Hall G M 1981 the effect of high dose fentanyl anaesthesia on the metabolic and endocrine response to cardiac surgery. British Journal of Anaesthesia 53: 1153–1165

Walsh E S, Paterson J L, Mashiter K, Hall G M 1982 Effect of phentolamine on the metabolic response to gynaecological surgery. British Journal of Anaesthesia 54: 517

Weichselbaum T E, Margraf H W, Elman R 1953 Quantitative determination of 17 hydroxycorticosteroids and 21 hydroxy 20 ketosteroids in the peripheral blood of humans before and

after operative trauma. Federation Proceedings 12: 287
Williamson D H, Farrell R, Kerr A 1977 Muscle protein catabolism after injury in man, as measured by urinary encretion of 3-methylhistidine. Clinical Science Molecular Medicine 52:527
Wilmore D W, Moyaln J A, Bristow B F, Mason A D, Pruitt B A 1974 Anabolic effects of human growth hormone and high caloric feelings following thermal injury. Surgery, Gynecology and Obstetrics 138: 875
Wise L, Mangraf H W, Ballinger W F 1972 Adrenocorticol function in severe burns. Archives of Surery 105: 213–220
Woolfson A M J, Heatley R V, Allison S P 1979 Insulin to inhibit protien catabolism after injury. New England Journal of Medicine 300:14
Yaksh T L, Rudy T A 1976 Analgesia mediated by a direct spiral action of narcotics. Science 192: 1357–1358

Paediatric anaesthesia and intensive care (1)

THE PRE-TERM INFANT

Over the last decade the prognosis for a prematurely born infant (less than 38 weeks' gestation) has continued to improve, whereas 20 years ago very few babies survived with birth weights below 1500 g. These infants survive because of the increased knowledge concerning immaturity of various organ systems. Many pre-term infants require surgery in the early post-natal period for conditions such as necrotizing enterocolitis, inguinal hernia, hydrocephalus and patent ductus arteriosus, and the expertise of the anaesthetist is required to supervise the care of this vulnerable group of patients.

Infant mortality in developed countries is now 7–12 per 1000 live births: since 1970 mortality has declined faster in the neonate compared with the post-neonatal group of infants. A further limited reduction in neonatal mortality is possible but can only be achieved at great expense (Boyle et al 1983, Bloom 1984). The cost of care for a 500–999 g baby may be up to 10 times greater than that for a baby over 1000 g, the costs increasing yearly. Walker et al (1984) analysed the cost-benefit for infants below 1000 g at birth and their subsequent development. 74% were normal or only minimally impaired, 10% were moderately handicapped while 16% were severely handicapped. The cost of care for a 900 g pre-term baby may be questioned on economic grounds. Saigal et al (1984) showed that prognosis is directly proportional to birth weight (Table 12.1).

Table 12.1 Progress of the pre-term infant in relation to birth weight

Birth weight (g)	Mortality (%)
501–600	97
601–700	69
701–800	51
801–900	38
901–1000	28

Neurological damage at birth or soon afterwards is probably the most important cause of handicap and may result, for example, in intraventricular cerebral haemorrhage. Care of pre-term babies involves minimizing the effects of such complications.

An accurate estimation of gestational age is important so that functional immaturity of physiological systems may be assessed in relation to identifying possible complications likely to arise during the course of anaesthesia.

Pulmonary maturity has been assessed by measuring the ratio of lecithin to sphingomyelin (L/S) in the amniotic fluid. An L/S ratio greater than 2 indicates pulmonary maturity with adequate surfactant and this is seen after the 35th week of gestation. Measurement of the surface active acid phospholipids, phosphatidyl inositol (PI) and phosphatidyl glycerol (PG) may predict more accurately the stage of lung development. PI reaches a peak at 35 weeks, but PG only appears at that stage and peaks at 40 weeks and is unaffected by, for example, maternal diabetes (Hallman et al 1977, O'Brien & Cefalo 1980, James et al 1984).

Ultrasonography for antenatal diagnosis of fetal defects is accurate even in the early stages of pregnancy (before 21 weeks) so that termination for anencephaly, for example, is both safe and legal (Gauderer et al 1984). Measurement of α-fetoprotein in maternal serum is used for screening for such neural tube defects (Persson et al 1983).

Congenital diaphragmatic hernia, oesophageal atresia, hydronephrosis, abdominal wall defects and hydrocephalus may also be diagnosed before birth with increasing accuracy as pregnancy proceeds. Such diagnosis allows the baby to be delivered at an optimal time for surgery in a unit in close proximity to, or even in, the regional paediatric centre. Surgery of the fetus is a possibility in some instances where the medical disorder may continue to damage the infant during the remainder of the pregnancy. For example, progressive hydrocephalus accentuates brain damage, while hydronephrosis leads to progressive renal damage.

Spielman et al (1984) described a technique for fetal surgery in utero under local analgesia. The mother was also given diazepam and morphine to reduce fetal movements. The incidence of induction of premature labour is high so β-methasone is given to accelerate fetal pulmonary development. Tocolytic agents such as ritodrine are not given as they are associated with maternal hypertension, dysrhythmia, pulmonary oedema and metabolic disturbances which may be transmitted to the fetus or the newborn if labour proceeds (Hermansen & Johnson 1984).

In fetal life breathing movements may be detected by ultrasonography. There is a diurnal rhythm as well as periods of breathing and periods of apnoea. Fetal breathing is reduced with hypoxia and hypoglycaemia and the pattern is modified with maternal barbiturates or general anaesthesia. It is possible that prolonged periods of fetal apnoea may result in apnoeic problems in neonatal life (Kaplan 1983). In premature labour, before 34 weeks' gestation, if no fetal breathing movements are detected, then delivery occurs within 48 hours, whereas if breathing movements are detected, the pregnancy will continue (Castle & Turnbull 1983).

After birth, clinical examination of the infant for assessment of gestational age is based on a percentile chart for weight at a particular gestational age (Lubchenco 1976) and clinical tests for passive tone as this changes with maturity (Smith & Smith 1982). The condition of a pre-term baby at birth is dependent on many factors such as maternal disease or drug ingestion and the type of delivery, with higher levels of fetal catecholamines after vaginal delivery (Hagnevik et al 1984). β-Blocking drugs taken during pregnancy may cause fetal growth retardation (Finnstrom et al 1984) and work on animals has shown that during maternal halothane anaesthesia fetal lambs suffer a marked fall in blood pressure (Biehl et al 1983).

Sykes et al (1983) have shown the need for continuous fetal heart monitoring together with frequent fetal blood sampling during delivery of pre-term babies. Clinical signs of fetal distress such as bradycardia are not as sensitive as biochemical determinations of fetal acidosis.

The pre-term baby has similar responses to the term baby to acute hypoxia by increasing perfusion to vital organs (Block et al 1984). The pre-term baby also responds to the stress of delivery with graded catecholamine release and though there is an increased adrenaline secretion in the pre-term baby, the catecholamine pattern is similar to the term baby (Newnham et al 1984). Bistoletti et al (1983) showed that surges of catecholamine release occur if the fetal pH falls below 7.25 causing abnormal fetal heart rate patterns. If bradycardia occurs the levels of noradrenaline are even higher, presumably putting the infant at an increased risk of intraventricular cerebral haemorrhage (see below).

PRE-TERM PHYSIOLOGY

The physiology of the newborn baby at term or prematurely born in relation to surgery and anaesthesia is reviewed (Hatch & Sumner 1985) but some aspects of the pre-term baby deserve closer attention. Immaturity of cardiorespiratory and metabolic functions complicates surgery in the peri-operative period, and respiratory function in ex-preterm babies may continue to be impaired during the first year of life, especially if the baby suffered from respiratory distress syndrome after birth (Steward 1982). The diaphragm of pre-term babies is particularly liable to fatigue, depending on the proportion of high oxidative type I muscle fibres present. Adults have 55% of these fibres whereas a full term infant has 25% and a pre-term baby before 30 weeks' gestation only 10% (Keens et al 1978).

Pre-term babies have difficulties in maintaining normal lung volumes, being likely to develop atelectasis with a marked increase in right–left intrapulmonary shunting as closing volume occurs during tidal breathing. The chest wall is very compliant and because the gas exchange units of the pre-term lung have a smaller diameter (75 μm) than the term (150 μm) or adult (250 μm), lung collapse will readily occur (Gregory & Stewart 1983). The high respiratory rate also helps to maintain the functional residual capacity (FRC) and during apnoea the FRC falls to very low levels as more gas has time to escape from the lungs (Gregory 1980). There is less efficient control of ventilation than for the term baby with a tendency to apnoea, together with the possibility of residual lung damage from mechanical ventilation earlier in life. Mild bronchopulmonary dysplasia is common and is manifested by mild tachypnoea with reduced lung compliance and oxygen dependency.

The pre-term cardiovascular system is immature and will not fully react to stress. The fetal myocardium develops less active tension during isometric contraction and only 30% of the myocardial muscle is contractile mass compared to 60% in the adult (Smith & Smith 1982) which allows these infants less capacity to increase stroke volume. For the cardiac output to increase there must be an increase in heart rate so that rates of up to 200/min are necessary to increase the cardiac output. Bradycardia, for example, in response to hypoxia, will cause a great fall in cardiac output. The effect of the sympathetic nervous system, which develops earlier in fetal life than the vagus, predominates in pre-term babies. The carotid sinus baroreceptors respond to acute haemorrhage but the resulting tachycardia only partially compensates for this and the blood pressure will fall.

Patent ductus arteriosus

Patent ductus arteriosus (PDA) is a very frequent finding in pre-term babies as the mechanism for its closure is immature and factors such as a labile pulmonary vascular resistance with transitional circulation, hypoxia and fluid overload tend to maintain its patency. The patent ductus should be routinely screened by echocardiography as no murmur may be present (Fox & Duara 1983, Archer et al 1984).

Neutral thermal environment

The neutral thermal environment for a low birth weight baby may be as high as 36°C and is explained by very high evaporative heat loss in the first week of life. These babies, if subject to a thermal stress, may not react by increasing oxygen consumption but by a change in body temperature. Sauer et al (1984) suggest a better definition for neutral thermal environment — it is the ambient temperature at which the core temperature of the infant at rest is between 36.7°C and 37.3°C and the core and mean skin temperatures are changing less than 0.2°C and 0.3°C per hour respectively. In the first week of life the neutral temperature depends on the gestational age and post-natal age, but after the first week depends more on the increased body weight and the post-natal age. Heat loss from radiation may be reduced by a secondary heat shield within the incubator. Because of the difficulty in maintaining body temperature of very small newborns in the operating theatre, Besag et al (1984) have suggested that surgery for such conditions as necrotizing enterocolitis should take place in an open incubator in the intensive care unit rather than involve a move to the operating theatre. Other advantages of this are decreased handling of the baby, no interruption of vital monitoring and a reduced risk of displacing the tracheal tube and arterial or venous lines.

Retrolental fibroplasia

The failure to eradicate retrolental fibroplasia (RLF) is still unexplained as the causal relationship with supplemental oxygen was suggested as long ago as 1956 (Silverman 1982). The increasing survival of babies below 1500 g birth weight probably accounts for the increase in the number of infants with the cicatricial form. Although Betts et al (1977) suggested that RLF could occur from exposure to excess oxygen during anaesthesia, Merritt et al (1981) pointed out that the condition was likely to have several causative factors. Flynn (1984) has shown, by the use of logistic analysis, that major surgery with anaesthesia did not contribute to the risk of cicatricial RLF but he wondered why the incidence of the condition appeared to be rising despite technological sophistication in the delivery and monitoring of oxygen. Until recently it has proved impossible to use an animal model to induce scarring lesions by over-exposure to oxygen alone. However Bougle et al (1982) showed that in the retina of kittens, hyperoxia led to a fall in the enzyme superoxide dismutase which protected against the toxic effects of oxygen radicals, although this fall may be partially prevented by pretreatment with tocopheral (vitamin E). It was noticed by Phelps & Rosenbaum (1982) that the infants with scarring RLF had lower Pa_{O_2} than those with simple RLF and the proposal that relative hypoxia after hyperoxia leads to scarring may be borne out by animal work. Flower & Blake (1981) have produced cicatricial lesions experimentally in puppies by preventing oxygen induced vasoconstriction with aspirin which blocks the synthesis of prostaglandin so that retinal damage seemed to occur only where there was inadequate vasomotor tone to protect immature vessels. Thus scarring of the retina may occur without exposure to supplemental oxygen, possibly due to increased blood flow and raised transluminal pressure in the development of retinal vasculature.

INTENSIVE THERAPY

Respiratory support continues to be a key part of intensive care for the pre-term baby. Respiratory pathology is the major cause of morbidity and mortality in this age group. High frequency ventilation is established for use in pre-term babies and may have particular value in patients with air leaks — pneumothorax, pneumopericardium or pneumoperitoneum (Pokora et al 1983). Using high frequency jet ventilation the air leak was markedly reduced in 7 out of 9 patients, with reduction in Pa_{CO_2} and A-aDO_2. Gas mixing occurred throughout the tracheobronchial tree so there was no 'dead space' as such, but there was a continuous CO_2 gradient from the alveoli to the periphery. The jet stream with inadequate humidity may cause rapid mucosal damage and tracheal obstruction occurred in 3 out of 6 patients exposed to this type of ventilation for more than 20 hours. Vincent et al (1984) using high frequency ventilation at 6–7 Hz following cardiac surgery in infants, found that it allowed a reduction of peak ventilatory pressure at airway opening by 19% and peak tracheal pressure by 42% with favourable effects on the cardiovascular pressures. Franz et al (1983) showed that adequate gas exchange at low tracheal pressures was possible using high frequency ventilation in premature infants with primary lung disease. The effect on gas exchange may be greater on CO_2 reduction than increasing Pa_{O_2} and Truog et al (1984) found no change in the natural history of experimental hyaline membrane disease in premature primates. High frequency jet ventilation may not be suitable for all types of lung pathology. Mammel et al (1983) found that conventional ventilation was superior for experimental meconium aspiration. Jet ventilation caused an increased A-aDO_2, increased pulmonary vascular resistance and increased pulmonary artery pressure.

Complications of mechanical ventilation which may be life threatening are mediastinal air leaks and bronchopulmonary dysplasia. The use of pancuronium may prevent pneumothorax in very sick pre-term babies breathing against the ventilator (Greenough 1984). However useful relaxants are in this group of pre-term infants, they can produce complications. Runkle & Bancalari (1984) showed that overall oxygenation improved in a group of pre-term infants after the administration of pancuronium, the effect being most marked in those with meconium aspiration. In patients with hyaline membrane disease the Pa_{O_2} actually tended to fall. Pancuronium has cardiovascular side effects with a consistent rise in heart rate and blood pressure which lasted for 30–50 minutes after administration (Cabal et al 1985). Such sympathetic activity may predispose to intraventricular cerebral haemorrhage.

Suctioning is important to maintain the patency of very small endotracheal tubes. It should be used to remove secretions which become retained because of the absence of the normal expulsive mechanisms.

If enteral feeding is possible this should be done by the jejunal route as gastric contents are freely regurgitated in pre-term babies and will be aspirated around the non cuffed tracheal tube, even at the clinical levels of the distending pressure of 4–8 cm H_20 of CPAP (Goodwin et al 1984). If enteral feeding is impossible then total parenteral nutrition should be undertaken using peripheral veins on a rotational basis.

Total parenteral nutrition (TPN) for infants has been reviewed by Hatch & Sumner (1985). The regime is computerized and an aseptic technique is used for preparing the fluids in the hospital pharmacy. A central venous catheter of the Hickman type is implanted at open operation if TPN is required for prolonged periods.

Respiratory distress syndrome

Pulmonary function in respiratory distress syndrome (RDS) progressively deteriorates until a diuresis occurs and the functional residual capacity increases by up to 40% at the time of the maximum diuresis (Heaf et al 1982). The diuresis may represent the removal of excess lung fluid which is necessary for improvement in the respiratory distress syndrome.

Green et al (1983) have shown that if there is no spontaneous diuresis by the 2nd or 3rd day of life then frusemide therapy may improve the survival from RDS, possibly independent of its function as a diuretic. Frusemide does dilate the pulmonary vascular bed and in some cases may maintain the patency of the ductus arteriosus.

Trials of heterologous natural surfactants are encouraging (Gitling et al 1984) and the idea of replacing surfactant is an attractive one. However, the mortality is low with conventional supportive therapy and no further treatment seems necessary. There is evidence that a patent ductus arteriosus which requires closure may be a complication of artificial surfactant therapy.

Monitoring

New techniques for non-invasive monitoring of pre-term babies both in the operating theatre and intensive care unit continue to be developed. Direct monitoring, although invaluable, may be limited by difficulties with vascular access particularly over a long period of intensive care. Transcutaneous oxygen electrodes ($TcPO_2$) have been adopted by all workers in this field, although the use of carbon dioxide electrodes is limited by leakage of air which nullifies the readings. Modern pulse oximetry may prove to be a valuable alternative to $TcPO_2$ (Yelderman & New 1983).

A new non-invasive technique for the monitoring of cerebral oxygenation in pre-term babies has been described by Brazy et al (1985). The technique relies on transilluminating the anterior cerebral field with near infra-red light which undergoes differential absorption with changes in oxidation and reduction levels of cytochrome aa_3 in haemoglobin of tissue blood. The levels correlate well with transcutaneous PO_2 readings and show that even a brief bradycardia causes a precipitate fall in reduction of cytochrome aa_3.

REFERENCES

See end of chapter 13.

Paediatric anaesthesia and intensive care (2)

INTRAVENTRICULAR HAEMORRHAGE

Intraventricular haemorrhage (IVH) is the commonest serious neurological event of the neonatal period, affecting approximately 40–50% of all pre-term infants under 35 weeks' gestational age (Volpe 1981). This incidence increases as gestational age decreases and an incidence of 61% has been reported in infants born before 33 weeks (Ment et al 1984). The lesions are less severe in infants born in a perinatal unit (Clark et al 1981, Dolfin et al 1983) and it has been suggested that 'at-risk' infants should only be delivered in these special units. Pre-natal events, particularly the duration and course of labour may also be contributory factors (Meidell et al 1985): the incidence of IVH is apparently higher after vaginal delivery than Caesarean section (Greisen & Petersen 1983).

As may be expected from its prevalence in pre-term infants, there is a high association with the respiratory distress syndrome (RDS) and IVH is the commonest neuropathological finding in infants dying with this disorder (Leech et al 1979). Other associated factors include hypoxia, hypercarbia, acidosis, high ventilatory requirements and pneumothoraces (Lipscombe et al 1981, Levene et al 1982), although these must in part reflect the severity of the RDS. Severe acidosis appears to be an independently acting contributory factor. Sudden rises in blood pressure, particularly after a period of relatively low pressure, may also lead to IVH (Fujimura et al 1979).

The study of IVH, which usually occurs within 72 hours of birth, has been greatly helped in recent years by the introduction of computerized axial tomography and especially by portable real time ultrasonography. The initial lesion is bleeding into the highly vascular periventricular germinal matrix, typically over the head of the caudate nucleus (Leech & Kohnen 1974). In the pre-term infants of less than 28 weeks' gestational age, the vulnerable site is over the body of the caudate nucleus (Hambleton & Wigglesworth 1976). With increasing maturity the germinal matrix disappears and there is a more pronounced arterialization of the cerebral cortex and adjacent white matter. Haemorrhage in near term infants is thus more likely to occur from the choroid plexus (Donat et al 1978).

Although numerous theories have been proposed for the aetiology of IVH, several recent observations suggest an arterial mechanism. Pape & Wigglesworth (1979) have shown the periventricular capillary bed to be essentially an immature vascular rete.

These vessels cannot be categorized on light microscopy, and consist only of a layer of endothelium without smooth muscle, collagen or fibrin (Haruda & Blanc 1981). The metabolic activity of brain capillary endothelial cells suggests that they are particularly dependent on oxidative mechanisms (Goldstein 1979) and may easily be damaged by hypoxic events. Lou et al (1979) and Milligan (1980) have demonstrated a failure of autoregulation of cerebral blood flow in distressed pre-term infants and this may be of more importance. These infants are often hypotensive and hypoxic with maximal cerebral vasodilatation and it has been postulated that any rise in cerebral blood flow, particularly if sudden, may rupture the fragile, unsupported vascular matrix. This may occur with hypercarbia or acidosis, or following therapeutic measures such as the rapid infusion of blood volume expanders (Goldberg et al 1980) or the use of hyperosmolar solutions such as glucose or sodium bicarbonate (Papile et al 1978b). Events that raise systemic blood pressure may also be detrimental. Endotracheal suctioning for example has been shown to produce a marked systemic pressor response with a prominent and consistent rise in anterior cerebral artery blood flow (Perlman & Volpe 1983). This must raise doubts about the safety of awake intubation in sick pre-term infants.

Anterior cerebral blood flow patterns in pre-term infants ventilated in the treatment of severe RDS have been shown to be either fluctuating or stable (Perlman et al 1983a). 21 out of 23 infants with fluctuating cerebral flow developed IVH, while only seven out of 27 infants with a stable flow pattern did so. The flow pattern reflected the simultaneously recorded blood pressure and correlated with the severity of the RDS. Mean peak airway pressure was higher in the IVH group. Paralysing the infants resulted in the fluctuating flow pattern becoming stable. The presence of a patent ductus arteriousus has also been shown to produce abnormal cerebral blood flow patterns (Martin et al 1982) which must predispose to IVH, particularly as there is often an acute rise in blood pressure as the ductus is ligated (Marshall et al 1982).

It is uncertain how the presence of a pneumothorax predisposes to IVH. It may be due to a moderate rise in diastolic blood pressure due to an increase in peripheral resistance (Hill et al 1982). However, it has recently been shown in newborn dogs that the rapid evacuation of a pneumothorax leads to a precipitate rise in blood pressure and cerebral blood flow to supranormal levels (Batton et al 1984). Periventricular capillary pressure may also be raised when venous pressure is raised, for example, during positive pressure ventilation.

Abnormalities of coagulation have also been implicated in the pathogenesis of newborn IVH. McDonald et al (1984) have recently documented a significant association between hypocoagulability in the first few hours of life in pre-term infants with subsequent onset of progression of IVH. It is not yet known whether early and aggressive correction of this coagulopathy will reduce the morbidity and mortality of IVH.

There are numerous ways of classifying IVH, but that proposed by Papile et al (1978a) is usually used. In mild cases (grade 1), the bleeding is confined to the periventricular germinal matrix. Frequently however this periventricular haemorrhage (PHV) ruptures through the ependyma into the ventricles producing the more severe IVH (grade 2). In grade 3 IVH, there is associated ventricular dilatation, and in the severe lesions there appears to be extension into the cerebral parenchyma (grade 4). Recent studies would suggest however that this intraparenchymal lesion is a concomitant haemorrhagic infarction rather than a simple extension of the germinal matrix bleed (Flodmark et al 1980).

Treatment

Attempts to reduce the incidence of IVH have included the prophylactic use of drugs such as phenobarbitone which prevents sharp increases in blood pressure (Wimberley et al 1982). Ninan et al (1985) reported that intravenous phenobarbitone (10 mg/kg) reduced the increases in heart rate, blood pressure and intracranial pressure and the fall in oxygenation following endotracheal suctioning in pre-term infants. However although the lesions were less severe, the drug had no effect on the incidence of IVH (Bedard et al 1984).

A significant reduction in IVH following the use of tocopheral (vitamin E) has also been reported (Speer et al 1984). This agent, an antioxidant, may protect endothelial cell membranes thereby limiting the magnitude of haemorrhage in the germinal matrix. Unfortunately its use is associated with an increased incidence of necrotizing entercolitis (NEC) and generalized sepsis, presumably by interfering with oxygen dependent antimicrobial defences (Johnson et al 1985). This side effect does not occur if blood levels are kept below 3.5 mg/dl.

Ethamsylate, a capillary stablizing drug which has been used to limit bleeding in a number of surgical procedures, may also be useful (Cooke & Morgan 1984) but further studies are necessary.

Progressive haemorrhage increases morbidity and mortality and it is therefore important to prevent or limit the extend of IVH. Thorburn et al (1981) reported a mortality of over 50% in severe bleeding with a third of the survivors having a major neurodevelopmental handicap. Williamson et al (1983) found that 50% of the survivors at the age of 3 years had moderate or severe neurological abnormalities and 52% were intellectually impaired. The poor outcome would appear to be directly related to the magnitude of the underlying haemorrhage (Papile et al 1983) although there may be some contribution from the chronic ventricular dilatation that usually occurs after IVH. This has been attributed to an obliterative arachnoiditis (Larroche 1972) or less often to obstruction of the flow of cerebrospinal fluid (CSF) by necrotic debris within the ventricles at the aqueduct of Sylvius (Hill et al 1984). Ventricular dilatation is often managed conservatively and only rarely does hydrocephalus lead to increased intracranial pressure which requires a shunt (Allan et al 1984).

Intraventricular haemorrhage (IVH) is not the only problem associated with failure of autoregulation of cerebral blood flow in pre-term infants. Intracerebellar haemorrhage may occur in 15–22% of patients, although this is more difficult to detect (Perlman et al 1983b) and is presumably also due to hyperperfusion. Hypoperfusion of boundary zones between different arterial territories which may occur during hypotensive episodes, may cause infarction within the periventricular white matter — periventricular leukomalacia (PVL). This can lead to cystic degeneration (Levene et al 1983) often affecting the pyramidal tracts as they pass from the motor cortex through the internal capsule. The fibres affecting distribution to the leg, and which are closer to the ventricle, are more likely to be damaged resulting in spastic diplegia which is a significant handicap.

It is important therefore to ensure that meticulous attention is paid to these patients at risk, avoiding as far as possible fluctuations in blood pressure and cerebral blood flow. Hypotension should be avoided by early blood transfusion, care being taken to avoid the dangers of rapid transfusion.

APNOEA

Apnoeic episodes occur frequently in pre-term infants and, although incompletely understood, the underlying mechanisms are becoming clearer. Apnoea must be distinguished from the periodic respiration which is commonly seen in all newborn infants. This is associated with ventilatory pauses of less than 10 seconds, without bradycardia or cyanosis, and is of no pathological significance. True apnoea is usually defined as cessation of breathing for 20 seconds or more (Rigatto 1982) and is often accompanied by bradycardia and a fall in oxygenation. The incidence and severity of apnoea increase with decreasing gestational age, so prematurity is one of the main predisposing factors. In many cases the episodes can be attributed to insults such as infection, metabolic disturbances, or IVH, but in many cases the aetiology is unknown and is attributed to immaturity of the brain stem centres. Early studies suggest that apnoea was precipitated by hypoxia but this has been discounted by Gerhardt & Bancalari (1984) who found no difference in oxygenation and pulmonary mechanisms between pre-term infants with or without apnoea. They demonstrated significantly decreased inspiratory effort in the infants with apnoea, with alveolar hypoventilation and hypercapnia. This evidence of decreased respiratory centre activity was confirmed by a CO_2 response curve which is flattened and shifted to the right. CNS immaturity is also reflected by the decreased number of synaptic connections, incomplete dendritic arborization and the poor myelination seen in the pre-term brain (Schulte 1977). This results in decreased afferent traffic to, and a decreased state of excitation of, the reticular formation and respiratory centre. This is supported by the clinical observation that various external stimuli can increase respiratory activity and reduce the incidence of apnoea. Furthermore, auditory evoked brain stem conduction time is prolonged in pre-term infants and shortens with advancing gestational age, due to improving synaptic efficiency and myelination (Henderson-Smart et al 1983). This prolongation of auditory evoked brain stem conduction time correlates strongly with apnoea and confirms that brain stem immaturity underlies apnoea of prematurity.

Some of the repiratory reflexes are also immature in the pre-term infant. For example, the Hering-Breuer inflation reflex is poorly developed at 28–35 weeks' gestation and does not reach maximal strength until term (Gerhardt & Bancalari 1981). This reflects a decreased vagal input which would normally occur with each breath and contributes to the establishment of regular breathing. The intercostal phrenic inhibitory reflex, which may terminate inspiratory effort when distortions of the chest wall occur (Knill & Bryan 1976), is particularly active in pre-term infants (Thach et al 1978). Chest wall distortion in newborns is reportedly increased during REM sleep, possibly due to central inhibition of intercostal muscle tone (Schulte et al 1977). This may explain the increase of apnoeic episodes seen during REM sleep (Steinschneider & Weinstein 1983). The amount of REM sleep falls with increasing age as does the incidence of apnoea.

Pre-term infants are at a further disadvantage if subjected to increased respiratory loads, such as obstruction, as much of the extra effort is dissipated in deformation of their soft and compliant chest wall. Apnoea thus readily follows airway obstruction which is common in these infants. This is frequently a pharyngeal problem (Mathew et al 1982) and may be partly due to reduced genioglossus muscle tone (Dransfield et al 1983). CPAP is well established treatment for apnoea but a recent paper suggests that it selectively reduces apnoea with an obstructive component, possibly by splinting the pharyngeal airway (Miller et al 1985). It may also act by stabilizing the chest wall thereby eliminating the intercostal phrenic inhibitory reflex. CPAP does not appreciably alter the ventilatory response to CO_2 (Durand et al 1983) and since hypoxia is not a cause of apnoea it presumably does not act by improving oxygenation.

Aminophylline is widely used in the treatment of idiopathic apnoea and is more effective than CPAP (Jones 1982). The mechanism is probably through inhibition of phosphodiesterase with increased levels of cyclic AMP. Cyclic AMP plays an important role in the action of a variety of neurotransmitters, and is also increased by catecholamines. Aminophylline may therefore compensate for the deficiency of catecholamines seen in pre-term infants with apnoea (Kattwinkel et al 1976). There is an increase in the sensitivity of the respiratory centre to CO_2 (the slope is increased and shifted to the left) with increased minute ventilation and decreased arterial CO_2 (Gerhardt et al 1979). Aminophylline also increases the strength of the Hering-Breuer reflex indicating an increase in vagal afferents from pulmonary stretch receptors. It is not clear whether this increased central stimulation is due to increased sensitivity of peripheral receptors or a facilitation of afferent signals or both. The ability to compensate for increased loads in pre-term infants is also increased (Gerhardt et al 1983).

Pre-term infants with a history of apnoea are more likely than full term infants to have apnoeic episodes following anaesthesia (Steward 1982). Indeed in one study, all prematurely born infants with a history of apnoea operated on before 41 weeks' gestational age required post-operative respiratory support (Liu et al 1983). This was irrespective of surgical procedure or anaesthetic technique. All infants with a history of apnoea, particularly those of less than 46 weeks' gestational age, should therefore be closely monitored for 24 hours post-operatively.

SUDDEN INFANT DEATH SYNDROME

The sudden infant death syndrome (SIDS) occurs more frequently in premature infants. The condition is a distinct clinical entity and is diagnosed by unexpected death from which the post-mortem examination fails to reveal an adequate cause for death and accounts for approximately 1500 deaths per year in the United Kingdom. In addition there is a group of infants who suffer a severe episode of apnoea and cyanosis, the 'near miss' SIDS, some of whom may die subsequently. This group of infants has been the subject of considerable physiological study as it was assumed that the 'near miss' is related to SIDS, because its peak age distribution was slightly earlier than that of SIDS and because of the sudden subsequent death of many 'near miss' patients.

Although the syndrome may be multifactorial, current research focuses on possible defective control of ventilation in these infants (Leading Article 1984) and abnormal ventilatory responses have been detected in the parents of SIDS babies (Schiffman et al 1980). There is an increased frequency of apnoeic pauses in a group of infants some of whom were SIDS victims later (Steinschneider et al 1982). Jeffery et al (1983) investigated 58 infants with 'near miss' SIDS and 6 twins of SIDS victims and found that some had idiopathic apnoea, minimal tracheomalacia, aberrant innominate arteries or temporal lobe seizures, but 55 had gastro-oesophageal reflux.

It has been shown that reflux precedes apnoea and that this could be induced by instilling dilute acid (not water or milk) on to the lower oesophagus (Herbst et al 1979). Simultaneous tracings of oesophageal pH, heart rate, impedence pneumography and nasal airflow showed that apnoea did not settle until surgical or medical treatment for reflux was undertaken. Reflux appeared to be a common factor in very many 'near miss' SIDS infants. Reflux may not be diagnosed on barium swallow, but requires the use of a milk scan (radioisotope gastroesophageal scintingraphy) (MacFayden et al 1983).

The phase of active sleep may be associated with depressed reflexes and therefore a vulnerability to asphyxia in infants (Jeffery et al 1980). The response to mild respiratory obstruction or liquid in the pharynx may be reflex apnoea but no arousal occurs because the ventilatory responses to CO_2 retention and hypoxia are also depressed. This forms the basis of the sleep apnoea theory for SIDS, but there may be also a further defect in the neurochemical control of respiration which allows non-arousal to occur during the sleep apnoea.

Recent investigation has concerned chemoreceptor activity in the carotid body which triggers acute responses to hypoxia. Perrin et al (1984) found that the carotid bodies of infants with SIDS had increased catecholamine levels including a ten-fold increase in dopamine when compared with infants dying from other defined causes.

Olson et al (1982) found that in adults, dopamine infusion may impair the ventilatory response to hypercapnia and hypoxia. It is thus possible that the high concentration of dopamine within the carotid bodies hampers the response of the infant to hypoxia and it is thus possible that there is a neurochemical cause of SIDS. An 'at-risk' infant could become severely asphyxiated during active sleep from very many minor problems such as upper respiratory tract infection, nasal obstruction or gastro-oesophageal reflux.

The prevention of SIDS is a controversial topic. Carpenter et al (1983) have shown that keeping a close watch at home on babies at risk will reduce mortality. They developed a scoring system which depends on maternal age, previous pregnancies, length of labour and gestational age. There is, however, a continuing mortality from SIDS. Home monitoring of apnoea and/or ECG, has been undertaken by Duffty et al (1982) in babies who have suffered 'near miss' SIDS and in siblings of SIDS victims. They used apnoea alarms of the transducer pad or chest impedence type or heart rate monitors for at least 2 months. The monitors were set to alarm after 20 seconds' apnoea or at a heart rate below 80. Many episodes of apnoea and bradycardia were detected, some being multiple and some serious. At least one patient later succumbed to SIDS. Simpson (1983) has reviewed the difficulties of home monitoring. The presence of the monitor at home may induce parental neurosis, although in practice the machines are well accepted. The selection of the patients may be difficult and although siblings of SIDS victims and those with 'near miss' are included, those with low birth weight from special care baby units, with bronchopulmonary dysplasia and those from narcotic dependent mothers should also be included. This would make for a large group requiring expensive machines. There is also concern about the efficacy of the monitors. Apnoea alarms are unreliable and many only detect central but not obstructive apnoea and breathing movements may continue until the moment of death.

There is a great deal of knowledge concerning the aetiology of this tragic cause of infant death, but its prevention still remains to be elucidated.

REFERENCES

Allan W C, Dransfield D A, Tito A M 1984 Ventricular dilation following periventricular-intraventricular hemorrhage: outcome at age 1 year. Pediatrics 73: 158–162

Archer L N J, Glass E J, Godman M J 1984 Silent ductus arteriosus in idiopathic respiratory distress syndrome. Acta Paediatrica Scandinavica 73: 652–656

Ariagno R L, Guilleminault C, Korobkin R, Owenboeddiker M, Baldwin R 1983 Near miss for sudden infant death syndrome infants — a clinical problem. Pediatrics 71: 726–736

Batton D G, Hellman J, Nardis E E 1984 Effect of pneumothorax-induced systemic blood pressure alterations on the cerebral circulation in newborn dogs. Pediatrics 74: 350–353

Bedard M P, Shankaran S, Slovis T L, Pantoja A, Dayal B, Poland R 1984 Effect of prophylactic phenobarbital on intraventricular hemorrhage in high-risk infants. Pediatrics 73: 435–439

Besag F M C, Singh M P, Whitelaw A G L 1984 Surgery of the ill, extremely low birth weight infant: should transfer to the operating theatre be avoided? Acta Paediatrica Scandinavica 73: 594–595

Betts E K, Downes J J, Schaffer D B, Johns R 1977 Retrolental fibroplasia and oxygen administration during general anesthesia. Anesthesiology 47: 518–520

Biehl D R, Côté J, Wade J G, Gregory G A, Sitar D 1983 Uptake of halothane by the fetal lamb in utero. Canadian Anaesthetists' Society Journal 30: 24–27

Bistoletti P, Nylund L, Lagercrantz H, Hjemdahl P, Ström H 1983 Fetal scalp catecholamines during labor. American Journal of Obstetrics and Gynecology 147: 785–788

Block B S B, Llanos A J, Creasy R K 1984 Responses of the growth retarded fetus to acute hypoxemia. American Journal of Obstetrics and Gynecolgoy 148: 878–881

Bloom B S 1984 Changing infant mortality: the need to spend more while getting less. Pediatrics 73: 862–866

Bougle D, Vert P, Reichart E, Hartemann D Heng E L 1982 Retinal superoxide dismutase activity in new born kittens exposed to normobaric hyperoxia: effect of vitamin E. Pediatric Research 16: 400–402

Boyle M H, Torrance G W, Sinclair J C, Horwood S P 1983 Economic evaluation of neonatal intensive care of very low birth weight infants. New England Journal of Medicine 308: 1330–1337

Brazy J E, Lewis D V, Mitnick M H, Van der Vliet F J 1985 Non-invasive monitoring of cerebral oxygenation in preterm infants: preliminary observations. Pediatrics 75: 217–225

Cabal L A, Siassi B, Artal R, Gonzalez F, Hodgman J, Plajsteck C 1985 Cardiovascular and catecholamine changes after administration of pancuronium in distressed neonates. Pediatrics 75: 284–287

Carpenter R G, Gardner A, Jepson M, Taylor E M, Salvin A, Sunderland R, Emery J L et al 1983 Prevention of unexpected infant death. Lancet i: 723–727

Castle B M, Turnbull A C 1983 The presence or absence of fetal breathing movements predicts the outcome of preterm labour. Lancet 2: 471–472

Clark C E, Clyman R I, Roth R S, Sniderman S H, Lane B, Ballard R A 1981 Risk factor analysis of intraventricular hemorrhage in low-birth-weight infants. Journal of Pediatrics 99: 625–628

Cooke R W I, Morgan M E I 1984 Prophylactic ethamsylate for periventricular haemorrhage. Archives of Disease in Childhood 59: 82–83

Dolfin T, Skidmore M B, Fong K W, Hoskins E M, Shennan A J 1983 Incidence, severity, and timing of subependymal and intraventricular hemorrhages in preterm infants born in a perinatal unit as detected by serial real-time ultrasound. Pediatrics 71: 541–546

Donat J F, Okazaki H, Kleinburg H, Reagan T J 1978 Intraventricular hemorrhages in full-term and premature infants. Mayo Clinic Proceedings 53: 437–441

Dransfield D A, Spitzer A R, Fox W W 1983 Episodic airway obstruction in premature infants. American Journal of Diseases of Children 137: 441–443

Duffty P, Bryan M H 1982 Home apnoea monitoring in 'near miss' sudden infant death syndrome (SIDS) and in siblings of SIDS victims. Pediatrics 70: 69–74

Durand M, McCann E, Brady J P 1983 Effect of continuous positive airway pressure on the ventilatory response to CO_2 in preterm infants. Pediatrics 71: 634–638

Finnstrom O, Ezitis J, Ryden G, Wichman K 1984 Neonatal effects of beta blocking drugs in pregnancy. Acta Obstetrica et Gynecologica Scandinavica (suppl.) 118: 91–93

Flodmark O, Becker L E, Harwood-Nash D C, Fitzhardinge P M, Fitz C R, Chuang S H 1980 Correlation between computed tomography and autopsy in premature and full-term neonates that have suffered perinatal asphyxia. Radiology 137: 93–103

Flower R W, Blake D A 1981 Retrolental fibroplasia: evidence for a role of the prostaglandin cascade in the pathogenesis of oxygen-induced retinopathy in the newborn beagle. Pediatric Research 15: 1293–1302

Flynn J T 1984 Oxygen and retrolental fibroplasia: update and challenge. Anesthesiology 60: 397–399

Fox W W, Duara S 1983 Persistent pulmonary hypertension in the neonate: diagnosis and management. Journal of Pediatrics 103: 505–514

Frantz I D, Werthammer J, Stark A R 1983 High frequency ventilation in premature infants with lung disease: adequate gas exchange at low tracheal pressure. Pediatrics 71: 483–488

Fujimura M, Salisbury D M, Robinson R O, Howat P, Emerson P M, Keeling J W, Tizard J P M 1979 Clinical events relating to intraventricular haemorrhage in the newborn. Archives of Disease in Childhoo 54: 409–414

Gauderer M W L, Jassani M N, Izant R J 1984 Ultrasonographic antenatal diagnosis: will it change the spectrum of neonatal surgery? Journal of Pediatric Surgery 19: 404–407

Gerhardt T, Bancalari E 1981 Maturational changes of reflexes influencing inspiratory timing in newborns. Journal of Applied Physiology 50: 1282–1285

Gerhardt T, Bancalari E 1984 Apnea of prematurity: 1. Lung function and regulation of breathing. Pediatrics 74: 58–62

Gerhardt T, McCarthy J, Bancalari E 1979 Effects of aminophylline on respiratory center activity and metabolic rate in premature infants with idiopathic apnea. Pediatrics 63: 537–542

Gerhardt T, MCarthy J, Bancalari E 1983 Effects of aminophylline on respiratory center and reflex activity in premature infants with apnea. Pediatric Research 17: 188–191

Gitlin J D, Parad R, Taeusch H W 1984 Exogenous surfactant therapy in hyaline membrane disease. Seminars in Perinatology 8: 272–282

Goldberg R N, Chung D, Goldman S L, Bancalari E 1980 The association of rapid volume expansion and intraventricular hemorrhage in the preterm infant. Journal of Pediatrics 96: 1060–1063

Goldstein G W 1979 Pathogenesis of brain edema and hemorrhage: role of the brain capillary. Pediatrics 64: 357–360

Goodwin S R, Graves S A, Haberkern C M 1984 Aspiration in intubated premature infants. Pediatrics 75: 85–88

Green T P, Thompson T R, Johnson D E, Lock J E 1983 Diuresis and pulmonary function in premature infants with respiratory distress syndrome. Journal of Pediatrics 103: 618–623

Greenough A, Wood S, Morley C J, Davis J A 1984 Pancuronium prevents pneumothoraces in ventilated premature babies who actively expire against positive pressure inflation. Lancet 1: 1–3

Gregory G A 1980 Respiratory care of the child. Critical Care Medicine 8: 582–587

Gregory G A, Steward D J 1983 Life threatening perioperative apnea in the ex-'premie'. Anesthesiology 59: 495–498

Greisen G, Petersen M B 1983 Intraventricular hemorrhage and method of delivery of very low birth weight infants. Journal of Perinatal Medicine 11: 495–498
67–73

Hagnevik K, Faxelius G, Irestadt L, Lagercrantz H, Lundell B, Persson B 1984 Catecholamine surge and metabolic adaptation in the newborn after vaginal delivery and caesarian section. Acta Paediatrica Scandinavica 73: 602–609

Hallman M, Feldman B H, Kirkpatrick E, Gluck L 1977 Absence of phosphatidylglycerol (PG) in respiratory distress syndrome in the newborn. Pediatric Research 11: 714–720

Hambleton G, Wigglesworth J S 1976 Origin of intraventricular haemorrhage in the preterm infant. Archives of Disease in Childhood 51: 651–659

Haruda F, Blanc W A 1981 The structure of intracerebral arteries in premature infants and the autoregulation of cerebral blood flow. Annals of Neurology 10: 303

Hatch D J, Sumner E 1985 Neonatal anaesthesia and perioperative care. Arnold, London

Heaf D P, Belik J, Spitzer A R, Gewitz M H, Fox W W 1982 Changes in pulmonary function during diuretic phase of respiratory distress syndrome. Journal of Pediatrics 101: 103–107

Henderson-Smart D J, Pettigrew A G, Campbell D J 1983 Clinical apnea and brain stem neural function in preterm infants. New England Journal of Medicine 308: 353–357

Herbst J J, Minton S D, Book L S 1979 Gastro esophageal reflux causing respiratory arrest and apnea in newborn infants. Journal of Pediatrics 95: 763–768
Hermansen M C, Johnson G L 1984 Neonatal supraventricular tachycardia following prolonged maternal ritodrine adminstration. American Journal of Obstetrics and Gynecology 149: 798–799
Hill A, Perlman J M, Volpe J J 1982 Relationship of pneumothorax to occurrence of intraventricular hemorrhage in the premature newborn. Pediatrics 69: 144–149
Hill A, Shackleford G D, Volpe J J 1984 A potential mechanism of pathogenesis for early posthemorrhagic hydrocephalus in the premature newborn. Pediatrics 73: 19–21
James D K, Chiswick M L, Harkes A, William S M, Tindall V R 1984 Maternal diabetes and neonatal respiratory distress. Maturation of fetal surfactant. British Journal of Obstetrics and Gynaecology 91: 316–324
Jeffery H E, Reid I, Rahilly P, Read D J C 1980 Gastro-oesophageal reflux in 'near miss' sudden infant death infants in active but not quiet sleep. Sleep 3: 393–399
Jeffery H E, Rahilly P, Read D J C 1983 Multiple cause of asphyxia in infants at high risk of sudden infant death. Archives of Disease in Childhood 58: 92–100
Johnson L, Bowen F W, Abbasi S, Herrmann N, Weston M, Sacks L, et al 1985 Relationship of prolonged pharmacologic serum levels of vitamin E to incidence of sepsis and necrotising enterocolitis in infants with birthweight 1500 grams or less. Pediatrics 75: 619–638
Jones R A K 1982 Apnoea of prematurity. A controlled trial of theophylline and facemask continuous positive airways pressure. Archives of Disease in Childhood 57: 761–765
Kaplan M 1983 Fetal breathing movements. American Journal of Diseases of Children 137: 177–181
Kattwinkel J, Mars T T, Fanaroff A A, Klaus M H 1976 Urinary biogenic amines in idiopathic apnea of prematurity. Journal of Pediatrics 88: 1003–1006
Keens T G, Bryan A L, Levison H, Ianuzzo D C 1978 Development pattern of muscle fiber types in human ventilatory muscles. Journal of Applied Physiology 44: 909–913
Kiely E 1984 One hundred consecutive central venous catheters in children. Zeitschrift Für Kinderchirurgie 39: 332–336
Knill R, Bryan A C 1976 An intercostal-phrenic inhibitory reflex in human newborn infants. Journal of Applied Physiology 40: 352–356
Larroche J C 1972 Post-haemorrhagic hydrocephalus in infancy: anatomical study. Biology of the Neonate 20: 287–299
Leader 1984 Ventilatory dysfunction and sudden death syndrome. Lancet ii: 558–559
Leech R W, Kohnen P 1974 Subependymal and intraventricular hemorrhages in the newborn. American Journal of Pathology 77: 465–475
Leech R W, Olsson M I, Alvord E C 1979 Neuropathologic features of idiopathic respiratory distress syndrome. Archives of Pathology and Laboratory Medicine 103: 341–343
Levene M I, Fawer C-L, Lamont R F 1982 Risk factors in the development of intraventricular haemorrhage in the preterm neonate. Archives of Disease in Childhood 57: 410–417
Levene M I, Wigglesworth J, Dubowitz V 1983 Hemorrhagic periventricular leucomalacia in the neonate: a real-time ultrasound study. Pediatrics 71: 794–797
Lipscombe A P, Thorburn R J, Reynolds E O R, Stewart A L, Blackwell R J, Cusick G, Whitehead M D 1981 Pneumothorax and cerebral haemorrhage in preterm infants. Lancet i: 414–416
Liu L M P, Cote C J, Goudsouzian N G, Ryan J F, Firestone S, Dedrick D F et al 1983 Life threatening apnea in infants recovering from anesthesia. Anesthesiology 59: 506–510
Lou H C, Lassen N A, Friis-Hansen B 1979 Impaired autoregulation of cerebral blood flow in the distressed newborn. Journal of Pediatrics 96: 119–121
Lubchenco L O 1976 The high risk infant. Saunders, Philadelphia
MacFadyen U M, Hendry G M A, Simpson H 1983 Gastro-oesophageal reflux in near miss sudden infant death syndrome or suspected recurrent aspiration. Archives of Disease in Childhood 58: 87–89
Mammel M C, Gordon M J, Connett J E, Boros S J 1983 Comparison of high frequency jet ventilation and conventional mechanical ventilation in a meconium aspiration model. Journal of Pediatrics 103: 630–634
Marshall T A, Marshall F, Reddy P P 1982 Physiologic changes associated with ligation of the PDA in preterm infants. Journal of Pediatrics 101: 749–753
Martin C G, Snider R, Katz S M, Peabody J L, Brody J P 1982 Abnormal cerebral blood flow patterns in preterm infants with a large PDA. Journal of Pediatrics 101: 587–593
Mathew O P, Roberts J L, Thach B T 1982 Pharyngeal airway obstruction in preterm infants during mixed and obstructive apnea. Journal of Pediatrics 100: 964–968
McDonald M M, Johnson M L, Rumack C M, Koops B L, Guggenheim M A, Babb C, Hathaway W E 1984 Role of coagulopathy in newborn intracranial hemorrhage. Pediatrics 74: 26–31
Meidell R, Marinelli P, Pettet G 1985 Perinatal factors associated with early-onset intracranial

hemorrhage in premature infants. American Journal of Diseases of Children 139: 160–163
Ment L R, Duncan C C, Ehrenkranz R A et al 1984 Intraventricular hemorrhage in the preterm neonate: timing and cerebral blood flow changes. Journal of Pediatrics 104: 419–425
Merritt J C, Sprague D N, Merritt W E, Ellis R A 1981 RLF : A multifactorial disease. Anesthesia and Analgesia 60: 109–111
Miller M J, Carlo W A, Martin R J 1985 Continuous positive airway pressure selectively reduces obstructive apnea in preterm infants. Journal of Pediatrics 106: 91–94
Milligan D W A 1980 Failure of autoregulation and intraventricular haemorrhage in preterm infants. Lancet i: 896–898
Newnham J P, Marshall C L, Padbury J F, Lam R W, Hobel C J, Fisher D A 1984 Fetal catecholamine releases with preterm delivery. American Journal of Obstetrics and Gynecology 149: 888–893
Ninan A, O'Donnell M, Hamilton K, Sankaran K 1985 Physiological changes induced by endotracheal instillation and suctioning in critically ill preterm infants with and without sedation. Pediatric Research 19: 355A (No. 1468)
O'Brien W F and Cafalo R C 1980 Clinical applicability of amniotic fluid tests for fetal pulmonic maturity. American Journal of Obstetrics and Gynecology 136: 135–144
Olson L G, Hensley M J, Saunders N A 1982 Ventilatory responsiveness to hypercapnic hypoxia during dopamine infusion in humans. American Review of Respiratory Disease 126: 783–787
Pape K W, Wigglesworth J S 1979 Haemorrhage, ischaemia and the perinatal brain. In: Clinics in Developmental Medicine, Nos. 69/70. Spastics International Medical Publications, William Heinemann, London
Papile L A, Burstein J, Burstein R, Koffler H 1978a Incidence and evolution of subependymal and intraventricular hemorrhage: a study of infants with birthweights less than 1500 gms. Journal of Pediatrics 92: 529–534
Papile L A, Burstein J, Burstein R, Koffler H, Koops B 1978b Relationship of intravenous sodium bicarbonate infusions and cerebral intraventricular hemorrhage. Journal of Pediatrics 93: 834–836
Papile L A, Munsick-Bruno G, Schaefer A 1983 Relationship of cerebral intraventricular hemorrhage and early childhood neurologic handicaps. Journal of Pediatrics 103: 273–277
Perlman J M, Volpe J J 1983 Suctioning in the preterm infant: effects on cerebral blood flow velocity, intracranial pressure and arterial blood pressure. Pediatrics 72: 329–334
Perlman J M, McMenamin J B, Volpe J J 1983a Fluctuating cerebral blood flow velocity in respiratory distress syndrome. Relation to the development of intraventricular hemorrhage. New England Journal of Medicine 309: 204–209
Perlman J M, Nelson J S, McAlister W H, Volpe J J 1983b Intracerebellar hemorrhage in a premature newborn: diagnosis by real-time ultrasound and correlation with autopsy findings. Pediatrics 71: 159–162
Perrin D G, Cutz E, Becker L E, Bryan A C, Madapallimatum A, Sole M J 1984 Sudden infant death syndrome: increased carotid-body dopamine and noradrenaline content. Lancet ii: 535–537
Persson P H, Kullander S, Gennser G, Grennert L, Laurell C B 1983 Screening for fetal malformations using ultrasound and measurements of alpha-fetoprotein in maternal serum. British Medical Journal 286: 747–749
Phelps D L, Rosenbaum A L 1982 The effect of marginal hypoxemia during the recovery period in oxygen-induced retinopathy in the kitten. Clinical Research 30: 146A
Pokora T, Bing D, Mammel M C, Boros S J 1983 Neonatal high-frequency jet ventilation. Pediatrics 72: 27–32
Rigatto H 1982 Apnea. Pediatric Clinics of North America 29: 1105–1116
Runkle B, Bancalari E 1984 Acute cardiopulmonary effects of pancuronium bromide in mechanically ventilated newborn infants. Journal of Pediatrics 104: 614–617
Saigal S, Rosenbaum P, Stoskopf B, Sinclair J C 1984 Outcome in infants 501–1000 g birth weight delivered to residents of the McMaster Health Region. Journal of Pediatrics 105: 969–976
Sauer P J J, Dane H J, Visser H K A 1984 New standards for neutral thermal environment of healthy very low birthweight infants in week one of life. Archives of Disease in Childhood 59: 18–22
Schiffman P L, Westlake R E, Santiago T V, Edelman N H 1980 Ventilatory control in parents of victims of sudden infant death syndrome. New England Journal of Medicine 302: 486–491
Schulte F J 1977 Apnea. Clinics in Perinatology 4: 64–76
Schulte F J, Busse C, Eichhorn W 1977 Rapid eye movement sleep, motoneurone inhibition and apneic spells in preterm infants. Pediatric Research 11: 709–713
Silverman W A 1982 Retinopathy of prematurity: oxygen dogma challenged. Archives of Disease in Childhood 57: 731–733

Simpson H 1983 Sudden unexpected infant death. Home monitoring. Archives of Disease in Childhood 58: 469–471
Smith P C, Smith N T 1982 The special considerations of the premature infant. In: Steward D J (ed) Some Aspects of Paediatric Anaesthesia. Elsevier, Amsterdam
Speer M E, Blifeld C, Rudolph A S, Chadda P, Holbein M E B, Hittner H M 1984 Intraventricular hemorrhage and vitamin E in the very low-birth-weight infant: evidence for efficacy of early intramuscular vitamin E administration. Pediatrics 74: 1107–1112
Spielman F T, Seeds J W, Corke B C 1984 Anaesthesia for fetal surgery. Anaesthesia 39: 756–759
Steinschneider A, Weinstein S 1983 Sleep respiratory instability in term neonates under hyperthermic conditions — age, sex, type of feeding, and rapid eye movements. Pediatric Research 17: 35–41
Steinschneider A, Weinstein S L, Diamond E 1982 The sudden infant death syndrome and apnea/obstruction during neonatal sleep and feeding. Pediatrics 70: 858–863
Steward D J 1982 Preterm infants are more prone to complications following minor surgery than are term infants. Anesthesiology 56: 304–306
Sykes G S, Molloy P M, Johnson P, Stirral G M, Turnbull A C 1983 Fetal distress and the condition of newborn infants. British Medical Journal 287: 943–945
Thach B T, Frantz I D, Adler A M, Taeusch H W 1978 Maturation of reflexes influencing inspiratory duration in human infants. Journal of Applied Physiology 45: 203–211
Thorburn R J, Lipscombe A P, Stewart A L, Reynolds E O R, Hope P L, Pape K E 1981 Prediction of death and major handicap in very preterm infants by brain ultrasound. Lancet i: 1119–1121
Truog W E, Standaert T A, Murphy J H, Woodrum D E, Hodson W A 1984 Effects of prolonged high-frequency oscillatory ventilation in premature primates with experimental hyaline membrane disease. American Review of Respiratory Disease 130: 76–80
Vincent R N, Stark A R, Lang P, Close R H, Norwood W I, Casteneda A R et al 1984 Hemodynamic response to high-frequency ventilation in infants following cardiac surgery. Pediatrics 73: 426–430
Volpe J J 1981 Neonatal intraventricular hemorrhage. New England Journal of Medicine 304: 886–891
Walker D-J B, Feldman A, Vohr B R, Oh W 1984 Cost-benefit analysis of neonatal intensive care for infants weighing less than 1000 g at birth. Pediatrics 74: 20–25
Williamson W D, Desmond M M, Wilson G S, Murphy M A, Rozelle J, Carcia-Prats J A 1983 Survival of low-birth-weight infants with neonatal intraventricular hemorrhage. American Journal of Diseases of Children 137: 1181–1184
Wimberley P D, Lou H C, Pedersen J, Hejl M, Lassen N A, Friis-Hansen B 1982 Hypertensive peaks in the pathogenesis of intraventricular hemorrhage in the newborn. Abolition by phenobarbitone sedation. Acta Paediatrica Scandinavica 71: 537–542
Yelderman M, New W 1983 Evaluation of pulse oximetry. Anesthesiology 59: 349–352

14

C. F. Mackenzie

Advances in trauma emergency care

INTRODUCTION

Trauma kills more people under 14 years of age in the USA compared with the combined total who die as a result of heart disease, cancer, pneumonia, intestinal disease and meningitis (Cowley & Trump 1971). It is the leading cause of death in those under 38 years of age and it is the fourth commonest cause of death for the entire population (Chicago National Safety Council 1982). Trauma is responsible in economic costs (1982 dollars) for 6.9% of health care expenditures and 2.3% of the United States gross national product. Over 61 billion dollars was spent on trauma in fiscal 1982 of which 19.3 billion dollars were treatment related expenses and 41.7 billion dollars were forgone earnings (Munoz 1984). Fatalities cost over twice the amount of non fatalities. Advances in trauma emergency care are important, therefore, both from the medical and economic standpoint (Norman & Moles 1977). This review describes the concept of regional trauma care and outcome evaluation and prediction. Systematic approaches to the management of patients with massive blunt trauma are discussed and advances in emergency care that increase the likelihood of survival are identified.

REGIONAL TRAUMA CARE

Data from several trauma centres in the USA suggest that fatalities can be prevented by implementation of regional trauma systems (Boyd 1973, Cowley 1975, Gill et al 1976, West et al 1979, Lowe et al 1983, Cales 1984, Wright et al 1984). Potentially salvageable patients are more likely to die in centres where facilities for the treatment of trauma are inadequate (West et al 1979, Lowe et al 1983, Cales 1984, Wright et al 1984). In one study, 25% of the fatalities and 16% of the results in non-trauma centres were considered inappropriate for the severity of injury incurred (Lowe et al 1983). In addition, small hospitals (less than 200 beds) had a higher percentage of early deaths from trauma than large hospitals. The age of those dying and the injury severity scores were higher after implemtation of regional trauma centres (Cales 1984). There was an improvement in trauma care and death rate from motor vehicle accidents as demonstrated when a 24% drop in mortality was reported after an emergency care system was started in Jacksonville, Florida (Waters & Wells 1973). In several states and regions in the USA, graded echelon trauma care systems have been developed. The first of these was the Maryland emergency medical services graded echelon system established in 1973. The major elements of such trauma care systems are shown in Table 14.1. These requirements are described in full by the American College of Surgeons Committee on Trauma Care (American College of Surgeons 1976, 1979, 1980). The commitment of an area wide emergency medical service can best be described by one such as the Maryland Emergency Medical Services System which is outlined in Table 14.2 The expertise, facilities and cost of a level 1 trauma centre is summarized in Table 14.3. Further details of the patient population,

Table 14.1 Major elements of a graded-echelon trauma care system

Central emergency telephone number
Centralized dispatch of ambulances and helicopters
Rapid field stabilization and resuscitation
Paramedic triage with field hospital communication
Rapid transport with ongoing resuscitation to a designated hospital
Designation and grading of standard of specified receiving hospitals
Ongoing training programs for medical personnel and the public

Table 14.2 Maryland emergency medical services (EMS) system

Population	4.25 million (3.1 million > 18 years) 3 054 000 registered motor vehicles
Roads	26 631 miles of State roads including 362 miles of motorway
Traffic accidents	130 009 592 were disabling and 650 people died (1984)
Trauma centers	Level 1 (Shock Trauma) + four Level 2 in Baltimore City; in each of four other EMS regions in State, one Level 2 regional trauma center
Telecommunications	Posts in Baltimore City and each of 23 counties
Transport	Helicopters: 5 State Police, 2 State Park, 1 Army Ambulances: Local, State and City

Table 14.3 Shock trauma — Level 1 Trauma Centre, Baltimore City (73 beds attached to a 785 bed University Hospital; 24 hour consultant and junior staff in-house coverage)

	Consultants	Fellows
Surgeons	11	10
Anesthesia/critical care	9	5
Neurosurgeons	3	4
Medical	2	
Nurses	207	
Annual operating costs and salaries		$22.4 million
Field operations		$2.7 million

mortality (Mackenzie et al 1979, 1982, 1983, 1984) and respiratory management (Mackenzie et al 1981) are described elsewhere.

OUTCOME, EVALUATION AND PREDICTION

Assessment of injury is essential for the appropriate allocation of therapeutic resources, for evaluation of the patient's status, prediction of outcome and for comparison of trauma care delivery. Blunt non-penetrating trauma, resulting from high speed motor vehicle injuries, rapid deceleration, high velocity missiles or blast injuries may cause massive multisystem tissue disruption and has a less favourable outcome than penetrating trauma. Penetrating trauma, occuring from low velocity missiles such as knife and hand gun injuries, or falls resulting in isolated bony injuries, presents a specific, easily defined problem. Single organ injury frequently occurs and the comparatively little systemic disturbance that ensues often allows hospital discharge within a few days of injury. Several indices of injury are currently used to allow comparisons of the extent of, and outcome from, injury. These include the Glasgow Coma Scale (Teasdale & Jennett 1974), Injury Severity Score (Baker & O'Neill 1976), Anatomic Index (Champion et al 1980), Trauma Score (Champion et al 1983) and Acute Physiology and Chronic Health Evaluation Index (APACHE) (Knaus et al 1985). These indices make numerical descriptions of the overall severity of injury possible in patients who have received multiple injuries and physiological derangements. The Glasgow Coma Scale (GCS) is incorporated into many of the other indices and, although it has limitations, it is generally considered a good predictor of outcome from head injury. The Trauma Score, based on systolic blood pressure, respiratory rate, respiratory effort, capillary refill and the GCS was shown to be a good predictor of survival from blunt trauma. It is thought to be a useful mechanism for assessment of patient triage (decision on urgency of treatment) and to identify anomalous outcomes in the management of the patients with multiple sites of trauma. The Injury Severity Score excludes those patients dead on arrival and has successfully been used to compare outcome from trauma in different states and countries. Patients with injury severity scores in excess of 30 should receive specialized trauma care. However, the objections to Injury Severity Score are that ranking of severity is based on subjective impressions and it is correlated with outcome only in patients with low mortality. Combinations of moderately severe injuries may result in a higher score than a fatal head injury. The Anatomic Index was developed to eliminate these problems and correlated with outcome when mortality was in excess of 20% (Champion et al 1980). The Anatomic Index is most useful when assessing patients with blunt trauma and head injury such as may occur following motor vehicle injuries.

Twelve variables make up the APACHE 2 scoring system. The score and the acute risk of death rises on the basis of initial physiological abnormality, with chronic health problems at advanced age. Since trauma mortality and morbidity are functions of both injury severity and quality of medical care, survival rates and the quality of care in two facilities, systems or countries can only be compared when patient injury severity is controlled. These indices are, therefore, a major development in emergency trauma care that enable clinicians, epidemiologists and health service researchers to obtain objective evidence for allocation and evaluation of emergency medical services.

SYSTEMATIC APPROACH TO THE MANAGEMENT OF MASSIVE BLUNT TRAUMA

The patient subjected to massive trauma is difficult to assess when admitted to hospital or even at the scene of injury for often no history is obtainable and the patient may be unconscious, unresponsive or under the influence of alcohol or other drugs. No past medical history is available and since trauma is unique to each individual, the extent and the site of injuries in unknown when the patient is first seen. The traditional management approach of history taking, physical examination and establishment of a diagnosis before starting therapy are clearly inappropriate in the management of massive trauma. Systematic approaches with use of treatment protocols and alogarithms to determine management options are familiar to the military forces and are advantageous in the management of the severely injured patient. As a result of treatment protocols it is thought that time is not wasted by the trauma team, which consists of anaesthetists, surgeons and nurses in determining possible management plans. Communication between the medical and nursing personnel is simplified, because each member of the resuscitation team knows their role, and can function independently during the period immediately after injury or reception of the injured patient. The therapeutic and diagnostic approach to the patient must be coordinated if survival is to occur. Protocols provide a simple coordinated approach to patient management, greatly simplify training of staff, facilitate research by establishing a standardized data base, and allow for evaluation of the changes in the protocols by comparison with previous practices (Cowley & Dunham 1982a).

The major importance of these systematic approaches are that (1) priorities of management are identified and may be executed in an orderly fashion, (2) the likelihood of omission in examination, investigation or therapy, is reduced, and (3) treatment is not delayed until the diagnosis is complete but investigation and therapy occur simultaneously guided by protocol priorities. The following guidelines were developed at the Maryland Institute of Emergency Medicine (Shock Trauma) and have been annually updated and revised. Similar management protocols are used and advocated at other trauma centres (Hassett et al 1984) and they illustrate a protocol approach to management of massive blunt trauma that has reduced mortality from 25.4% in 1972 to 11.7% of admissions in 1984 (Fig. 14.1). Protocols may readily be developed into alogarithms with treatment/diagnosis options (Gill & Long 1979) that may be useful in less well equipped or staffed medical facilities and may also be computerized.

First priorities

1. Establish an airway and provide adequate ventilation with 100% oxygen. Auscultate the chest and confirm bilateral and equal breath sounds.
2. Control external haemorrhage with pressure. Order blood from blood bank, establish intravenous lines and begin volume infusion.

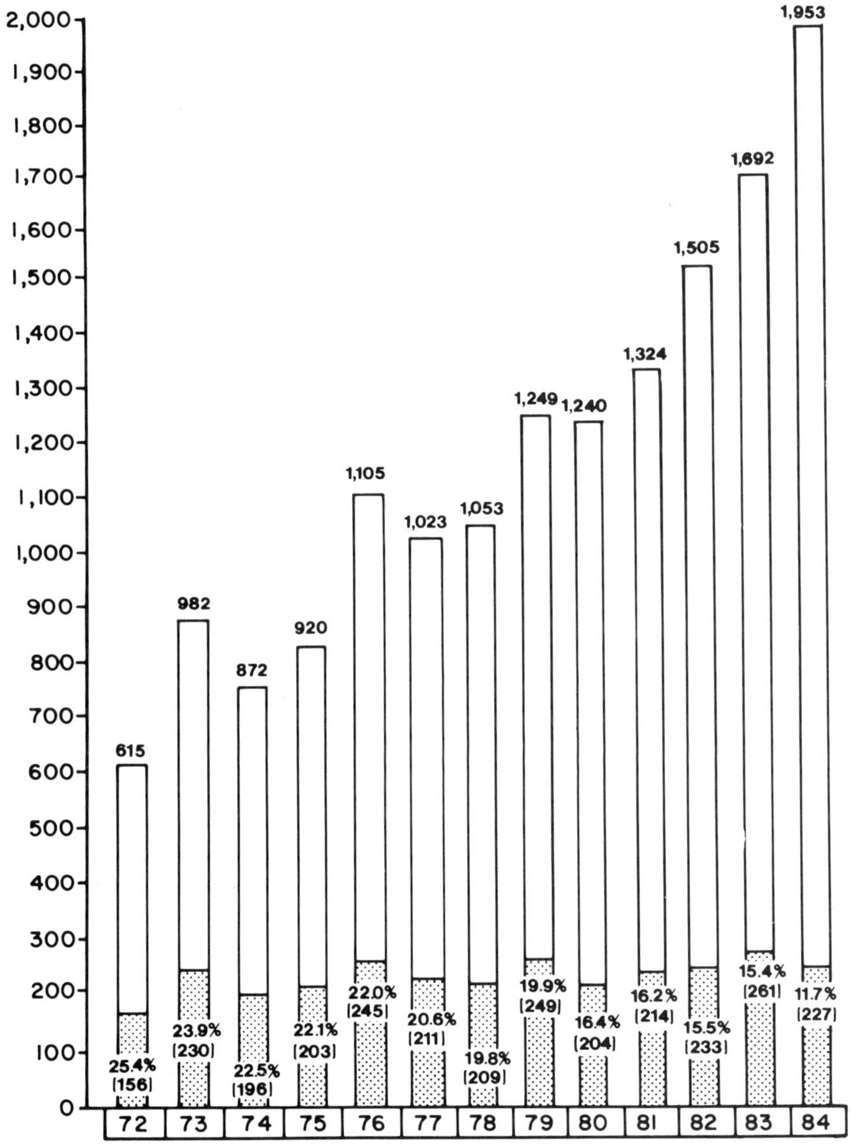

Fig 14.1 Number of patients admitted to the Maryland Institute for Emergency Medical Services (Shock Trauma) for fiscal years 1972–84. Mortality is shown as the dotted portion of the histogram. The percentage mortality varies from 25.4% to 11.7%. The number of patients this mortality represents is shown in brackets.

3. Two minute evaluation in which the central nervous system is examined (follows commands, speaks, moves all extremities, note extremity response to noxious stimuli, pupil size — equality and light reaction). Pulse and blood pressure are measured and an inspection of the naked patient (front and back) is rapidly carried out to identify the visible extent of trauma. The head, chest, abdomen, pelvis and extremities are briefly examined.

4. Baseline blood samples to include haemoglobin, haematocrit, white blood cell and platelet count, urea, electrolytes, glucose, creatinine, osmolality, lactate and a coagulation profile (PT, PTT, fibrinogen) are made on 70 ml of blood drawn on insertion of a central venous monitoring and infusion catheter. An arterial blood gas is obtained by percutaneous femoral artery sampling. Results are sent by computer and are available within 5–20 min depending on the investigation.
5. Monitor patient with ECG.
6. Pass nasogastric tube.

Second priorites

1. Emergency investigations.

X-ray. (a) All motor vehicle accident and major trauma victims receive a cervical spine X-ray to include C7. (b) Once spinal injury and fractures are excluded a true erect chest X-ray is taken with the patient sitting up. This identifies a haemo/pneumothorax; tracheal tube, nasogastric tube and central venous catheter placement; ruptured diaphragm, bony fractures and aortic rupture. Failure to identify the aortic arch or widening of the mediastinum on a true erect chest X-ray is an indication for an aortogram. (c) A pelvic X-ray is taken.

Peritoneal lavage. 1 litre of normal saline is infused by peritoneal dialysis catheter through a periumbilical incision while the patient is tilted head up and then head down (to detect a bleeding ruptured diaphragm or pelvic haematoma). The fluid is siphoned off, and the finding of frank blood or inability to read newsprint through the lavage tubing or bottle is a positive result, making exploratory laparotomy mandatory. More quantitative analysis of the lavage fluids, showing an erythrocyte count $> 100\,000$ mm^3 or leucocyte count greater > 500 mm^3, presence of gastrointestinal contents or an elevated amylase are also positive results (Cowley & Dunham 1982b).

Pass a urinary catheter and send urine sample for analysis of urine electrolytes, creatinine and test for blood, protein and glucose. Haematuria requires intravenous pyelography if the blood pressure is at least 70 mmHg systolic. A cystogram is performed when haematuria occurs with a major pelvic fracture.

2. Splint extremity fractures. Air inflatable or rigid splints may be used.
3. A brief and pertinent history is obtained when available.
4. An arterial catheter is inserted if indicated for blood pressure and sample monitoring.

Third priorities

1. Systematic examination includes the face and scalp, the extremities, the back as well as rectal, pelvic and perineal examinations.
2. Additonal systematic investigations may include specific X-rays, computerized tomographic (CT) scans and contrast studies, if indicated.
3. Speciality consultation is obtained from neurosurgeons, orthopaedic surgeons, urologists, etc.
4. A multidisciplinary discussion then takes place with the anaesthetist, surgeon, nurse and consultants' participation and subsequent management is determined.

Despite this approach to the management of trauma victims, mortality still ranges from 24–11.7% in trauma centres (Fischer et al 1984, Geritsen et al 1984) (see Fig. 14.1). In Maryland, State laws are very supportive of the Medical Examiners or Coroner's office and a high autopsy rate is mandatory by law. Of 2320 motor vehicle accident victims who were admitted to the Maryland Institute of Emergency Medicine in a four year period, 1703 came directly by helicopter from the scene of injury and 383 (22.4%) of the direct admissions died. Autopsies were performed on 366 (95.6%) of these deaths (Mackenzie et al 1982). If only the deaths occurring within 24 hours of a motor vehicle accident are considered, there was a 98.3% (300:305) autopsy rate (Mackenzie et al 1984). From these data the commonest cause of death within 24 hours of injury is craniocerebral trauma which accounted for 40.3% (123:305) of all deaths. Haemorrhage was the second commonest cause of death, accounting for 30.2% (92:305) of all deaths; and cervical spine injury was the third commonest cause of death, accounting for 12.5% (38:305) of all deaths. Unconsciousness on admission was the most sensitive indicator of a fatal prognosis. Management of head injured patients included tracheal intubation, mechanical hyperventilation, routine intracranial pressure monitoring, corticosteroids and for one of the four years, barbiturate therapy for persistent intracranial pressure greater than 25 mmHg (Mackenzie et al 1982). This latter barbiturate intervention did not alter death from head injury compared to prior years.

Despite multiple long bone, pelvic and other bony fractures fat embolus was extremely rare, the syndrome being detected in only one patient in 5 years of admissions. This may be related to early reduction of fractures with internal fixation of femurs (Riska et al 1980, Browner et al 1984) and use of external Hoffman type fixation of the tibial, humeral and pelvic fractures. These techniques allow early mobilization of the trauma victim and are thought to reduce post-operative pulmonary complications (Mackenzie et al 1981, Browner et al 1984).

Surgical intervention is carried out after resuscitation on admission, since operating conditions, because of oedema, haematoma and sepsis, are frequently less optimal 1 week or more later. Once again priorities are established, but all surgery is carried out in one session. This may mean that several teams of surgeons may operate simultaneously on the same patient. All surgical procedures are completed before the patient is transferred to the critical care unit having had all the general surgical, orthopaedic, neurosurgical and plastic surgery necessary for recovery. While this approach results in operating and anaesthesia times of 8–24 hours, it saves repeated subsequent visits for surgery and provides for optimum management on admission and may prevent the development of pulmonary complications, fat emboli and sepsis.

ADVANCES IN VENTILATION, INFUSION AND PUMPING

Advances in emergency trauma care that increase the chance of survival are discussed in the context of Weil & Shubin's (1969) VIP approach (ventilation, infusion, pumping) to the management of shock.

Airway ventilation

Advances in airway ventilation management are outlined in Table 14.4. The oesophageal obturator has been modified since its introduction including the design

Table 14.4 Advances in airway management

Esophageal obturator
Pharyngeo-tracheal lumen airway
Cricothyroidotomy
Jet ventilation

of an oesophageal gastric tube airway. However, it is still reported to be associated with oesophageal rupture, inadvertent tracheal intubation and inadequate CO_2 removal (Bryson et al 1978, Taryle et al 1979, Smith et al 1983). However, the obturator does protect the airway from aspiration of gastric contents and oxygenation is usually adequate. The obturator is, therefore, an improvement on simple oropharyngeal airways, although non anaesthesia personnel have difficulty with the mask fit. New mask designs include a 'jellyfish' mask (Respironics Corporation) which is reported to provide maximum tidal volume at two different lung compliances with minimum leak in comparison to two alternative mask designs, one having an inflatable cuff rim (Stewart et al 1984). The pharyngotracheal lumen (PTL) airway has a two tube, two cuff, system that is inserted blind and it functions as a tracheal tube if the trachea is entered or as an oesophageal obturator with oesophageal intubation. It protects against aspiration, gastric dilatation and inflation and provides similar oxygenation and CO_2 removal to mechanical ventilation through a conventional orotracheal tube (Niemann et al 1984). There are limited clinical data on the use of the PTL airway and conventional tracheal intubation is still the management of choice when the necessary expertise is available.

Cricothyroidotomy is an emergency surgical procedure that may be life saving and indicated with acute upper airway obstruction or when orotracheal intubation cannot be accomplished. A minitracheostomy kit facilitates the performance of a cricothyroidotomy (Portex). However, the long term morbidity from laryngeal granuloma is disturbing when these stoma are used for prolonged tracheal intubation. For this reason a cricothyroidotomy should be converted to a translaryngeal or tracheostomy intubation as soon as possible once the initial airway emergency is overcome. Cannulae passed through the cricothyroid membrane may be used for O_2 insufflation or for ventilation by means of a jet device that interrupts the 3.3 kPa (50 psi) oxygen pressure source intermittently (Sanders 1967). Oxygen insufflation with as little as 1 l/min may maintain O_2 levels for 10–30 min whereas the jet ventilator also removes CO_2 (similar to the technique of ventilation during shared airway endoscopy procedures). The jet ventilator can provide adequate oxygenation and ventilation in animals in shock with an open thorax and aortic cross clamp (Jorden et al 1984) and in humans in the presence of large airway leaks (Turnbull et al 1981). The cricothyroid membrane puncture may also be used to facilitate orotracheal intubation and avoid tracheostomy by passage of a guide wire in a retrograde manner through the larynx and out of the mouth. An orotracheal tube is then directed into the larynx down the guide wire which is removed when the tube enters the trachea. A long Intracath substitutes for a guide wire if this is not available.

Infusion

Advances in infusion techniques relate to the rapidity and type of fluid replacement. Two new techniques can greatly increase the infusion of intravenous (i.v.) fluids based on Poiseuilles law. Large bore intravenous tubing (5.0 mm ID compared to standard 3.2 mm ID) in conjunction with a 10 French (Fr) gauge short i.v. catheter or 8 Fr pulmonary artery catheter introducer enabled infusions of 1200–1400 ml/min of crystalloid or whole blood to be made (Millikan et al 1984). The ability to replace fluids rapidly is frequently the limiting factor in survival of trauma patients. Multiple i.v. sites may hinder movement around the patient, although multiple i.v. sites above and below the diaphragm on the right and left sides of the patient are also advocated. Multiple i.v. sites ensure circulatory volume replacement and avoid expansion of an undetected extravascular haematoma that may have occurred as a result of vessel rupture. Iserson & Reeter (1984) developed a reservoir that allows up to five individual infusion bags to be run simultaneously. They feed through a single large diameter tube to a 4.5 mm ID catheter which provides a maximum of 650 ml/min gravity flow and a pressurized flow of more than 1600 ml/min.

The delay while awaiting for cross matching of blood in the bleeding patient who cannot be adequately resuscitated with crystalloid or colloid infusion may result in exsanguination. Type O blood can be transfused without fear of major incompatability reactions; however the red cell does contain antibodies than cause minor transfusion reactions (Gervin & Fischer 1984). To avoid Rh sensitization in Rh negative patients low titre O blood with no Rh antigen may be used. This blood is extemely scarce and when O Rh positive packed cells were transfused no haemolytic transfusion reactions occurred. Absence of reactions was found even though 170 of the 343 patients transfused with 1945 units of group O Rh positive blood during a 22 month period were of blood groups other than O. However, of the 47 Rh negative patients 36 developed anti-Rh (D) antibody (Sohmer et al 1979). Resuscitation of trauma patients with type specific uncrossmatched blood also resulted in lack of transfusion reactions. Subsequent major crossmatch failed to identify either blood incompatibility or significant antibodies in 236 patients who received 1141 units of blood in a 3 year period (Gervin & Fischer 1984).

Pumping

Whether or not pneumatic trousers are beneficial in the prehospital management of hypovolaemic shock remains controversial. Several authors have found no increase in cardiac filling pressures with application of military anti-shock trousers (MAST) and in one controlled study of their field use there was no significant improvement in blood pressure, mortality or trauma score in patients who had MAST (Bukell et al 1984). There was no demonstrable benefit of MAST in patients with cardiac arrest (Mackersie et al 1984) although others report increased survival (Mahoney & Murick 1983). Further prospective randomized studies are required to establish the usefulness of external counterpressure.

After remaining unchanged for 20 years, cardiopulmonary resuscitation (CPR) techniques have undergone recent major changes. The new era of research into CPR began with the suggestion that alterations in pleural pressure and not direct cardiac compression are the cause of blood flow during CPR (Criley et al 1976, Chandra et al 1981, Weisfeldt 1983). Elevations in pleural pressure are transmitted to all the chambers of the heart and vascular structures in the chest. Because of the unique valvular arrangements in the heart that only permits forward flow and because there are competent venous valves at the thoracic inlet and the pulmonary valve remains closed, changes in pleural pressure are transmitted to the extra thoracic arteries resulting in forward flow of blood. In most adults during CPR, chest compression results in a pressure gradient between arteries and veins outside the thorax, due to the pleural pressure elevations transmitted to the heart. Children with compliant chest walls or thin adults may be exceptions (Rogers 1985).

Pleural pressure may be elevated to obtain maximum cardiac output by synchronizing chest compression and ventilation during CPR (Chandra et al 1981, Weisfeldt 1983). However, simultaneous compression and ventilation or 'new' CPR results in higher intracranial pressures than seen with conventional CPR. Although carotid blood flow increases, the benefit, in terms of cerebral perfusion pressure (mean arterial - mean intracranial pressure) with simultaneous chest compression and ventilation (SCV–CPR) is not as great as was initially hoped. However, cerebral perfusion pressure is still increased in comparison to conventional CPR. Use of an abdominal binder or simultaneous abdominal compression further augments the pleural pressure changes and carotid blood flow during SCV–CPR (Chandra et al 1981).

Pharmacological intervention following cardiac arrest has also changed. Cerebral perfusion may be improved by increasing resistance in extracerebral vessels with α agonist drugs such as adrenaline in high doses (Michael et al 1984). Since there are not thought to be α adrenergic receptors active in the cerebral vessels, blood flow is diverted to the cerebral circulation. Other α agonists may also be useful and are presently being investigated (Rogers 1985). Calcium entry blocking drugs such as nimodipine (Steen et al 1985), lidoflazine and verapamil (Vaagnes et al 1984) improve outcome following cardiac arrest, possibly by preventing vascular smooth muscle vasospasm resulting in improved post-ischaemic cerebral blood flow. Recent data implicate the calcium ion as a triggering element in a number of adverse reactions in a wide variety of tissues after shock, sepsis, trauma and anoxia. Reports have also linked ionic calcium shifts to abnormalities in cellular metabolism, intracellular release of free fatty acids, and production of oxidative free radicals. Calcium and the prostaglandins are also involved in the non-reflow phenomenon that occurs with cerebral vascular constriction after cardiac arrest. All of these factors are implicated in neuronal injury after ischaemic anoxia and the use of calcium blockers and other pharmacological agents in post-resuscitation brain injury clearly requires further investigation (White et al 1983, Shapiro 1985). While outcome from ventricular fibrillation cardiac arrest is quite favourable, much improvement is required in asystolic cardiac arrest. The ability to improve myocardial perfusion during resuscitation may be crucial in determining a successful outcome. It seems likely in the future that not one but several CPR techniques will be used to resuscitate patients depending on the cause and type of cardiac arrest. To prevent neurological disability calcium channel blockers may be used alone or in combination with other agents such as indomethacin, barbiturates, free radial scavengers (White et al 1983) and α agonists (Michael et al 1984).

REFERENCES

American College of Surgeons 1976 Optimal hospital resources for care of the seriously injured. Bulletin ACS 61(9): 15–22
American College of Surgeons Committee on Trauma. 1979 Hospital resources for optimal care of the injured patient. Bulletin ACS 64(8): 43–48
American College of Surgeons Committee on Trauma Care 1980 Appendix A, C1, C2, D, E, F. Bulletin ACS 65(2): 9–35
Baker S P, O'Neill B 1976 The injury severity score: an update. Journal of Trauma 16: 882–885
Boyd D R 1973 A symposium on the Illinois trauma program. A systems approach to the care of the critically injured. Journal of Trauma 12: 275–276
Browner B D, Burgess A R, Robertson R J et al 1984 Immediate closed antegrade Ender nailing of femoral fractures in polytrauma patients. Journal of Trauma 24: 921–927
Bryson T K, Benumof J F, Ward C F 1978 The esophageal obturator airway: a clinical comparison to ventilation with a mask and oropharyngeal airway. Chest 74: 537–539
Bukell W H, Pepe P L, Applebaum D J et al 1984 Effect of antishock trousers on the trauma score. A prospective analysis (abstract). Annals of Emergency Medicine 12: 402
Cales R H 1984 Trauma mortality in Orange County: the effect of implementation of a regional trauma system. Annals of Emergency Medicine 13: 1–10
Champion H R, Sacco W J, Lepper R C et al 1980 An anatomic index of injury severity. Journal of Trauma 20: 197–202
Champion H R, Sacco W J, Hunt T R 1983 Trauma severity scoring to predict mortality. World Journal of Surgery 7: 4–11
Chandra N, Weisfeldt M L, Tschik J et al 1981 Agumentation of carotid flow during CPR by ventilation at high airway pressure simultaneous with chest compression. American Journal of Cardiology 48: 1053–1063
Chicago National Safety Council 1982 Accident facts
Cowley R A 1975 Total emergency medical system for State of Maryland. Maryland State Medical Journal 24: 37–45
Cowley R A, Dunham C M (eds) 1982a Shock trauma/ critical care manual. University Park Press, Baltimore, p XII
Cowley R A, Dunham C M (eds) 1982b Shock trauma/critical care manual. University Park Press, Baltimore, p146
Cowley R A, Trump B 1971 Todays neglected disease — trauma. Bull. University Maryland School of Medicine 56: 19–25
Criley J M, Blarfuss A H, Kissel G L 1976 Cough-induced cardiac compression. Journal of the American Medical Association 236: 1246–1250
Fischer R P, Flynn T C, Miller P W 1984 Urban helicopter response to the scene of injury. Journal of Trauma 24: 946–951
Geritsen S M, Loenhoul T Van, Gunbrere J S F 1984 Prognostic signs and mortality in multiply injured patients. Injury 14: 89–92
Gervin A S, Fischer R P 1984 Resuscitation of trauma patients with type specific uncrossmatched blood. Journal of Trauma 24: 327–331
Gill W, Champion H R, Long W B et al 1976 A clinical experience of multiple trauma in Maryland. Maryland State Medical Journal 25: 55–58
Gill W B, Long W B 1979 Shock trauma manual. William and Wilkins, Baltimore
Hassett J, LaDuca J, Seibel R, Border J R 1984 Priorities in multiple injuries: a brief review. Injury 14: 12–16
Iserson K V, Reeter A K 1984 Rapid fluid replacement. A new methodology. Annals of Emergency Medicine 12: 97–100
Jorden R C, Moore E E, Marx J A et al 1984 Percutaneous transtracheal ventilation in a canine shock model with an open thorax. Annals of Emergency Medicine 13: 22–25
Knaus W A, Draper E A, Wagner D P et al 1985 APACHE II — A severity of disease classification system. Critical Care Medicine 13: 818–829
Lowe D K, Gatley H L, Goss J R et al 1983 Patterns of death, complication and error in the management of motor vehicle accident victims. Implication for a regional system of trauma care. Journal of Trauma 23: 503–509
Mackenzie C F 1981 History and literature review of chest physiotherapy, chest physiotherapy program, patient population and respiratory care at MEIMSS. In: Mackenzie C F (ed) Chest physiotherapy in the intensive care unit. Williams and Wilkins, Baltimore, ch 1, p 1–26
Mackenzie C F, Shin B, Fisher R et al 1979 Two year mortality in 760 helicopter transported patients direct from the road accident scene. American Surgeon 45: 101–108

Mackenzie C F, Shin B, Fisher R et al 1982 Four year mortality of trauma victims admitted directly from the accident by helicopter. Anesthesiology 57: A96
Mackenzie C F, Shin B, Fisher R et al 1983 Transports des accidentes de la voie publique (vehicules a moteur): mortalite pour 1703 primaries en 4 ans. Convergences Medicales 2: 427–431
Mackenzie C F, Shin B, Sodestrom C et al 1984 Would field deployment of physicians reduce deaths within 24 hours of road traffic accidents. Anesthesiology 61: A93
Mackersie R C, Christensen J M, Lewis F R 1984 The pre hospital use of external counter pressure. Does MAST make a difference? Journal of Trauma 24: 882–888
Mahoney B D, Murick M J 1983 Pneumatic trousers in refractory prehospital cardiopulmonary arrest. Annals of Emergency Medicine 12: 8–12
Michael J R, Gueria A D, Koehler R C et al 1984 Mechanisms whereby epinephrine augments cerebral and myocardial perfusion during cardiopulmonary resuscitation in dogs. Circulation 69: 822–835
Millikan J S, Cam T L, Hansborough J 1984 Rapid volume replacement for hypovolemic shock. A comparison of techniques and equipment. Journal of Trauma 24: 428–431
Munoz E 1984 Economic cost of trauma, United States, 1982. Journal of Trauma 24: 237–244
Neimann J T, Rosborough J P, Myers R A M et al 1984 The pharyngeotracheal lumen airway: preliminary investigation of a new adjunct. Annals of Emergency Medicine 13: 591–596
Norman J, Moles M 1977 Trauma and immediate care: editorial. British Journal of Anaesthesia 49: 641–642
Riska E B, Bonsdorff H von, Hakkinen S et al 1980 Prevention of fat embolism by early internal fixation of fractures in patients with multiple injuries. Injury 8: 110–116
Rogers M C 1985 Cardiopulmonary resuscitation — present and future. IARS Review Course Lectures. Presented at the 159th International Anesthesia Research Society Congress, Houston Texas, 10–13 March, p 124–126
Sanders R D 1967 Two ventilating attachments for bronchoscopes. Delaware Medical Journal 39: 170–175
Shapiro H M 1985 Post cardiac arrest therapy: calcium entry blockade and brain resuscitation. Anesthesiology 62: 384–387
Smith J P, Bodai B I, Seifkin A et al 1983 The esophageal obturator airway. A review. Journal of the American Medical Association 250: 1081–1084
Sohmer P R, Etter M, Shin B et al 1979 Rh sensitization subsequent to transfusion with uncrossmatched Rh positive packed red cells (abstract). Critical Care Medicine 7: 144
Steen P A, Giswold S E, Milde J H et al 1985 Nimodipine improves outcome when given after complete cerebral ischemia in primates. Anesthesiology 62: 406–414
Stewart R D, Kaplan R, Thompson F et al 1984 Influence of mask design on bag-mask ventilation (abstract). Annals of Emergency Medicine 13: 404
Taryle D A, Chandler J E, Good J T et al 1979 Emergency room intubations. Complication and survival. Chest 75: 541–543
Teasdale G, Jennett B 1974 Assessment of coma and impaired consciousness. Lancet ii: 81–84
Turnbull A D, Carlon G, Howland W S et al 1981 High frequency jet ventilation in major airway or pulmonary disruption. Annals of Thoracic Surgery 32: 468–474
Vaagnes P, Cantadore R, Safar P et al 1984 The effect of lidoflazine and verapamil on neurologic outcome after 10 minutes ventricular fibrillation cardiac arrest in dogs (abstract). Critical Care Medicine 12: 228
Waters J M, Wells C H 1973 The effects of a modern emergency medical care system in reducing automobile crash deaths. Journal of Trauma 13: 645–647
Weil M H, Shubin H 1969 The 'VIP' approach to the bedside management of shock. Journal of the American Medical Association 207: 337–340
Weisfeldt M L 1983 Augmentation of cerebral perfusion by simultaneous chest compression and lung inflation with abdominal binding following cardiac arrest in dogs. Circulation 67: 266–275
West J G, Trunkey D D, Lim R C 1979 System of trauma care. A study of two counties. Archives of Surgery 114: 455–460
White B C, Windegar C D, Wilson R F et al 1983 Possible role of calcium blockers in cerebral resuscitation: a review of the literature and synthesis for future studies. Critical Care Medicine 11: 202–207
Wright C S, McMurty R Y, Pickard J 1984 A postmortem review of trauma mortalities — a comparative study. Journal of Trauma 24: 67–68

15

R. A. Green

Medico-legal aspects of anaesthesia

INTRODUCTION

When the author began in anaesthetic practice over three decades ago, an unexpected death or misadventure which occurred during anaesthesia and surgery was viewed by the patient's family and by the public at large as a tragic event which was often unavoidable and one of the accepted risks of surgery. 'Doctors are only human and are doing their best', was a common reaction to unfortunate events.

At the present time the attitude of the general public has altered in that not only do they expect a first class medical service but also in the event of a complication arising, they are entitled to compensation. There is no shortage of skilled lawyers available to facilitate the process of litigation for negligence while doctors are often called upon to testify against their colleagues. It is not suggested that gross carelessness or lack of knowledge does not occasionally lead to damage, nor that under such circumstances the patient should not receive adequate compensation, but the majority of anaesthetic mishaps although often avoidable are due to normal human error or lack of judgement rather than negligence. Considering the calculated risks anaesthetists have to take every day, the number of serious mishaps which do occur are remarkably few. Even so, every mishap is one too many and continuing efforts must be made to reduce the incidence of such events by improving the supervision and training of anaesthetists and the quality of equipment.

The changing public attitude to medical mishaps is clearly unpleasant and may eventually have some damaging effect on medical care, in that the doctor is forced into defensive medicine. There is evidence that this has already happened in some countries, but in the UK there has been little development in that direction so far. It is believed that some benefit has accrued from the increase in public scrutiny. We seem to be more aware of the weaknesses in our professional standards and more willing to learn from our own and our colleagues mistakes, thus improving our overall standard of care.

This chapter presents a study of the anaesthetic mishaps which have occured over the last 10 years and which have been reported to The Medical Protection Society (MPS). This study should highlight the nature and magnitude of the problem and suggest possible ways of reducing the incidence of mishaps and of mitigating the difficulties involved in dealing with claims for damages when they occur.

It is probably fair to say that the anaesthetist more than any other medical practitioner is, during his active professional life, in a position where a lapse of concentration, error of technique or lack of knowledge can have sudden and devastating consequences. It is these more serious consequences of error to which attention will be paid but it must be remembered that anaesthetists are often assessed by their ability to avoid minor injuries such as broken teeth, sore throat, muscle pains and bruising at injection sites. The patient judges our skills by our ability to prevent minor insults rather than our professional knowledge and expertise. Similarly the surgeon is often judged by the neatness of his scar rather than his technical dexterity within the abdomen.

STUDIES OF ANAESTHETIC MISHAPS

Studies of anaesthetic mishaps are often difficult and incomplete, as collecting information depends upon the cooperation of so many professional people. Since 1949 the Association of Anaesthetists has attempted to acquire accurate information on the causes of mortality for anaesthesia on a number of occasions. The first of these was published by Edwards et al (1956). This study surveyed 1000 deaths and found that aspiration of vomit was the major cause of death. Dinnick (1964) reported on a further 600 cases and observed that the major cause of death was hypovolaemia. Following the publication of the first report and the widespread attention drawn to it the incidence of aspiration of vomit has declined. In 1982 the results of a further study on mortality related to anaesthesia were published and it was noted that aspiration of vomit and hypotension resulted in 30% of the deaths (Lunn & Mushin 1982).

A further study by the Association of Anaesthetists and the Association of Surgeons have recently been set up to assess morbidity and mortality in relation to surgical procedures. Bearing in mind the potential seriousness of anaesthetic mishaps it is fortunate that such events are relatively infrequent. In a study set up in New South Wales (1959) and covering a period of 20 years, a mortality rate of 1:30 000 anaesthetics administered was reported. In the 1982 study edited by Lunn & Mushin, a death rate of 1:10 000 directly attributable to anaesthesia was reported but this study included deaths up to 6 days after operation. Both studies indicated the expected mortality rate from anaesthesia but did not attempt to give any indication of anaesthetic morbidity. Serious complications such as brain damage and major peripheral nerve damage were excluded as were the minor hazards associated with anaesthesia. Information on the incidence of major anaesthetic mishaps is difficult to collect, including those which might have resulted in death (near miss). It is relatively easy, however, to acquire data on those cases in which a suit for damages has been filed. As a member of the Council of the Medical Protection Society the author has been able to review such cases which have been considered by the Society during the last 10 years. It is from this source that the problems involved will be discussed. The figures presented do not in any way represent the overall incidence of anaesthetic complications but they do give some insight into the number of claims made against anaesthetists who are members of the Medical Protection Society and outlines the nature of the mishaps which are encountered.

Figure 15.1 shows a steady increase in the number of claims made against anaesthetists from the period 1974–83. The reason for this increase is complex but for the most part must represent a trend towards more litigation rather than a deterioration in anaesthetic standards or an increase in the number of anaesthetists who are members of the Society. Whatever the cause, it is certain that these mishaps lead to intense suffering for patients and their relatives while the anaesthetist also suffers considerable psychological trauma.

In a recent study in the USA, Sollazzi & Ward (1984) recorded a ratio of suicide or attempted suicides of one in every 45 anaesthetists who were sued for negligence. The claims also represent a greatly increasing financial burden on our medical protection societies. It is thus of paramount importance that an attempt should be made to reduce the incidence of errors by improvements in technique and monitoring as well as being aware of possible hazards that have already been alluded to in the anaesthetic literature.

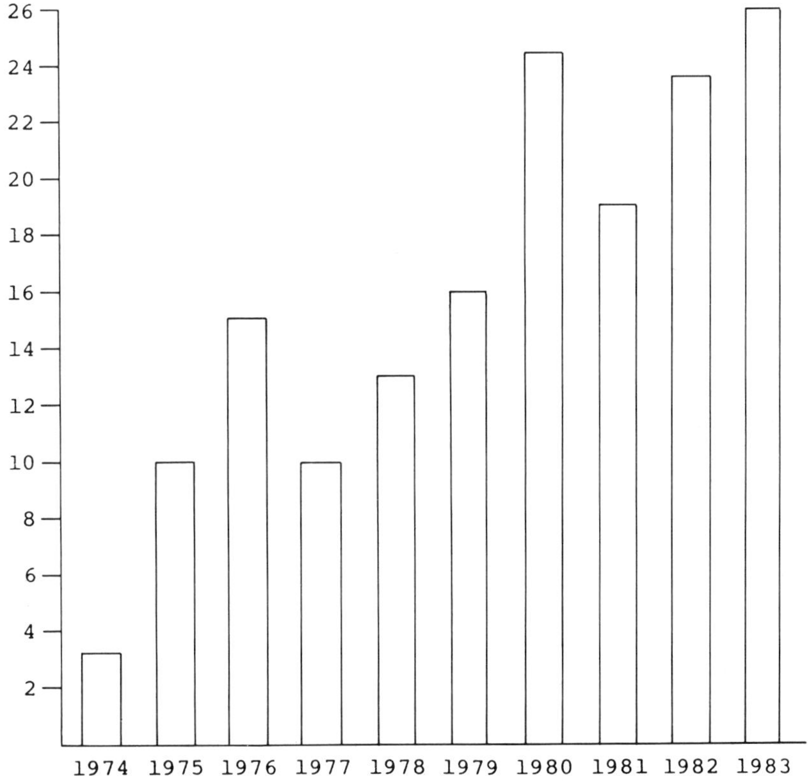

Fig. 15.1 Number of claims made against anaesthetists 1974–83.

MAJOR ANAESTHETIC MISHAPS

Table 15.1 represents the primary cause of mishaps during anaesthesia or in the recovery period and which leads to death or serious neurological damage.

Table 15.1 Primary causes of mishaps resulting from anaesthesia leading to death or serious neurological damage

Cause of mishap	Number of cases	Percentage of major mishaps
Respiratory obstruction	19	18.6
8 Recovery room		
11 Theatre		
Respiratory insufficiency	12	11.9
9 Recovery room		
Oesophageal intubation	12	11.9
Aspiration of vomit	8	7.8
Disconnection of apparatus	5	4.9
Difficult intubation	3	2.9
Endobronchial intubation	1	1.0
Transposition of gases	1	1.0
Hypotension	9	8.8
4 Hypotensive anaesthesia		
3 Regional anaesthesia		
2 Anterior spinal artery syndrome		
Hypovolaemia	5	4.9
Halothane jaundice	4	3.9
Malignant hyperpyrexia	3	2.9
Equipment failure	4	3.9
Myocardial infarct	5	4.9
Anaphylaxis	1	1.0
Dental surgery anaesthesia	7	6.8
5 Operator anaesthetist		
2 Independent anaesthetist		
Unknown cause	3	
Total	102	

Respiratory obstruction

Respiratory obstruction was the commonest cause of a major catastrophe during the 10 year period under review and accounted for 18.6% of all major claims. Slightly less than 50% of these episodes occurred in the recovery period when the patients were being supervised by nursing staff (see below). The remainder occured immediately after induction or during the course of the operation. Two cases, which resulted in severe brain damage, were due to severe bronchospasm, and may be said to have been unavoidable but all the others were almost certainly avoidable and could have been prevented if constant vigilance had been exercised by the anaesthetist. In four of these cases the patient had been left unattended by the anaesthetist when the incident occurred, a situation which is certainly negligent and may even be regarded as criminally negligent by some courts. Recently, a judge pronounced that such cases might in the future carry a verdict of manslaughter and many anaesthetists would accept this view.

The tragedies resulting from patients being left unattended poses the problem of delegation of patient care during the course of operation. Is there any justification for leaving a nurse or an ODA in charge of an anaesthetized patient while the anaesthetist is called upon to attend to other possible problems outside the operating theatre. The answer must be an emphatic negative and there is little doubt that the courts would take the same view unless the anaesthetist could prove convincingly that his absence from the theatre was necessary to save another life. Often the anaesthetist is summoned from the operating theatre to take or make an 'urgent' telephone call. Anaesthetists often work singlehanded, are frequently called upon to assist with emergencies elsewhere and may be under considerable pressure to leave the patient in the care of untrained staff. The author recommends that all anaesthetic trolleys should be equipped with a telephone or that during prolonged surgery the anaesthetist should have an assistant trained in anaesthesia.

Respiratory depression

It is often difficult from the reports available to distinguish between events which are due to unrecognized and untreated respiratory depression or obstruction. Where there was clear evidence of untreated drug excess or failure to adequately reverse muscle relaxants, the cases were classified as due to respiratory insufficiency (see Table 15.1).

Twelve such cases leading to severe brain damage were reported to the Society. In nine of these, cardiac arrest occurred during the recovery period, whilst the patient was in the charge of nursing staff. In every case death or brain damage was clearly avoidable. In many instances there was clear evidence that the anaesthetist delegated the care of a patient who was still in an unsafe condition to nursing staff who were inadequately trained to recognize respiratory problems. In addition there was a failure in some of the cases to give specific instructions as to the degree of supervision required when the patient was still under the influence of respiratory depressant drugs.

Disconnection of apparatus

Unfortunately, by modern technical standards, much of the anaesthetic equipment in constant use in our hospitals falls below acceptable safety standards. For example, methods used for connecting patients to ventilating circuits are unstable and frequently fall apart. Constant vigilance by the anaesthetist in charge should of course avoid a tragedy from this cause but such tragedies do still occur. Five such cases were reported to the Society in the 10 year period under review. In one case the anaesthetist was known to have been absent from the theatre at the time of the event while in another the anaesthetist, who had no trained assistant, was setting up a CVP line in an emergency when the disconnection occurred and was undetected.

There is little excuse for failing to fit airway pressure alarms on all ventilator circuits, but this is still not the routine practice in the UK. These devices are readily available and reasonably reliable and should therefore be considered standard equipment. Their use would certainly reduce the incidence of unrecognized disconnections but cannot and should not replace constant vigilance by the anaesthetist.

Intubation problems

Problems in performing tracheal intubation was the second commonest cause of mortality or serious morbidity during anaesthesia in this series, accounting for 15% of all major claims. Although intubation problems will occur from time to time during anaesthesia and failure to intubate successfully may be unavoidable, it is seldom possible to defend any case where a patient dies or suffers brain damage as a direct result of unsuccessful tracheal intubation. It is only in the most exceptional case that a competent anaesthetist will be unable to maintain adequate oxygenation with a mask during attempts at intubation.

Oesophageal intubation

A discussion of the hazards of oesophageal intubation with most anaesthetists produces a fairly standard answer — 'it commonly occurs but it is easy to recognize and should never be missed'. Is this always the case? Howells & Reithmuller (1982) described a case in which great difficulty was experienced in recognizing the mistake and the author has on record from MPS files 12 cases of oesophageal intubation in which cardiac arrest or brain damage occurred before the error was recognized. Five of these cases were in dark skinned patients in whom cyanosis was less readily detectable. In three of these cases more than one experienced anaesthetist confirmed the presence of tracheal intubation before cardiac arrest intervened and the tube was subsequently found to be in the oesophagus. In all cases clear respiratory sounds were said to be present on auscultation. The implication of these reports is that even a conscientious and careful anaesthetist may be unable to distinguish between a tracheal and oesophageal intubation by the commonly employed methods. It is possible that monitoring the end expired carbon dioxide is the only certain way of providing a clear differential diagnosis.

We can learn three things from these observations.

1. We cannot rely upon auscultation of the chest and epigastrium to make the correct diagnosis.
2. If there is a failure to maintain oxygenation immediately after attempted tracheal intubation, then oesophageal intubation must be suspected, the tube withdrawn and the patient ventilated with a mask. Only in the event of a firm diagnosis of some other cause for cyanosis should artificial respiration be continued through the tube. If intubation has been difficult, then the tube may be kept in situ and lung inflation achieved with a mask placed over the tube.
3. Special care must be taken with dark skinned patients.

Unsuccessful intubation

Difficult or impossible intubation will occur from time to time and no anaesthetist should be criticized for failing to intubate a patient but failure to maintain adequate oxygenation of the patient during attempts at intubation cannot be defended. In this series there were three such cases leading to cardiac arrest or severe brain damage. In none of them was difficulty anticipated as a result of the pre-operative history. In each case many attempts at intubation were made using repeated doses of suxamethonium accompanied by periods of hypoxaemia.

These rare tragedies could have been avoided if the anaesthetist had abandoned his endeavours after the second or third attempt. There are few operations which cannot be carried out without intubation or postponed until alternative procedures have been considered. Even emergency caesarian section or laparotomy can be performed more safely under general anaesthetia using a face mask and oesophageal tube rather than exposing the patient to considerably greater risk of repeated attempts at intubation.

Aspiration of vomit

Regurgitation with the inhalation of gastric contents can occur at any time during anaesthesia but death or brain damage from this cause is commonest during late pregnancy. Eight cases were reported to the Society during the period 1973–84, seven of which occurred during the induction of anaesthesia for operative obstetrics. In four of these cases both cricoid pressure and an adequate antacid therapy were reported as having been used. In the other four cases either cricoid pressure was not used or it was not reported as having been used. Since the introduction of cricoid pressure by Sellick (1961) the incidence of this complication has undoubtedly decreased, but despite these precautions, regurgitation and inhalation does still occur. This may well be due to the unwelcome fact that obstetric anaesthesia is still being administered by junior anaesthetists without adequate supervision. It would seem that an improvement in our anaesthetic technique for these vulnerable patients is still necessary (Green 1978).

Hypotension

Uncontrolled drug induced hypotension accounted for nearly 9% of the cases reported to the Society. Four were associated with controlled hypotensive anaesthesia. These cases have caused particular concern as all the patients were undergoing cosmetic surgery in which the degree of hypotension used was not considered to be essential for the success of the operation. The other four cases followed epidural or spinal anaesthesia. In two of these cases the regional anaesthesia resulted in permanent paralysis from anterior spinal artery thrombosis and two were maternity cases which suffered cardiac arrest following epidural anaesthesia for delivery (one vaginal delivery and the other for caesarean section).

OBSTETRIC ANAESTHESIA

It is not the intention in this chapter to single out any particular subspeciality of anaesthesia for discussion, but obstetric anaesthesia does merit our special attention for two reasons. The first is that it represents 12% of all anaesthetic related claims reported and secondly because the anaesthetist has dual responsibility for mother and child. Errors in technique and adverse reactions involving the mother can adversely affect the baby.

Five claims were for minor injury such as retained epidural catheters, post-spinal headache and awareness. The remaining 15 were either death or severe brain damage. Two of the major tragedies involved epidural anaesthesia, but the remaining 13 resulted from difficult intubation, oesophageal intubation or chemical pneumonitis as the result of inhaled gastric contents. The significance of these hazards during general anaesthesia in the obstetric patient has been emphasized in the confidential report into maternal deaths in the UK (1979). During 1976–79 there were 30 maternal deaths due directly to the administration of anaesthesia in pregnancy (17.2

deaths per million pregnancies). Eleven of these patients died as the direct result of inhalation of gastric contents and 16 from the complications associated with intubation. These figures are disturbing and have led to a considerable increase in the number of operative deliveries performed under epidural anaesthesia in the last 5 years. It remains to be seen whether this move towards regional rather than general anaesthesia reduces the hazards of operative obstetrics (Green & Taylor 1982).

Experience of claims against anaesthetists for episodes which occurred during general anaesthesia for operative obstetrics reinforce the importance of ensuring that a senior anaesthetist, experienced in obstetric anaesthesia, with a competent assistant, is always available for these patients. The recent trend to resort to epidural or spinal anaesthesia for operative obstetrics may reduce some of the hazards inherent in general anaesthesia but epidural anaesthesia for caesarean section may also introduce hazards such as hypotension and is not a technique to be delegated solely to junior anaesthetic staff.

MINOR ANAESTHETIC MISHAPS

The esteem of individual anaesthetists and the speciality in general is seldom judged by the occurrence of errors leading to a major catastrophe which are fortunately rare. Reputation is judged by the frequency of minor damage, such as bruises, cut lips, sore throats, corneal abrasions and muscle pains. Only a very small number of these minor injuries lead to claims for damages but nevertheless they result in considerable discomfort to patients. These comparatively minor mishaps can be avoided by the use of meticulous care and technique.

Dental damage

Damage to teeth and crowns represent by far the commonest minor injury leading to claims against the anaesthetist. Twenty-six claims for dental damage were reported (Table 15.2). This is a gross underestimate of the numbers that have occurred as many of these claims are considered without reference to the medical committee of the MPS and are not included in this series. The majority of these claims cannot be defended as it appears that the anaesthetists were unaware of the presence of crowns

Table 15.2 Minor claims against anaesthetists 1974–83

Cause of claim	Number of cases	Percentage of all claims
Dental damage	26	16.6
Peripheral nerve injury	9	5.8
Awareness	6	3.8
Extra vascular injection	4	2.6
Thrombophlebitis	4	2.6
Broken catheter in epidural space	2	1.3
Headache (spinal tap)	2	1.3
Cut cheek	1	0.6
Total	54	

in the upper jaw, had inserted an oral airway when a nasopharyngeal airway would have sufficed or had failed to use a crown guard during intubation.

Awareness

Awareness during anaesthesia is causing considerable concern as the incidence would seem to be increasing. In this series one of the five cases occurred during caesarean section and was successfully defended in court — the others could not be defended. Three cases arose during major abdominal surgery when the anaesthetic technique involved the use of a muscle relaxant, fentanyl, nitrous oxide and oxygen while one occurred during a difficult intubation. It is not always fully appreciated how close to awareness some patients are, when relaxant-narcotic techniques are employed and the extent of psychological trauma that results even after a short period of awareness. A recent award of £13 000 made in an English court, to a mother who experienced awareness during caesarean section might well be a forerunner to further claims.

MONITORING AND RECORD KEEPING

Monitoring

Despite the development during the last decade of many excellent monitors available for the anesthetized patient there is only one monitoring system that should be relied upon for the ultimate safety of the patient and that is the three senses of the well trained anaesthetist — sight, sound and touch. Any damage to a patient which is accompanied by a failure to apply these senses continuously during the course of an anaesthetic is unlikely to be defendable in a court of law. Fortunately, major anaesthetic tragedies are rare, but it may be this very infrequency of human error leading to major patient damage which lulls many anaesthetists into a sense of false security and allows him to relax the standard of vigilance that is needed to avoid the tragedies that do occur. If we were to extrapolate from the mortality figures reported by Lunn & Mushin (1982), in which they recorded 227 deaths related to anaesthesia in 1 147 000 operations, half of which were considered avoidable, we can expect to have one avoidable anaesthetic related death in every 10 000 anaesthetics administered. This is, on average, about one in every 10 years of an anaesthetist's professional career.

If individual human vigilance is not to be relied upon, then other supplementary monitoring and alarm systems must be employed. Each device has its own range of usefulness and no instrument on its own will cover all respiratory or circulatory situations. At the present stage of our knowledge of monitoring techniques and the ever increasing liability of being involved in litigation, some if not all the following 'fail safe' non-invasive monitoring devices should be considered mandatory in all but very short minor cases:

Automatic sphygmomanometer	(with high–low level alarm)
Digital pulse monitor	(with high–low rate alarm)
Electrocardiogram	(with high–low rate alarm)

Capnometer	(with high–low CO_2 and respiratory rate alarm)
Disconnection alarm	(on every ventilating system)
Oxygen analyser	(with high–low O_2 alarm)

Unfortunately the most readily available monitoring devices do not give a sufficiently rapid indication of the commonly occurring ventilation problems. For example, the ECG, pulse monitors and automatic sphygmomanometer will not alert the anaesthetist to oesophageal intubation, disconnection, kinked tube or anoxic mixtures until long after the observant anaesthetist has located the problem or the patient has already been irreparably damaged. The oesophageal intubation requires a capnograph for rapid diagnosis of the problem: the disconnection — an incircuit airway pressure alarm and the kinked tube or anoxic mixture — an O_2 analyser, in order to alert the anaesthetist in time.

Mishaps may occur when the anaesthetist has become fatigued during a prolonged or protracted operating list and cannot be deemed to be negligent. It is to protect the patient in this situation that monitoring devices with alarms are essential. It is however imprudent to impose minimal requirements for monitoring as any firm recommendation will tend to become mandatory when judgements in law are involved. The type of operation may dictate the nature of the monitoring which undoubtedly would be more extensive for complex cardiac surgery than that for minor operative procedures. In some countries the use of routine temperature monitoring would be considered essential for the early detection of malignant hyperpyrexia. The introduction of numerous alarm systems into the operating theatre may make the noise emitted by these warning devices difficult to interpret (Kerr 1985). Nevertheless the use of a blood pressure recorder, pulse monitor and perhaps an electrocardiogram on all patients requiring anaesthesia for more than a few minutes should be considered essential.

Record keeping

One of the most common difficulties encountered by those trying to defend the anaesthetists against negligence claims made by their patients, is the lack of a proper record of the events which took place. Contemporaneous record keeping is often difficult or impossible during anaesthesia especially during a crisis, but there is absolutely no merit in distorting the account of events to ameliorate the situation. Attempts at transforming an indefensible case to a defensible one can readily be detected by a discerning prosecuting counsel, adding to the torment and anguish of the anaesthetist.

PATIENT RECOVERY

The recovery room is now an integral part of the operating theatre suite and no anaesthetist would question the value of the facilities they offer. He must always be aware however that patient safety during the recovery period can only be judged by the efficiency of the staff who run them. In this survey of claims 20% of the major injuries resulting from anaesthesia (death or brain damage) occurred during the recovery period, and most of these in a properly designed recovery room.

In a survey of events which occurred in the recovery room Eltringham (1979) noted that cardiovascular complications were the most common cause for concern. It is therefore interesting to observe that in this series where claims for damages were involved, 15 out of the 21 events which occurred in the recovery period were respiratory problems in which the nursing staff failed to respond to the situation. In eight cases the respiratory problem was due to uncorrected respiratory obstruction. In the remaining nine cases there was clear evidence of an unacceptable degree of respiratory depression when patient care had been transferred to the recovery ward staff. In a significant number of these cases the anaesthetist had already left the theatre suite when cardiac arrest and/or subsequent brain damage occurred.

These rare but tragic events inevitably lead to a claim for damages which can seldom be defended. This poses the question of liability after patient care had been delegated to nursing staff. At present in the UK, the courts are likely to take the view that the anaesthetist must accept the major responsibility for the care of his patient during the recovery period until that patient is conscious and able to control his own vital functions. Should the evidence show that the nurse in charge has fallen short of her expected skills, then the hospital authorities may have to accept some of the responsibility, but the major liability will always remain with the anaesthetist. As improved recovery facilities are developed and higher standards for training of recovery ward staff are promoted, this legal attitude may change. In Canada and the USA where recovery room services have been established for over 25 years a different view is often held and incidents leading to patient damage which occur in the recovery rooms are considered to be the primary responsibility of the hospital authority nursing staff, and not the anesthesiologist (Farman 1979).

STATUS OF ANAESTHETIST

In the UK the National Health Service aims to provide a trained anaesthetist (Consultant or Senior Registrar) for the majority of routine surgical procedures performed under general anaesthesia whereas in the private sector fully trained anaesthetists are practically always involved in providing anaesthesia. Despite these overall principles 60% of the claims against anaesthetists which reached the Society were against junior anaesthetists working without supervision. One of the most disturbing features arising out of the analysis of these claims is that in many cases the anaesthetist was clearly insufficiently trained to manage the particular case by himself. An inadequate staff structure was often the reason quoted for persuading junior staff to undertake work beyond their capabilities. More often it was the failure of the consultant in charge of administration to ensure that suitably trained staff were available and assigned to operating lists appropriate to the stage of their training.

CONCLUSION

It is hoped that this analysis of cases will be helpful in clarifying the problems of morbidity and mortality in relation to anaesthesia since most of the cases were uncomplicated without coexisting or life threatening disease. Claims against such doctors are not usually made when serious complications arise in patients with pre-existing disability.

It is also hoped that a review of a few of the mishaps which have occurred during the last decade will alert anaesthetists to the problem and help to prevent some of the mishaps occurring in the future.

'Where the consequence of error is certain to be disastrous it is impossible to be too careful.'

REFERENCES

Dinnick O P 1964 Deaths associated with anaesthesia: a report of 600 cases. Anaesthesia 19: 536–556

Edwards G, Morton H J V, Pask E A, Wylie W D 1956 Deaths associated with anaesthesia: a report of 1000 cases. Anaesthesia 11: 194–220

Eltringham R J 1979 Complications in the recovery room. Journal of the Royal Society of Medicine 72: 278–280

Farman J V 1979 Do we need recovery rooms? Journal of the Royal Society of Medicine 72: 270–272

Fisher J L 1970 Recovery from anaesthesia. Canadian Medical Association Journal 109: 348–350

Green R A 1978 Anaesthesia for caesarian section. Anaesthesia 33: 70–71

Green R A, Taylor T H 1984 Anaesthesia mishaps in the UK. International Anesthesiology Clinics 22: 73–89

Holland R 1984 Anaesthesia related mortality in Australia. International Anesthesiology Clinics 22: 61–71

Howells T H, Reithmuller R J 1980 Signs of endotracheal intubation. anaesthesia 10: 984–986

Kerr J H 1985 Warning devices. British Journal of Anaesthesia 57: 696–708

Lunn J N, Mushin W W 1982 Mortality associated with anaesthesia. Nuffield Provincial Hospital Trust, London

Report on Confidential Enquiries into Maternal Deaths in England and Wales 1970–72, 1975 and 1979. H M Stationary Office, London.

Sellick B A 1961 Cricoid pressure to control regurgitation of stomach contents during the induction of anaesthesia. Lancet ii: 404–406

Solazzi R W, Ward R J 1982 The spectrum of medical liability cases. International Anesthesiology Clinics 22: 43–59

A. C. Wainwright

Anaesthesia and laser surgery

The problem created for the anesthetist by the introduction of the surgical laser is the risk not only of the combustion of volatile anaesthetic agents but also the ignition of equipment such as plastic endotracheal tubes which readily ignite in the presence of oxygen. Laser light, unlike ordinary light, retains a high intensity of energy at great distances from its source. It is said to be coherent in that the light is not only of a single wavelength but also oscillating in time. Thus the essentials of laser light are that it is monochromatic and appears as a non-divergent pencil beam of light. In contrast ordinary light is a mixture of many wavelengths and is emitted in all directions. Lasers are named after the materials from which the light is emitted. The material determines the laser's wavelength, which in turn governs the absorption of the light in tissues and hence the use of that particular laser. At present the most widely used lasers in medicine are the carbon dioxide, argon and Nd-Yag (neodymium-yttrium aluminium garnet) lasers.

CARBON DIOXIDE LASER

The wavelength of light from the carbon dioxide laser is 10.6 μ, which is in the far infra-red. The light from the carbon dioxide laser is absorbed by water and glass. In the tissues light energy is strongly absorbed by cellular water, causing it to boil, and this bursts the cell. Thus the cell temperature does not exceed 100°C, causing minimal heating of adjacent cells. This in turn produces very little oedema so that the carbon dioxide laser is now widely used in laryngeal surgery. It is in the larynx in particular that the laser beam can come into contact with the endotracheal tube.

All plastics and rubbers are heated by the carbon dioxide laser at a rate of approximately 5000°C per second, thus causing conflagration in an atmosphere enriched by oxygen or nitrous oxide. It should not be forgotten that nitrous oxide supports combustion more vigorously than 100% oxygen (Leonard 1975, Hirshman & Smith 1980, Chilcoat et al 1983). The ignition of the endotracheal tube is instantaneous, very vigorous and occurs without warning. Combustion is similar in appearance to a magnesium flare; toxic fumes are also emitted. If this happens at operation it is highly unlikely that the patient will survive. Any flammable anaesthetic agents such as diethyl ether or cyclopropane are absolutely contra-indicated when lasers are used. Earlier work (Leonard 1975) suggested that halothane, enflurane and isoflurane were not flammable in the concentrations used in anaesthesia.

There are a number of methods for avoiding ignition of the endotracheal tube although none is perfect (Hermens et al 1983, Gupta et al 1984). It should be stressed again that ignition of the endotracheal tube is to be avoided at all costs, otherwise results are likely to be catastrophic. However, with due care and attention accidents can be prevented.

Adults

There are three methods of preventing ignition of the endotracheal tube:

1. By protecting the standard tube.
2. By the use of a specially designed laser proof tube.
3. By avoiding the use of an endotracheal tube.

Protected standard endotracheal tube.

Three methods have been suggested for protecting standard tubes. The most widely used is half inch (1.25 cm) wide adhesive aluminium tape which is wound spirally around the tube so that it just overlaps, from the upper edge of the cuff for a distance of approximately 4 in (10 cm). The winding starts at the cuff in order to prevent the beam from getting under the edge of the tape (Fig 16.1). The optimum size of tube is a 5 mm microlaryngeal tube which allows a tolerably good view of the vocal cords and also protects the airway. Artificial ventilation is effective with this tube but a disadvantage is that, although the wrapped portion is laser proof, it is virtually rigid, can kink easily and the edges are traumatic to the vocal cords. This is the reason for limiting the protected area of the tube to 4 inches.

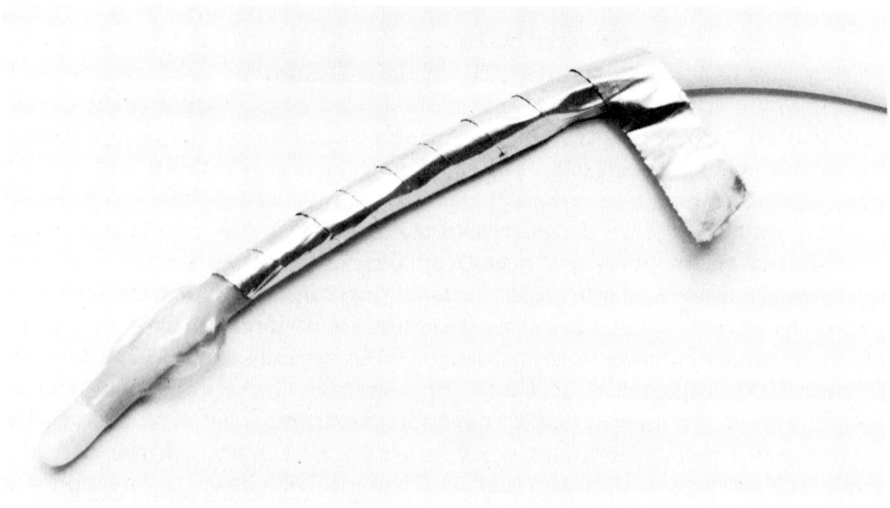

Fig. 16.1 Aluminium protected standard endotracheal tube.

During laser surgery it is essential to protect the cuff by inserting a pledget of wet cotton wool between the vocal cords and the cuff. As this pledget readily dries out it is frequently replaced by the surgeon to keep the area moist. It is also advantageous to fill the cuff with saline instead of air: this allows a leak in the cuff to be readily identified and at the same time reduces the likelihood of ignition. It is inadvisable to attach the tube firmly to the patient because in the event of ignition the tube should be removed as quickly as possible. Incandescant particles have been reported to have caused ignition of a tube on one occasion (Hirshman & Smith 1980).

The second method of protecting the tube involves the use of wrappings of thin aluminium foil. The aluminium foil consists of the leader portion of recording tapes which is not only thin and difficult to apply but is laminated with a thin sheet of plastic which is also flammable.

The third method suggested is the use of wet gauze but this is unwieldy as it has to be wrapped evenly around the tube. It also has to be kept in position and must be wet but not moist, otherwise it will be just as inflammable. A tube prepared in this way is also very bulky. These alternative methods cannot be recommended as they are less effective than the use of aluminium tape in protecting the tube.

There has been considerable debate as to whether tubes made of plastic are safer than those made of rubber. The use of either material can be dangerous. Although the flammability and penetration of rubber are slightly less, the vapours emitted from rubber are more toxic than from plastic. There is a minor advantage in the use of PVC in that combustion is self extinguishing if there is no more oxygen (Russell 1983).

Pashayan & Gravenstein (1985) have recently shown that a mixture of 40% oxygen and 60% helium increases the mean time to ignition to 42.6s, or 25.3s with 2% halothane, at a laser power of 10 W. It has therefore been suggested that the duration of each burst of laser activity should be restricted to less than 10s.

Specially designed endotracheal tubes

Norton & De Vos (1978) have produced a laser proof endotracheal tube which so far has proved most successful. It is made of stainless steel, is flexible and is relatively non-traumatic to the vocal cords. It is completely laser proof but unfortunately is thick walled and has no cuff. A small tube has to be used to obtain a good view of the vocal cords but the resistance to expiration is high. It can be used in conjunction with an injector technique, especially in patients with chronic pulmonary disease or obesity (see below).

An attempt has been made to produce a laser proof cuffed tube that is flexible and soft with thin walls. Tubes were coated with aluminium flakes, except for the cuff, and then covered with a thin reflective layer of aluminium, silver or gold. This was applied by vacuum extraction of metal vapour and resulted in a soft and flexible standard tube with a high degree of reflective surface. On inspection with the naked eye the tube appeared to be satisfactory but unfortunately laser resistance was present on only 90% of the surface. Reluctantly, the project had to be abandoned (Russell 1983).

A further attempt to produce a laser proof tube has resulted in the manufacture of a silicone tube which is largely covered by aluminium paste. In an atmosphere of less than 25% oxygen in nitrogen it will not fully ignite. When the laser beam impinges on its surface it temporarily ignites producing silicone dioxide which forms a flame-shield (Gabba et al 1984). Thus the tube has the advantage that in air it is laser resistant but not laser proof, provided it is not hit repeatedly by the laser beam. The silicone tube is soft and flexible with a cuff like an ordinary endotracheal tube. Unfortunately it must only be used in the presence of air as it ignites like PVC if the oxygen concentration is greater than 25%. Nitrous oxide is also not permissible as it supports combustion even better than oxygen. Once this tube does ignite it is not self extinguishing in air. Very few patients who require laser surgery to the larynx are fit and healthy, and since the anaesthetic techniques employ supplementary oxygen the use of the silicone tube is limited. The tube may also be used with pulsed lasers and at a maximum energy level of 3900 W/cm^2.

The conditions under which silicone tubes can be used for laser surgery are clearly stated on the packaging and these must be strictly adhered to otherwise unnecessary fatalities may arise.

General anaesthesia without an endotracheal tube

The high pressure Venturi injector, which has been widely used for many years for bronchoscopy, offers an attractive alternative to the use of an endotracheal tube. The normal surgical laryngoscope is tubular and acts as an attachment for the injector (Fig 16.2). Ventilation of the patient is adequate in the majority of patients provided the tip of the laryngoscope is near the cords. The laryngoscope is completely laser proof, it gives a clear view of the larynx, it is not traumatic and during the procedure a high percentage of oxygen may be given. As with bronchoscopy, general anaesthesia is

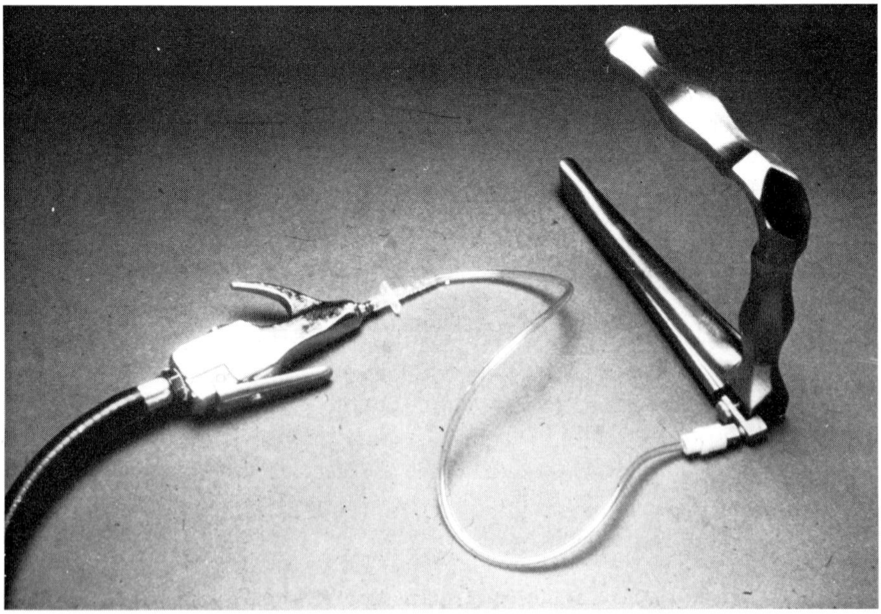

Fig. 16.2 Normal surgical laryngoscope acting as attachment for injector.

maintained intravenously. The author can only recall one obese patient who was difficult to ventilate adequately and who had two strictures of the trachea, one of which was subglotic and the other further down the trachea. In such circumstances a smaller size of Norton tube may be used as an extension to the injector. Suggestions that the injector might be used with other plastic endotracheal extensions such as the Bennett tube are untenable as any plastic or rubber which comes within the operative field must be laser proof.

The possible disadvantages of the injector are twofold. The slight movement of the vocal cords between inspiration and expiration produced by the change in gas flow may result in small lesions of the cords moving out of view of the operating microscope. In practice this can be overcome by keeping the respiration regular so that the surgeon can predict the movement of the cords. The other theoretical disadvantage is that where a lesion is on the medial edge of the cords, the trachea below this is unprotected. In practice this does not seem relevant.

For the majority of adult patients it is the author's preference to use the injector technique. Laryngoscopy is performed with either a wrapped tube or an unwrapped tube in situ, and anaesthesia is maintained with a combination of inhalational agents and muscle relaxants. After the lesion has been assessed by the surgeon and laser therapy is indicated, the tube is removed and the injector is applied. Inhalational agents are withdrawn and anaesthesia is maintained by intravenous drugs. Close cooperation between the surgeon and anaesthetist is particularly important when carbon dioxide lasers are applied to the larynx (Conacher et al 1985). The use of high frequency ventilation may have a place in laser surgery.

Children

In children where the larynx is so much smaller, a technique without an endotracheal tube becomes even more attractive. Much has been written about the advantages and disadvantages of using injectors in children, especially the dangers of causing pneumothorax, but despite this the injector has its advocates (Scamman & McCabe 1984).

The carbon dioxide laser is the treatment of choice for juvenile viral papillomata as it does not stimulate further profusion of the growth. This unpleasant condition may present in young children of 1 or 2 years of age in whom the small larynx becomes invisible and impossible to intubate. The author's preference is to anaesthetize these children with deep inhalational anaesthesia with spontaneous respiration throughout (Rita et al 1983). Anaesthesia is induced by either intravenous or inhalational methods and maintained with oxygen and halothane. Halothane is preferred to enflurane as the end-tidal carbon dioxide is less under deep anaesthesia. When the level of anaesthesia is adequate for laryngeal surgery to be tolerated an 8 or 10 French gauge suction catheter is passed through the nose into the nasopharanx, with a marker 3–4 cm from the tip to ensure that it does not protrude from the nasopharanx into the operating field. High flows of 6–8 l/min of oxygen are insufflated down the tube, 3% halothane being required to maintain the correct depth of anaesthesia. A high flow is also necessary to prevent incandescant particles from becoming lodged in the catheter during expiration (Hirshman & Smith 1980). This technique results in low arterial PCO_2 levels and may even cause apnoea (Van Hasselt et al 1985).

Tracheostomy tubes

Tracheostomy tubes in either adults or children need to be protected in the same way as laryngeal tubes. This is best done by changing to a silver Negus tracheostomy tube or some such similar metal tube. As this tube is metal it is laser proof. If the patient already has a fenestrated Negus tube in position it should be changed for a non-fenestrated one in order to facilitate ventilation. As a stricture or stenosis is lasered there may be problems of excessive leakage causing difficulties with ventilation, which may be overcome with the Venturi injector as above.

It is important to have metal connectors joining the tracheotomy tube to the anaesthetic circuit. There is a danger too that if a fenestrated tube is inadvertently used plastic or rubber connections are a risk. A metal connector suitably wedged forms a better and safer connection. Anaesthesia is maintained by inhalational agents but in adults muscle relaxants are also used to reduce movement of the vocal cords.

Oral lesions

These are also increasingly treated with the carbon dioxide laser. Although there remains a risk that the endotracheal tube may come into the field of the laser, protection is easier. An ordinary full size endotracheal tube with a metal connection may be wrapped with aluminium tape, leaving 3 cm clear above the cuff so that the larynx is not damaged. If the lesion concerned extends anywhere near the larynx, it should be regarded as a laryngeal lesion and treated as such. Wrapping of the tube must start at the lowest point and work upwards and over the connector so that no plastic is showing in the surgical field. It is advisable to move the tube to the opposite side of the mouth from the lesion. With the airway thus secured any suitable general anaesthetic may be administered.

THE ND-YAG LASER (Neodymium-yttrium aluminium garnet)

The laser works in the near infra-red range and therefore has the same theoretical risks as the carbon dioxide laser. The principle difference is that the light can be transmitted down fibre-optic pathways and can therefore be applied more directly to the lesions. There should be no flammable materials between the end of the fibre-optic instrument and the area to which it is directed. If there is any doubt, similar precautions should be taken as detailed for the carbon dioxide laser. It is fairly easy to arrange in vitro tests to assess flammability if there is further doubt.

ARGON LASER

This laser does not generally produce any problems for the anaesthetist. It produces visible light in the blue green spectrum and is used where it may be absorbed by red or black pigments. It is advocated for treatment of port wine stains of the face, where it may possibly come in contact with the endotracheal tube and cause ignition of a red rubber tube. Although in the majority of cases this is unlikely, it is prudent to use a plastic disposable tube wrapped in aluminium tape as outlined above.

REFERENCES

Chilcoat R T, Byles P H, Kellamn R M 1983 The hazard of nitrous oxide during laser endoscopic surgery. Anesthesiology 59: 258

Conacher I D, Paes M C, Morritt G N 1985 Anesthesia for carbon dioxide laser surgery on the trachea. British Journal of Anaesthesia 57: 448–450

Gabba D M, Hayes D M, Goode R L 1984 Incendiary characteristics of a new laser-resistant endotracheal tube. Anesthesiology 61: A147

Gupta B, Lingham R P, McDonald J S, Gage F 1984 Hazards of laser surgery. Anesthesiology 61: A146

Hermens J M, Bennett M J, Hirshman C A 1983 Anesthesia for laser surgery. Anesthesia and Analgesia 62: 218–229

Hirshman C A, Smith J 1980 Indirect ignition of the endotracheal tube during carbon dioxide laser surgery. Archives of Otolaryngology 106: 639–641

Kroll D A, Morris M D, Norton M L 1984 Hazards of laser degradation of methylmethacrylate. Anesthesiology 61: 115–116

Kumar A, Frose E 1981 Prevention of fire hazard during laser microsurgery. Anesthesiology 54: 350

Leonard P F 1975 Lower limits of flammability of halothane, enflurane and isoflurane. Anesthesia and Analgesia 54: 238–240

Norton M L, De Vos P 1978 New endotracheal tube for laser surgery of the larynx. Annals of Otology, Rhinology and Laryngology 87: 554–557

Pashayan A G, Gravenstein J S 1985 Helium retards endotracheal tube fires from carbon dioxide lasers. Anesthesiology 62: 274–277

Rita L, Seleny F, Holinger L D 1983 Anesthetic management and gas scavenging for laser surgery of infant subglottic stenosis

Rogers R C, Gibbons J, Cosgrove J, Copple D L 1985 High-frequency jet ventilation for tracheal surgery. Anaesthesia 40: 32–36

Russell C A 1984 Tracheal tubes for laser surgery. Anaesthesia 39: 293–294

Scammen F L, McCabe B F 1984 Evaluation of supraglottic jet ventilation for laser surgery of the larynx. Anesthesiology 61: A447

Van Hasselt G, Wainwright A C, Carruth J A S 1985 Personal Communication

17 *D. C. White*

Some aspects of the use of narcotics in general anaesthesia

INTRODUCTION

An opiate or narcotic analgesic is a drug (synthetic or naturally occurring) having, to a greater or lesser extent, morphine like properties. The term opioid was coined by Acheson in 1957 and defined as a synthetic morphine substitute. The meaning has now widened to include any substances which bind to opioid receptors and may therefore include compounds having no analgesic action.

Analgesia

Analgesia is defined as a painless state and this is reflected in the demotic expression 'pain killer'. In common medical usage an analgesic drug is one that reduces the sensation of pain. There is a difficulty here because, if the subject feels any pain at all, he cannot be in the anaesthetic state which implies the absence of awareness. However, as will be described below, it has been shown that analgesic drugs can significantly decrease the concentration of inhalational agents required to produce anaesthesia and therefore the anaesthetic state can be regarded as having an analgesic component. At least that is one interpretation of the findings.

Narcotics

Narcotics were used before the introduction of general anaesthesia and continue to be used as adjuncts either as premedicant agents or to allay post-operative pain. Smith (1908), in a paper on morphine-scopolamine anaesthesia, cited 157 references on the subject. Scrutiny of the paper showed that morphine and scopolamine alone was used in only four cases and having been found to be unsatisfactory the two drugs were thereafter used as supplements to chloroform.

Crile and Lundy, who wrote classical papers on the anaesthetic state, considered that the desirable analgesic component of that state was best achieved with the use of local anaesthetic agents and, indeed, recent work has confirmed their value in suppressing the metabolic response to surgery. Abolition of the autonomic reflex response to surgical stimulus was not considered an integral part of general anaesthesia until the publiction of a paper entitled 'Changing concepts concerning depth of anesthesia' by Woodbridge (1957). But before this date it had become apparent that nitrous oxide alone was not always able to provide adequate anaesthesia in the paralysed patient, and in 1947 Neff et al published the first paper describing the use of a narcotic analgesic —pethidine — as a supplement to nitrous oxide analgesia. This technique was introduced to the UK following a visit to Dr Neff at Stanford by Drs Mushin and Randell-Baker (1949) who advocated a method using 66% nitrous oxide with gallamine or d-tubocurarine and incremental doses of 25 mg of pethidine at 25–30 minute intervals. Techniques of this type immediately became very popular and have continued in widespread use ever since. Early work on the subject is reviewed by Siker (1956) and of interest is a paper describing laryngeal intubation under pethidine (Ruben & Andreassen 1951). Also of interest is a double blind comparison in 113 patients (Holmes 1976) of equianalgesic doses of pethidine, morphine, phenoperidine and fentanyl as a supplement to nitrous oxide anaesthesia. Very little difference was found between the four opiates and Bouill et al (1984) have commented that it is a characteristic of opiates that when they are combined with anaesthetic agents differences between them tend to be obscured.

Reduction of the amount of anaesthetics required

Claude Bernard, in a lecture published in 1869, stated that morphine injected into dogs before anaesthesia reduced by half the amount of chloroform needed for surgical anaesthesia (Schrier 1982). A similar view was expressed on the effect of morphine on cyclopropane anaesthesia by Waters & Schmidt (1934). Experimental work in support of this is reviewed by Robbins (1958) in his monograph on cyclopropane. Morphine was found to produce marked reductions in the blood cyclopropane concentrations required for various levels of anaesthesia. Two groups of workers (Seevers et al 1934, Robbins et al 1939) found that although morphine reduced the blood concentration of cyclopropane necessary for anaesthesia, the concentration at which respiratory arrest occurred was not altered. It was therefore considered that morphine increased the safety margin in the use of cyclopropane.

In the human subject 10 mg of morphine given intravenously 10 minutes before anaesthesia was shown to reduce by 15% the blood ether concentration required for a given depth of anaesthesia as defined by electroencephalographic changes (Taylor et al 1957).

Later work has approached this subject by demonstrating reductions in maximum alveolar concentration (MAC) for various anaesthetic agents produced by narcotic analgesics. Reductions in MAC for human subjects given pre-anaesthetic doses of morphine in the range 8–15 mg have been shown for halothane to be —7% (Saidman & Eger 1964) and for fluroxene —20% (Munson et al 1965).

More recently experiments to measure the anaesthetic sparing effects of various doses of different narcotic analgesics have given interesting results. Initial work showed that the strong narcotic analgesics, morphine and pethidine (μ agonists) reduced the cyclopropane requirement for anaesthesia in rats by an amount directly proportional to the log dose of the analgesic, but the agonist/antagonist drug pentazocine showed a ceiling effect, in that at doses above 20 mg/kg no further reduction in anaesthetic requirement occurred (Hoffman & Difazio 1970). This finding for narcotic analgesics of the agonist/antagonist class has been confirmed in dogs for butorphanol with which maximum reduction of enflurane MAC was found to be 11% and nalbuphine, for which the maximum reduction in enflurane MAC was found to be 8% (Murphy & Hug 1982a). Of great interest is the finding by the same authors that if a sufficiently high dose is used a ceiling effect is found with morphine and also with fentanyl (Murphy & Hug 1982b). However large the dose of morphine or fentanyl the MAC could not be reduced by more than 65%.

Naloxone

The introduction of naloxone, an effective narcotic antagonist active at the μ receptor, promised a more flexible approach to effective analgesia. However, it soon became apparent that it was best reserved for emergency use. The duration of effective action of one bolus dose in the clinical range (0.1–0. 4 mg) does not usually exceed 30 minutes so that most patients who have received a relative overdose of any one of the commonly used narcotic analgesics require either a continuous slow infusion or repeated doses; both methods needing close supervision. An alternative method of supplemental intramuscular doses of naloxone has been advocated (Longnecker et al 1973) but there must always be a degree of uncertainty about the rate of absorbtion by this route.

Naloxone reverses analgesia to the same or similar degree that it reverses respiratory depression, but it is possible by judicious titration to reverse respiratory depression sufficiently while retaining a degree of analgesia (Krycke et al 1976, Drummond et al 1977). Because of the considerable differences between the kinetics of the drugs involved, such a titration technique requires very close supervision.

There are further objections to the routine use of naloxone; it may cause vomiting even with small doses (Longnecker et al 1973), restlessness and shivering (Tammisto & Tigerstedt 1979), pruritis and copious diuresis (Smith 1984), serious or indeed fatal ventricular dysrhymthias (Michaelis et al 1974, Andree 1980), acute left ventricular failure with severe pulmonary oedema (Flache et al 1977) and severe hypertension (Azar & Turndorf 1979, Estillo & Cottrell 1981). Most of these side-effects have been described in patients who were already seriously ill but Prough et al (1984) have recorded two cases of acute pulmonary oedema in healthy teenagers following small doses of naloxone given post-operatively to reverse doses of 0.5 mg of fentanyl given during the course of minor surgery. These authors consider that naloxone may cause neurogenic pulmonary oedema.

The severe cardiovascular effects sometimes seen when naloxone is used to reverse narcotics resemble those of massive catecholamine release (Tanaka 1974). Patschke et al (1977) observed increases in heart rate, cardiac output and blood pressure in anaesthetized dogs on administering naloxone after large doses of morphine: they considered that these effects might be due to an acute abstinence syndrome. These effects could not be due to stress and pain because the dogs remained anaesthetized while the effects were seen.

Finally, the work of Kruynack & Gintautas (1982) should be noted: they proposed that naloxone may govern the duration of narcosis through the actuation of an opposing arousal system in the CNS unrelated to pharmalogical competition for opiate receptors.

SEQUENTIAL ANALGESIA

In a classic paper Lasagna & Beecher (1954) showed that nalorphine, which had hitherto been regarded solely as an antagonist of morphine, did itself have analgesic properties in man, and the possibility that mixtures of morphine and nalorphine might be clinically useful was investigated by a number of workers. The object of these investigations was to see if it were possible by the use of such mixtures to separate, or at least diminish, the undesirable side-effects associated with narcotic analgesia, particularly respiratory depression. Nalorphine does oppose the respiratory depression produced by morphine (Bellville & Fleischli 1968), but the relationship in action between the two drugs proved to be of a complex biphasic nature (Houde & Wallenstein 1956) and it was these observations that led to the concept of 'receptor dualism' (Martin 1967).

Nalorphine

Nalorphine, in doses sufficient to have an analgesic action, also has a high incidence of psychotomimetic effects (dysphoria, delirium and hallucinations) but the introduction of similar compounds with a lower incidence of these σ-agonist actions makes possible a clinical use of the drug interactions described above.

Fentanyl

In 1968 de Castro & Viars described a technique in which high doses of fentanyl were used as the sole anaesthetic agent and the respiratory depressant action reversed by a large dose of pentazocine which left the patients breathing adequately but having analgesia for the immediate post-operative period from the pentazocine. They named this technique anésthesie analgésie sequentielle (AAS), a name which unfortunately embodies some confusion between analgesia and anaesthesia. Rifat (1972) described a series of elderly patients undergoing hip surgery who, after intravenous induction and intubation (using propranidid and suxamethonium), received fentanyl 25 μg/kg and alcuronium and were ventilated with 50/50 $N_20/0_2$. Additional doses of fentanyl 125 μg were given if required. At the end of the operation, after reversal of the relaxant and withdrawal of the nitrous oxide, 48 of the 52 patients studied remained unconscious and were apnoeic or ventilation was inadequate. The were given pentazocine 1 mg/kg and all resumed adequate ventilation and regained consciousness. After extubation all maintained adequate blood gases, blood pressure and central venous pressure and in only three patients was any further analgesic needed in the first five post-operative hours.

Pentazocine

Pentazocine, although more useful than nalorphine, is nevertheless an unsatisfactory drug in many ways. It has a weak analgesic action reaching a ceiling at a dose of about 1 mg/kg and at or above this level the incidence of psychotomimetic effects becomes unacceptably high, reaching 50% is some series (Wood et al 1974). Pentazocine also has undesirable haemodynamic effects and may increase heart rate and systemic and pulmonary blood pressure (Alderman et al 1972) due to, or at least associated with, catecholamine release not connected with hypercarbia (Tammisto et al 1979).

Nalbuphine

Nalbuphine appears considerably superior to pentazocine for use in sequential analgesia. It is considerably more potent than pentazocine as a μ antagonist, being about one fourth as potent as nalorphine in this respect (Jasinski & Mansky 1972). In common with other drugs in this class, both respiratory depression (Romagnoli & Keats 1980, Julien 1982) and analgesia (Gal et al 1982) appear to be limited, i.e. there is a ceiling effect, at about the same dosage level of approximately 0.15 mg/kg. At this dose the analgesic potency is equal to or slightly less than the same dose of morphine and has a similar duration of action (Beaver & Feise 1978). The incidence of psychotomimetic effects seen with nalbuphine is very much less than with pentazocine (Jasinski 1979, Stambaugh 1982).

Magruder et al (1982) reported a series of 15 patients having a wide variety of operations under anaesthesia by a nitrous oxide, narcotic and relaxant technique after thiopentone induction. The narcotic analgesic used was oxymorphone or hydromorphone and the dose given (0.05 mg/kg plus 0.05 mg) was equivalent to 30 mg of morphine in a 70 kg patient. At the end of the surgery, after reversal of the muscle relaxant and extubation, all the patients had inadequate ventilation confirmed by blood gas estimation and were given nalbuphine 0.1 mg/kg. The response was dramatic and in all patients blood gas estimation showed that ventilation had returned to normal. There were no episodes of renarcotization and analgesia remained adequate for an average period of 7 hours. Following this the authors adopted a routine of 0.1 mg/kg of nalbuphine intravenously and 0.2 mg/kg intramuscularly given post-operatively in 150 patients. They found that this provided protection against respiratory depression even after total morphine doses of 2–3 mg/kg. The only adverse effect observed was a transient pressor response to nalbuphine producing an increase in heart rate and mean arterial pressure of about 20% above control value.

Latasch et al (1984 described a series of 60 patients undergoing elective general surgery who were anaesthetized by a fentanyl–relaxant–nitrous oxide technique. The dose of fentanyl used was 7 μg/kg, plus a standardized dose of 0.2 mg every 15 minutes. At the end of the operation, after reversal of the relaxant, a further 0.2 mg of fentanyl was given to ensure apnoea during transfer to the recovery room where 20 mg of nalbuphine was given intravenously to all the patients. As in the previous series there was a dramatic and rapid response. In no patient was more than 1.5 minutes required from apnoea to ventilation adequate to maintain normal blood gas, and after 2 minutes all patients were so alert that they required immediate extubation. Pain was measured by a visual analogue scale and pain relief was found to be excellent throughout the following 3 hours without further nalbuphine. No renarcotization was seen in this series and the authors note that no significant changes in heart rate or blood pressure occurred. Side-effects included vomiting in 5 patients and shivering in 12 patients immediately after the nalbuphine. As already mentioned shivering is commonly seen when naloxone is administered.

Finally, Moldenhauer et al (1985) reported on 21 patients undergoing aorto-coronary bypass who were anaesthetized by a high dose fentanyl technique. In the first group of patients, who received a mean dose of 120 μg/kg of fentanyl, reversal by nalbuphine was carried out on the morning after the day of surgery. In the second group, who received a mean dose of 97 μg/kg of fentanyl, nalbuphine was given within 8 hours of the end of surgery. In this series nalbuphine was administered with great caution in 15 μg/kg increments (i.e. 1.05 mg for a 70 kg man) every 30–60 minutes until the Pa_{CO_2} decreased to <48 mmHg or until a total dose of 150 μg/kg had been given. The total dose of nalbuphine required for each patients was in the range 1–10 mg. Three patients in the first group experienced an immediate increase in pain on receiving nalbuphine which was relieved by giving additional nalbuphine. Four patients in the series experienced transient increases of more than 25% in mean arterial pressure after nalbuphine administration. Renarcotization (Pa_{CO_2} >55 mmHg) occurred in three patients of the second group and further nalbuphine was required 2–3 hours after the last dose. The object of treatment by nalbuphine in this series was to shorten the time to extubation which was carried out about 20 minutes after the effective or final dose of nalbuphine.

The successful use of nalbuphine in sequential analgesia has been demonstrated but clearly further study is required to determine the optimum dosage and timing. The transient rise in blood pressure is also a cause for concern.

Buprenorphine

Buprenorphine is the other clinically available drug which has similar actions to pentazocine and nalbuphine, i.e. antagonism at the μ receptor and partial agonist effects at the κ receptor. Its use in the technique of sequential analgesia was suggested by de Castro (1979). Results have not yet been reported but the interactions between fentanyl and buprenorphine on opioid receptors isolated from rat brain have been described by Boas & Villiger (1985). Buprenorphine was able to displace fenanyl from receptors in a concentration and time dependent manner. Buprenorphine was very slow in its action compared to fentanyl and appeared less selective than fentanyl. From the data in this paper it appears that buprenorphine may be of value in the technique of sequential analgesia, but its time of onset and offset is markedly different from nalbuphine and pentazocine and it is hardly at all antagonized by naloxone.

There is a further problem with buprenorphine. The dose response curve for analgesia, at least in rats and mice, has been clearly shown to be both biphasic and bell shaped. After attaining a peak of analgesia, increasing the dose results in the analgesia decreasing towards zero (Dum & Herz 1981).

The complexities of this subject are discussed by Hull (1985) and emphasized by a recent report (Schmidt et al 1985) which described a series of 12 patients given either 30 or 40 μ/kg of buprenorphine as a component of balanced anaesthesia for cholecystectomy. Six of these patients were in pain post-operatively and were given naloxone 0.04 mg/min (the maximum dose given was 0.44 mg). This dose of naloxone was found to give a prolonged period of pain relief. In these patients the buprenorphine produced respiratory depression when first given but the recorded respiratory rates post-operatively suggested that that respiratory depression was not present at that time and these rates were not affected by the naloxone. It is tempting to speculate that the naloxone pushed the patient's analgesic state back up the far side of the bell shaped curve.

The technique of sequential analgesia has the potential of overcoming one of the major disadvantages of using high doses of narcotic analgesics during anaesthesia, i.e. a prolonged post-operative respiratory depression. However, it is not yet clear whether, when an agonist/antagonist analgesic is used in this manner, it completely displaces the powerful agonist substituting its own more limited degree of analgesia or whether it only partially reverses the action of the more potent drug. As has already been described, by using naloxone, partial reversal of fentanyl is possible, but clearly the kinetics of these drug interactions are complex and they may prove to be unsuitable for routine clinical use. Further research may bring us closer to being able to produce profound analgesia without respiratory depression.

NARCOTICS AND THE STRESS RESPONSE

The stress response is the name given to the complex of hormonally regulated metabolic changes which occur in response to surgery and, to a much lesser extent, to anaesthesia. The subject is reviewed in this volume by Bailey & Child (see Ch. 11). There are reasons for thinking that the abolition or at least the reduction of some of the components of the stress response may be beneficial to the patient. For instance a prominent feature of the stress response is the release of catecholamines from the adrenal medulla with consequent stimulation of α and β receptors. This results in large increases in heart rate and blood pressure which may produce cardiac ischaemia in susceptible patients. It is not surprising therefore to find that it is the blocking of this response which has been chiefly studied. However, it is not at all clear whether it is desirable to supress many of the the components of the stress response. John Hunter thought not. In 1794 he wrote 'there is a circumstance attending accidental injury which does not belong to disease, namely that the injury done, has in all cases a tendency to produce, both the disposition and the means of cure' (Cuthbertson 1976). Other more recent writers have observed 'teleologically, sympathetic activity has relevance in enabling a stressed individual to survive a traumatic event such as injury after attack by animals. It is not clear whether the surgeon should be placed in this category' (Ellis & Humphrey 1982). Certainly some of the components of the response such as the adrenal cortical response and the liberation of growth hormone are concerned with maintenance of intravascular volume and substrate mobilization necessary to promote healing processes and clearly these should be preserved.

Abdominal surgery

In 1959 it was shown that morphine suppressed release of adrenocorticotropic hormone (ACTH) from the anterior pituitary (McDonald 1959). The effect of large doses of this drug on cortisol and growth hormone release were investigated by George et al (1974). They found that 1 mg/kg of morphine reduced, but did not abolish, the hormonal changes during abdominal surgery and that 4 mg/kg for cardiac surgery abolished responses only until the start of bypass. This finding has been confirmed by other workers. Large doses of fentanyl (50 μg/kg) were found by Hall et al (1978) to abolish the endocrine response to tubal microsurgery under halothane anaesthesia. But McQuay et al (1979) who studied patients undergoing more stressful major pelvic surgery found that the plasma cortisol response was not blocked by fentanyl. In major gastric surgery the same dose of fentanyl was found to reduce but not to abolish the stress response inter-operatively. All patients in this series required respiratory support post-operatively (Cooper et al 1981).

In another series of upper abdominal cases 50 μg/kg of fentanyl abolished the cortisol response but in this series no effect on the hyperglycaemic response was found (Haxholdt et al 1981). Alfentanil (150 μg/kg followed by infusion of 3 μg/kg/min) was found to inhibit increases in plasma cortisol and glucose during abdominal hysterectomy but the effect did not extend more than 3 hours into the post-operative period (Moller et al 1985).

The circulatory response to laryngoscopy and intubation has been found to be more easily blocked by narcotics. Martin et al (1982) found that 8 μ/kg of fentanyl greatly reduced the response, and Kautto (1982) observed that 6 μg/kg of this drug completely abolished changes in the blood pressure and pulse rate observed during laryngoscopy and intubation.

To conclude this aspect of the use of narcotics, Roisen et al (1981) determined the anaesthetic dose blocking the adrenergic cardiovascular responses to skin incision for various anaesthetic agents and for morphine. This dose was termed the MAC BAR. In a group of unpremedicated patients the dose of morphine required was found to be 1.13 mg/kg and this compared with a mean alveolar concentration of 1.1% of halothane.

Cardiac surgery

The era of narcotic anaesthesia for cardiac surgery was ushered in by the classic paper of Lowenstein et al (1969) which showed how slight were the effects of morphine (1 mg/kg) on cardiovascular function. It became apparent that very large doses of morphine, up to 3 mg/kg body weight, could be safely given to patients with cardiac disease and that these doses resulted in modification of the cardiovascular stress response.

The use of narcotic analgesics in connection with anaesthesia for cardiac surgery has generated a great deal of research and the subject has recently been comprehensively reviewed (Bovill et al 1984). A necessarily brief summary will be given. The frequent requirement of post-operative mechanical ventilation after cardiac surgery which necessitated retention of the endotracheal tube was, in practice, the major factor resulting in the introduction of large doses of morphine as part of the aneasthetic technique for cardiac surgery (Lowenstein & Philbin 1983). As attempts were made to achieve better results by using larger doses of morphine various difficulties became apparent. A fall in peripheral vascular resistance had been a feature noted in a pioneering paper of Lowenstein et al (1969) and indeed it had been considered a desirable feature in patients with congestive failure as it constituted a form of internal phlebotomy. But Stanley et al (1973), in a series of cardiac cases in which the average dose of morphine was 11 mg/kg, found that the requirement of blood to be excessively high both during and after surgery. It has also been shown that there was a requirement for a significant rate of transfusion volume during cardiac surgery when a more moderate dose of 3 mg/kg of morphine was used compared to the fluid requirements under halothane anaesthesia (Stanley et al 1974).

It seems that a large part, if not all, of this undesirable effect of high dose morphine is due to histamine release.

In a series of coronary artery bypass graft (CABG) patients, Rosow et al (1982) found that a dose of 1 mg/kg of morphine produced an average 750% peak increase in plasma histamine and that this was associated with a fall in systemic vascular resistance (SVR) and blood pressure. In contrast patients given fentanyl (50 μg/kg showed no increase in plasma histamine. Evidence suggesting that the cardiovascular changes were entirely due to histamine was provided by Philbin et al (1981) who found that the administration of a combination of an H_1 antagonist (diphenhydramine) and an H_2 antagonist (cimetidine) completely blocked the fall in SVR and diastolic blood pressure in CABG patients given 1 mg/kg of morphine.

As mentioned above, the synthetic narcotic analgesic fentanyl does not cause histamine release and for this and other reasons is now routinely use in anaesthesia for cardiac surgery in doses of 50–100 μ/kg. Two analogues of fentanyl, sufentanil and alfentanil, have also been used in high dosage for cardiac surgery. Their actions resemble fentanyl closely, but they differ in potency and duration of action. Sufentanil appears to be between five and seven times as potent as fentanyl and to have a similar duration of action (Rolly et al 1979, de Langa et al 1982) and alfentanil to have a potency and duration of action of approximately one-third that of fentanyl. Some of the problems associated with the use of high doses of narcotic analgesics will be briefly discussed below.

Awareness

Lowenstein et al (1969) noted that 1 mg/kg morphine often did not cause unconsciousness if adequate oxygenation and CO_2 excretion were maintained, and since then a number of cases of awareness during high dose fentanyl/oxygen anaesthesia have been reported. In one case (Mummaneni et al 1980) a patient given 75.8 μg/kg of fentanyl and 10 mg of diazapem for a cardiac operation had no awareness but for a further operation shortly afterwards the same patient was given 72 μg/kg of fentanyl and no diazepam and awareness and recall were reported. In another case (Hilgenberg 1981) in which a total of 90 μg/kg of fentanyl was given there was no sign of lightness of anaesthesia during the operation but there was undoubted recall, although this was only of hearing. In a third case, despite the patient being given a total dose of 96 μg/kg of fentanyl, diazepam 10 mg and 50% nitrous oxide for 25 minutes the stimulation of the incision, entering the chest and diathermy of the edges of the pericardium resulted in a hypertensive crisis requiring thiopentone, enflurane and other drugs, including 50% nitrous oxide for the rest of the operation (Mark & Greenberg 1983). The patient recalled the incident afterwards. These and other occurrences confirm that narcotic analgesics alone cannot be relied upon to produce anaesthesia and this view is expressed by Wong (1983) in an editorial robustly entitled, 'Narcotics are not expected to produce unconsciousness and amnesia'. Certainly general anaesthetic agents appear to depress the central nervous system in a fairly non-specific manner related to their lipid solubility whereas narcotic analgesics have a critical structure and bind specifically to localized receptors producing analgesia, respiratory depression and other specific effects. These receptors are currently being subdivided into various subgroups, none of which appear to subserve the functions of unconsciousness or amnesia. The failure of narcotic analgesics at what ever dose to reduce MAC by more than 65% (referred to previously) is a further indication that these drugs do not produce anaesthesia. The use of even more potent narcotic analgesics may be beneficial in that, since less of the drug is required, there is less likelihood of side-effects (Janssen 1982). But greater specificity is even less likely to include lack of awareness and absence of recall among the spectrum of activities. The contrary view has been expressed by Stanley (1983), who considers that the higher the dose the less likely is incomplete amnesia.

The subdivision of receptors referred to above is of great interest as it contains the possibility of a drug producing effective analgesia without respiratory depression or addictive liability.

Not least of the problems of preventing awareness with fentanyl/O_2 anaesthesia, is the finding that the addition of nitrous oxide in the presence of high concentrations of fentanyl and other narcotic analgesics produces significnt myocardial depression with increased systemic vascular resistance and lowered cardiac output and blood pressure (Wong et al 1973). This view has been challenged by Balasaraswathi et al (1981) and Michaels et al (1984). The direct action of nitrous oxide on the myocardium is depressant but this is usually compensated for by the sympathomimetic effects of the gas (Eisele 1985). Blocking of these effects by the narcotic may uncover the direct depressant action.

Cardiovascular depression is also observed when diazepam is added to high dose fentanyl (Reves et al 1984), and depressant interactions between morphine and halothane (Stoelting et al 1974) and fentanyl and enflurane (Bennet and Stanley 1979) have also been described. Despite these findings benzodiazepine and inhalational anaesthetic agents, particularly isoflurane, are widely used to ensure a lack of awareness when high dose narcotics analgesics are used. It seems likely that the extent of the depressant interactions on the myocardium between narcotic analgesics and other sedative or anaesthetic drugs depends very much on the state of the coronary circulation (Barash & Kopriva 1982).

Muscular rigidity

A peculiar feature of very large doses of narcotic analgesics is the production of muscular rigidity confined to the thorax and abdomen becoming apparent during induction. This effect, which appears supraspinal in origin but whose cause is unknown, was first noted by Hamilton & Cullen (1953) and with morphine by Freund et al (1973). With morphine the rigidity is relatively mild and manifests itself by expiratory grunting and restrictive expiration. If vigorously exhorted, conscious patients are able to overcome this by spontaneous effort (Lowenstein & Philbin 1983).

With fentanyl and the newer narcotic analgesics the rigidity may be much more severe and may prevent inflation of the lungs by intermittent positive pressure. It has been pointed out by Andrews & Prys-Roberts (1983) that there is no reason why abdominal or thoracic rigidity should prevent inflation of the lungs and that this must be due to closure of the glottis. Whatever may be the truth of this, the phenonemon requires the routine use of muscle relaxants to overcome it. In one large series (Grell et al 1970) muscle rigidity sufficient to impair intermittent positive pressure ventilation was seen when the dose of fentanyl exceeded 0.25 mg. It has been claimed that rigidity is not seen with slow infusion rates (Stanley & Webster 1978). An infusion rate of 1 mg/min of fentanyl to a total dose of 50 μg/kg produced truncal rigidity in 88% of patients which was reduced by pretreatment with small doses of pancuronium (12.2 μg/kg) or metocurine (50 μg/kg) (Jaffe & Ramsey 1983). Hill et al (1981), who found a high incidence of rigidity at the relatively slow fentanyl infusion rate of 3 μg/kg/min occurring after a mean dose of 14.6 μg/kg, considered that this could be prevented by simultaneous infusion of pancuronium at the rate of 12 μg/kg/min without the patient becoming aware of paralysis. Finally, it has been reported (Christian et al 1983) that three patients developed truncal rigidity between 5 and 8 hours after induction of anaesthesia. The dose of fentanyl in these cases was 75 or 115 μg/kg and the rigidity was immediately abolished by naloxone. The authors consider that acid-base changes had effected brain fentanyl concentrations. This effect has been shown to occur in dogs. Ainslie et al (1979) found marked increases in brain concentration with decreasing Pa_{CO_2}.

Despite, or because of, the great amount of work on high dose narcotic analgesics for cardiac surgery very little has been done to demonstrate that this technique is actually superior in results to any other. A recent paper (Fischerstrom et al 1985) describes results in a series of 20 unselected patients with severe angina undergoing coronary artery bypass surgery. They were randomly allocated to two groups, one group receiving nitrous oxide/halothane and the other nitrous oxide/fentanyl/diazepam. A benign and almost identical haemodynamic response to surgery and bypass was observed in the two groups. The dose of fentanyl used in this series was very moderate.

A careful review of the question of narcotic versus inhalation anaesthesia for cardiovascular surgery (Roizen 1984) concludes that no available data justify the belief that any narcotic or inhalational agent is superior in its effect on outcome when used in conjunction with cardiac or vascular surgery.

REFERENCES

Ainslie S G, Eisele J H, Corkill G 1979 Fentanyl concentrations in brain and serum during respiratory acid base changes in the dog. Anesthesiology 51: 293–297

Alderman E L, Barry W H, Graham A F, Harrison D C 1972 Haemodynamic effects of morphine and pentazocine differ in cardiac patients. New England Journal of Medicine 287: 623–627

Andree R 1980 Sudden death following naloxone administration. Anaesthesia and Analgesia 59: 782–784

Andrews C J H, Prys-Robert C 1983 Fentanyl — a review. Clinics in Anaesthesiology 1: 97–121

Azar I, Turndorf H 1979 Severe hypertension and multiple atrial premature contractions following naloxone administration. Anaesthesia and Analgesia 58: 524–525

Bailey P, Gerbode F, Garlington L 1958 An anesthetic technique for cardiac surgery which utilizes 100% oxygen as the only inhaland. Archives of Surgery 76: 437–440

Balasarasuathi K, Kumar P, Rao T, El Etr A A 1981 Left ventricular and diastolic pressure as an index for nitrous oxide use during coronary artery surery. Anesthesiology 55: 708–709

Barash P G, Koprina C J 1982 Narcotics and the circulation. In: Kitahata, Collins (eds) Narcotic Analgesics in Anesthesiology. Williams and Wilkins, Baltimore

Beaver W T, Feise G A 1978 A comparison of the analgesic effect of intramuscular nalbuphine and morphine in patients with postoperative pain. Journal of Pharmacology and Experimental Therapeutics 204: 487–496

Bennett G M, Stanley T H 1979 Cardiovascular effects of fentanyl during enflurane anesthesia in man. Anaesthesia and Analgesia 58: 179–182

Bellville J W, Fleischli G 1968 The interaction of morphine and nalorphine on respiration. Clinical Pharmacology and Therapeutics 9: 152–162
Boas R A, Villiger J W 1985 Clinical actions of fentanyl and buprenorphine. The significance of receptor binding. British Journal of Anaesthesia 57: 192–196
Bovill J G, Sebel P S, Stanley T H 1984 Opioid analgesics in anesthesia with special reference to their use in cardiovascular anesthesia. Anesthesiology 61: 731–755
Christian C C, Waller J L, Moldenhauer C C 1983 Postoperative rigidity following fentanyl. Anesthesia and Anesthesiology 58: 275–277
Cooper G M, Paterson J L, Ward I D, Hall G M 1981 Fentanyl and the metabolic response to gastric surgery. Anaesthesia 36: 667–671
Cuthbertson D P 1976 Surgical metabolism: historical and evolutionary aspects In: Wilkinson, Cuthbertson (eds) Metabolism and the Response to Injury. Tunbridge Wells
De Castro J 1979 British Journal of Clinical Pharmacology 7: 319S
De Castro J, Viars P 1968 Archives of Medicine 23: 170–171
De Langa S, Boscoe M J, Stanley T H, Pace N 1982 Comparison of sufentanil-0_2 and fentanyl-0_2 for coronary artery surgery. Anesthesiology 56: 112–118
Drummond G B, Davie I T, Scott D B 1977 Naloxone: dose dependant antagonism of respiratory depression by fentanyl in anesthetised patients. British Journal of Anaesthetics 49: 151–154
Dum J, Herz A 1981 In vivo receptor binding of opiate partial agonist buprenorphine correlated with its agonistic and antagonistic effects. Journal of Pharmacology 74: 627
Eiselle J H 1985 Cardiovascular effects of nitrous oxide. In: Eger E I (ed) Nitrous Oxide. Edward Arnold, London
Ellis R F, Humphrey D E 1982 Clinical aspects of endocrine and metabolic changes relating to anaesthesia surgery. In: Watkins (ed) Trauma, Stress and Immunity in Anaesthesia and Surgery. Butterworth, London
Estillo A E, Cottrell J E 1981 Naloxone, hypertension and ruptured cerebral aneurysm. Anesthesiology 54: 352
Fischerstrom A, Oliquist, Settergren G 1985 Comparison of fentanyl and halothane as supplement to nitrous-oxide-oxygen anaesthesia for coronary artery surgery Acta Anaesthesiologica Scandinavica 29: 16–21
Flache J W, Flache W E, Williams G D 1977 Acute pulmonary oedema following naloxone reversal of high dose morphine anaesthesia. Anesthesiology 47: 376–378
Freund F G, Martin W E, Wong K, Hornbein T F 1973 Abdominal muscle rigidity induced by morphine and nitrous oxide. Anesthesiology 38: 358–362
Gal T J, Difazio C A 1982 Analgesic and respiratory depressant activity of nalbuphine: a comparison with morphine. Anesthesiology 57: 367–374
George J M, Reier C E, Lanese R R, Rower J M 1974 Morphine anaesthesia blocks cortisol and growth hormone response to surgical stress in humans. Journal of Clinical Endocrinology and Metabolism 38: 736–739
Grell F L, Koom R A, Nedson J S 1970 Fentanyl in anesthesia. A report of 500 cases. Anesthesia and Analgesia 49: 523–532
Hall G M, Young C, Holdcroft A, Labgband-Zadeh J 1978 Substrate mobilisation during surgery. A comparison between halothane and fentanyl anaesthesia. Anaesthesia 33: 924–930
Hamilton W K, Cullen S C 1953 Effect of levallorphan tartrate upon opiate induced respiratory depression. Anesthesiology 14: 550–554
Haxoldt O S, Kehlet H, Dryberg V 1981 Effect of fentanyl on the cortisol and hyperglycaemic response to abdominal surgery. Acta Anaesthesiologica Scandavica 25: 434–436
Hilgenberg J C 1981 Intraoperative awareness during high dose fentanyl-oxygen anesthesia. Anesthesiology 54: 341–343
Hill A B, Nahrwold M L, Rosayro M De, Knight P R, Jones R M, Bottes R E 1981 Prevention of rigidity during fentanyl oxygen induction of anesthesia. Anesthesiology 55: 452–454
Hoffman J C, Difazio C A 1970 The anesthesia sparing effecting of pentazocine, meperidine and morphine. Archives Internationales de Pharmacodynamie et de Therapie 186: 261–268
Holmes C McK 1976 Supplementation of general anaesthesia with narcotic analgesics. British Journal of Anaesthesia 48: 907–913
Houde R W, Wallenstein S L 1956 Clinical studies of morphine-nalorphine combinations. Federation Proceedings 15: 440–441
Hull C J 1985 Receptor binding and its significance. British Journal of Anaesthesia 57: 131–133
Jaffe T B, Ramsey F M 1983 Attenuation of fentanyl-induced truncal rigidity. Anesthesiology 58: 562–564
Janssen P A S 1982 Potént new analgesics tailor made for different purposes. Acta Anaesthesiologica Scandanavica 26: 262–268

Jasinski D R, Mansky P A 1972 Evaluation of nalbuphine for abuse potential. Pharmacology and Therapeutics 13: 78–90
Jasinski D R 1979 Human pharmacology of narcotic antagonists. British Journal of Clinical Pharmacology 7: 287S
Julien R M 1982 Effects of nalbuphine on normal and onymorphone-depressed ventilatory responses to carbon-dioxide challenge. Anesthesiology 97: A320
Kaufman L 1982 Anaesthesia and the endocrine response. In: Kaufman L (ed) Anaesthesia Review 1, Churchill Livingstone, Edinburgh
Kaufman L 1984 Update. Anaesthesia and the endocrine response. In: Kaufman L (ed) Anaesthesia Review 2. Churchill Livingstone. Edinburgh
Kautto U M 1982 Attenuation of the circulatory resonse to laryngoscopy and intubation of fentanyl. Acta Anaesthesiologica Scandanavica 26: 217–221
Kraynack B J, Gintautas J G 1982 Nalaxone: analeptic action unrelated to opiate receptor antagonism. Anesthiology 56: 251–253
Krycke B J, Finck A J, Shah N K, Snow J C 1979 Naloxone antagonism after narcotic supplemented anaesthesia. Anaesthesia and Analgesia 55: 800–805
Lasagna L, Beecher H K 1954 The analgesic effectiveness of nalorphine and nalorphine-morphine combinations in man. Journal of Pharmacology and Experimental Therapeutics 122: 356–363
Latasch L, Probst S, Dudziak 1984 Reversal by nalbuphine of respiratory depression caused by fentanyl. Anaesthesia and Analgesia 63: 814–816
Longnecker D, Grazis P, Eggers G 1973 Naloxone for antagonism of morphine induced respiratory depression. Anaesthesia and Analgesia 52: 447-452
Lowenstein E, Hallowell P, Levina F H, Duggett W M, Austin G, Laver M B 1969 Cardiovascular response to large doses of morphine in man. New England Journal of Medicine 281: 1389–1393
Lowenstein E, Philbin D M 1983 Narcotic anaesthesia clinics. Anesthesiology 1: 5–15
McDonald R K, Evans F T, Weise V K, Patrick R W 1959 Effect of morphine and nalorphine on plasma hydrocortisone levels in man. Journal of Pharmacology and Experimental Therapeutics 125: 241–245
McQuay H J, Moore R E, Paterson G M C, Adams A P, 1979 Plasma fentanyl concentrations and clinical observations during and after operation. British Journal of Anaesthesia 515: 543–550
Magruder M R, Delaney R D, Difazio C A 1982 Reversal of narcotic-induced respiratory depression with nalbuphine hydrochloride. Anesthesiology 9: 34–37
Mark J B, Greenberg L M 1983 Intraoperative awareness and hypertensic crisis during high dose fentanyl-diazepam-oxygen anaesthesia. Anaesthesia and Analgesia 62: 698–700
Martin D E, Rosenberg H, Aukburg S F 1982 Low dose fentanyl blunts circulatory responses to tracheal intubation. Anaesthesia and Analgesia 61: 680–684
Martin W R 1967 Opioid antagonists. Pharmacology Review 10: 463–521
Michaels I, Trout J R, Barash P G 1984 In: Estafanous F G (ed) Opiods in Anesthesia. Boston, 256–260
Michaelis L L, Hickey P R, Clark T A 1974 Ventricular irritability associated with the use of naloxone hydrochloride. Journal of Thoracic Surgery 18: 608–614
Moldenhauer C C, Roach G W, Finlayson D C 1985 Nalbuphine antagonism of ventilatory depression following high-dose fentanyl anesthesia. Anesthesiology 62: 647–650
Moller I W, Krantz T, Wandall E, Kehlet H 1985 Effect of alfentanil anaesthesia on the adrenocortical and hyperglycaemic response to abdominal surgery. British Journal of Anaesthesiology 57: 591–594
Munson E S, Saidman L J, Eger E I 1965 Effect of nitrous oxide and morphine on the minimum anaesthetic concentration fluroxene. Anesthesiology 26: 134–139
Mummaneni N, Rao T L, Montoya A 1980 Awareness and recall with high dose fentanyl-oxygen anesthesia. Anaesthesia and Analgesia 59: 948–949
Murphy M R, Hug C C 1982a The enflurane sparing effect of morphine, butorphanol and nalbuphine. Anesthesiology 57: 489–492
Murphy M R, Hug C C 1982b The anesthetic potency of fentanyl in terms of its reduction of enflurane MAC. Anesthesiology 57: 485–488
Muskin W W, Rendell-Baker L 1949 Pethidine as a supplement to nitrous oxide anaesthesia. British Medical Journal 2: 472
Neff W, Mayer E C, De La Luz Perales M 1947 Nitrous oxide and oxygen anaesthesia with curare relaxation. California Medicine 66: 67–69
Patschke D, Eberlein H J, Tarnour J, Simmerman G 1977 Antagonism of morphine with naloxone in dogs: cardiomuscular effects with special reference to the coronary circulation. British Journal of Anaesthesia 49: 525–533
Philbin D M, Moss J, Akins C W 1981 The use of H_1 and H_2 histamine antagonists with morphine anesthesia. Anesthesiology 55: 292–296

Prough D S, Roy R, Bumgarner J, Shannon G 1984 Acute pulmonary oedema in healthy teenagers following conservative doses of IV naloxone. Anesthesiology 60: 485–486
Rifat K 1972 Pentazocine in sequential analgesic anaesthesia. British Journal of Anaesthesia 44: 175–182
Robbins B H, 1958 Cyclopropane anaesthesia, 2nd ed. Williams and Wilkins, Baltimore
Robbins B H, Baxter J H, Fitzhugh D G 1939 Studies of cyclopropane V. The effect of morphine, barbital and amytal upon the concentration of cyclopropane in the blood required for anesthesia and respiratory arrest. Journal of Pharmacology and Experimental Therapeutics
Roison M F 1984 Does choice of anesthetic (narcotic versus inhalational) significantly affect cardiovascular outcome after cardiovascular surgery? In: Estafanous F G (ed) Opioids in Anesthesia. p 180–189
Roison M F, Horrigan R W, Frazer B M 1981 Anesthetic doses blocking adrenorgic (stress) and cardiovascular responses to incision-MAC-BAR. Anesthesiology 54: 390–398
Romagnoli A, Keats A S 1980 Ceiling effect for respiratory depression by nalbuphine. Clinical Pharmacology and Therapeutics 27: 478–485
Rolly G, Kay B, Cock X 1979 A double blind comparison of high doses of fentanyl and sufentanil in man. Acta Anaesthesiologica Belgica 30: 247–254
Rosow C E, Moss J Philbin D M, Saverese J J 1982 Histamine release during morphine and fentanyl anaesthesia. Anesthesiology 56: 93–96
Ruben H, Andreassen 1951 Pharmacological effects of pethidine on the larynx seen during intubation. British Journal of Anaesthesia 23: 33–38
Saidman L J, Eger E I 1964 Effect of nitrous oxide and of narcotic premedication on the alveolar concentration of halothane required for anesthesia. Anesthesiology 25: 302–306
Schmidt J F, Chraemmer J, Orgensen B, Pederson J E, Risbo A 1985 Postoperative pain relief with naloxone. Severe respiratory depression and pain after high dose buprenorphine. Anaesthesia 40: 583–586
Schrier R I 1982 Narcotic analgesics for preoperative and postoperative medication. In: Kitahata L M (ed) Narcotic Analgesics in Anesthesiology. Williams and Wilkins, Baltimore, p 177–187
Seevers M H, Meek W J, Rovenstine E A, Stiles J A 1934 A study of cyclopropane anesthesia with especial reference to gas concentrations, respiratory and electrocardiographic changes. Journal of Pharmacology and Experimental Therapeutics 51: 1–17
Siker E S 1956 Analgesic supplements to nitrous oxide anaesthesia. British Medical Journal 2: 1326–1331
Smith R R 1908 Scopolamine-morphine anaesthesia. Surgeries in Gynaecology and Obstetrics 7: 414–420
Smith T C 1984 Opioid reversal and postoperative narcotic analgesia. In: Estafanous F G (ed) Opioids in Anaesthesia. Butterworths, Boston, p 297–301
Stambaugh J E 1982 Evaluation of nalbuphine. Current Therapeutic Research 31: 393–401
Stanley T H 1983 High dose fentanyl. Mt Sinai Journal of Medicine 50: 308–311
Stanley T H, Gray: N H, Stanford W, Armstrong R 1973 The effects of high-dose morphine on fluid and blood requirements in open heart procedures. Anesthesiology 38: 536–541
Stanley T H, Isern-Amaral J, Gray N H, Patton C P 1974 Comparison of blood requirements during morphine and halothane anaesthesia for open-heart surgery. Anesthesiology 41: 34–38
Stanley T H, Webster L R 1978 Anesthetic requirements and cardiovascular effects of fentanyl-oxygen and fentanyl-diazepam-oxygen anesthesia in man. Anaesthesia and Analgesia 57: 411–416
Stoelting R K, Creasser C E, Gibbs P S 1974 Circulatory effects of halothane added to morphine anaesthesia in patients with coronary artery disease. Anaesthesia and analgesia 53: 445–449
Tammisto T, Tigersted I 1979 Restlessness and shivering after naloxone reversal of fentanyl-supplemented anaesthesia. Acta Anaesthesiologica Scandinavica 23: 51–56
Tanaka G Y 1974 Hypertensive reaction to naloxone. Journal of American Medical Association 228: 25–26
Taylor H E, Doerr J C, Gharib A 1957 Effect of preanesthetic medication on ether content of arterial blood required for surgical anaesthesia. Anesthesiology 18: 849
Waters R M, Schmidt E R 1934 Cyclopropane anaesthesia. Journal of the American Medical Association 103: 975–983
Wong K C 1983 Narcotics are not expected to produce unconsciouness and amnesia. Anaesthesia and Analgesia 62: 625–626
Wong K C, Martin W E, Hornbein T F 1973 The cardiovascular effects of morphine sulfate with oxygen and with nitrous oxide in man. Anesthesiology 38: 542–549
Wood A J T, Moir D C, Campbell C 1974 Medicines, evaluation and monitoring group: central nervous system effects of pentazocine. British Medical Journal 1: 305–307
Woodbridge P D 1957 Changing concepts concerning depth of anaesthesia. Anesthesiology 18: 536–550

Recovery from neuromuscular blockade

INTRODUCTION

Many anaesthetists administer an anticholinesterase at the end of an operation to reverse the effects of non-depolarising neuromuscular blockade as otherwise the relaxant might still be occupying a variable but possibly significant number of receptor sites. In the absence of neuromuscular monitoring, the anaesthetist often equates neuromuscular function with tests of muscle strength such as head raising, hand grip strength and eye opening, or with respiratory measurements such as tidal volume, respiratory rate or inspiratory and expiratory airway pressures. Unfortunately tidal volume and respiratory rate are influenced by a number of factors unrelated to neuromuscular function, and the presence of spontaneous breathing is in itself no guarantee of adequate recovery from neuromuscular blockade (Ali et al 1975). Competitive neuromuscular blocking agents have been shown to have a sparing effect on the muscles of respiration compared with peripheral muscles (Foldes et al 1961, Johansen et al 1964, Gal & Smith 1976, Wymore & Eisele 1978) so that spontaneous breathing can occur in the presence of marked peripheral neuromuscular blockade. Although gas exchange may be satisfactory in a patient whose airway is safeguarded by an endotracheal tube, this degree of recovery may not leave enough margin of safety for an extubated patient who subsequently develops an obstructed airway. Two studies have questioned the adequacy of anaesthetists' clinical judgement. Harrison (1978) carried out a retrospective survey of anaesthetic deaths in his hospital in South Africa and found that 10 out of 53 were due to inadequate respiration following myoneural blockade. More recently Viby Mogensen (1979) used a nerve stimulator to assess patients post-operatively. These patients, who had been returned to the ward, had all been judged by the anaesthetist on clinical grounds to be adequately 'reversed'. He found that 42% of patients had a train of four ratio less than 0.7, and concluded that residual paralysis remained a problem in patients who had not been quantitatively assessed.

Neuromuscular monitoring

The need has evolved for precise monitoring during routine anaesthesia to reduce the risk of residual paralysis. The simplest method is to stimulate a peripheral nerve and

*'Reversal' — more correctly reversal of the neuromuscular blocking action of the drug but 'reversed' or 'reversal' appear to be in *common* usage.

quantify the response of the muscle supplied by that nerve before and after the administration of a neuromuscular blocking agent. The ulnar nerve at the wrist is often chosen because of ease of access, and following supramaximal stimulation the response of the adductor pollicis muscle is measured. The twitch response is a relatively insensitive test as 75–80% of receptors have to be occupied before there is any diminution of the control height (Paton & Waud 1967). The sensitivity can be increased by using tetanic stimulation at 50 Hz (Gissen & Katz 1969) or a train of four at 2 Hz (Ali et al 1970). A few studies have correlated tests of neuromusclar function with adequacy of ventilation and clinical signs of recovery. Walts and colleagues (1970) concluded that sustained muscular contraction in response to tetanic stimulation at 30 Hz for 5 seconds was useful because it correlated with 90% recovery of vital capacity in human volunteers. They concluded that head raising was unreliable as it did not return to control but perhaps this is because head raising is a more sensitive test. Johansen et al (1964) found that head lift and hand grip strength were 38% and 48% of control when both inspiratory and expiratory flow rates were more than 90% of control. Ali & Kitz (1973) found that when the vital capacity was more than 90%, tetanus at 50 Hz was fully sustained and the mean train of four ratio was 75% following block with tubocurarine and this ratio was found to be lower in conscious volunteers who fulfilled similar criteria (60%) (Ali et al 1975). Thus the train of four may be a more sensitive test of neuromuscular function than the tetanus performed at frequencies up to 50 Hz and the ratio need not recover to unity to be judged adequate. Miller (1976) collated data from several studies and suggested that the sensitivities of the tests were head lift > hand grip > inspiratory force, inspiratory and expiratory flow and normal train of four > sustained tetanus at 30 Hz,and normal vital capacity > normal tidal volume and twitch height. He concluded that even when the test was normal it could not be assumed that all receptors were free of relaxant. This underlines the importance of achieving the maximum possible recovery of neuromuscular function at the end of surgery.

Observation of the single twitch is not particularly useful as observer memory of the control twitch response may be unreliable. The train of four is independent of the control and therefore might be more useful. However, evaluation of the ratio of the train of four using a simple peripheral nerve stimulator even in expert hands is poor (Savarese & Ali 1977, Viby Mogensen et al 1983). A more precise evaluation can be obtained using a force transducer with recording apparatus (Ali & Savarese 1976). This provides both a record for the control single twitch and allows detailed analyses of fade of the tetanus or train of four. Alternatively the EMG can be recorded and simple EMG devices are now available which provide an analogue reading of the compound electromyogram with a meter display of the assessment of block (Lam et al 1981). Close correlation between this EMG measurement and that of the force transducer has recently been found for single twitch and train of four modes (Windsor et al 1985). These workers confirmed the increased accuracy of this method of monitoring over the simple nerve stimulator. It should be remembered that for equivalent degrees of depression of the single twitch response, the degree of fade of the train of four (or tetanus) will vary with different drugs as each drug has its own individual profile (Williams et al 1980). Hence the place of the ratio of the train of four as a measure of neuromuscular function has yet to be defined.

An assessment of the degree of neuromuscular block present during anaesthesia is important since the reversal agent is more effective if there is already some degree of spontaneous recovery (Katz 1967a, 1971, Kopman 1979). Thus Katz (1971) noted that if the twitch height was less than 20% of control following neuromuscular blockade with pancuronium, reversal with neostigmine could take 30 minutes. However, if the twitch height was at least 20–25% of control then reversal could be accomplished in under 10 minutes. The recovery time following neuromuscular blockade with atracurium and vecuronium has been shown to be considerably reduced (Baird et al 1982, Baird & Kerr 1983).

Neuromuscular function

During neuromuscular transmission, acetylcholine released from the nerve ending diffuses across the neuromuscular junction to the motor endplate where it brings about depolarization. It is then hydrolysed to choline and acetate by the action of acetylcholinesterase which is probably not a structural component of either the pre- or post-junctional membrane but rather coats them both. This reaction is completed within milliseconds and enables the endplate to become rapidly repolarized and responsive to subsequent nerve impulses at physiological rates up to 50 Hz. It has been estimated that at least 10 active acetylcholinesterase sites are available for each molecule of acetylcholine released. This explains the efficiency of destruction.

ANTICHOLINESTERASES

A single molecule of acetylcholinesterase appears to contain six binding and hydrolytic sites for acetylcholine (Wright & Plummer 1973). Each active centre consists of two subsites: one is known as the anionic site and bears an overall negative charge which binds the positively charged end of the acetylcholine molecule and orientates it properly for hydrolysis; the other is known as the esteratic site and is responsible for the actual cleavage of the molecule. Drugs that inhibit or inactivate acetylcholinesterase are called anticholinesterases and those currently available for their anti-relaxant action at the neuromuscular junction are neostigmine, pyriodostigmine and edrophonium. They act either by reversible occupation of the active site of the enzyme, e.g. edrophonium, or by acylation of the esteratic site, e.g. carbamates (physostigmine, pyridostigmine and neostigmine) and organophophates. Whereas edrophonium has a brief duration of action presumably owing to its reversible attachment and subsequent rapid renal clearance, deacylation of carbamylated and phosphorylated acetylcholinesterase takes longer and until this has taken place the enzyme is inhibited. Both neostigmine and pyridostigmine form the same carbamylated enzyme: thus the duration of enzyme inhibition produced by these drugs is the same and exceeds that produced by edrophonium.

There is still uncertainty as to whether the effect on neuromuscular transmission is due to inhibition of acetylcholinesterase. Hobbiger (1976), in a comprehensive review of the subject, classified only the carbamates as anticholinesterases as it was more difficult to show that the in vivo action of the 3- and 4-hydroxyanilinium ions, e.g. edrophonium, was the result of acetylcholinesterase inhibition. They are classed as anticholinesterases for the purpose of this review to distinguish them from other drugs with facilitatory actions at the neuromuscular junction whose mechanisms of action do not necessarily involve acetylcholinesterase inhibition. These drugs include guanidine, tetraethylammonium and 4-aminopyridine, all of which increase the prejunctional output of acetylcholine by blocking ion channels: they have been tried with varying degrees of success in disorders in which the output is absolutely or relatively low.

Actions of anticholinesterases

Much of the present controversy about the mode and site of action of anticholinesterases is attributable to the widely held view that the role of acetylcholinesterase is confined to terminating the action of acetylcholine at the postsynaptic membrane. Experimental evidence suggests that this is not the case and that when acetylcholinesterase is inhibited, acetylcholine gains access to nerve terminals and exerts actions there. The classic facilitatory effects of anticholinesterases were originally described by Brown and colleagues (1936). They showed that after physostigmine administration a single indirect stimulus produced repetitive firing in the muscle. Masland & Wigton (1940) reproduced these results with neostigmine. This repetitive firing increases the twitch tension (Feng & Li 1941). Not only does the muscle action potential become repetitive but so does the nerve action potential and this can be recorded antidromically. These nerve action potentials are associated with fasciculations which are a characteristic finding after anticholinesterase treatment in resting muscles (Masland & Wigton 1940, Feng & Li 1941, Eccles 1942, Riker & Wescoe 1946, Boyd & Martin 1956, Meer & Meeter 1956, Blaber & Goode 1968). The period of transmitter release is prolonged by anticholinesterases (Hubbard & Schmidt 1961). Probably the most satisfactory explanation for this repetitive firing is the existence of acetylcholine receptors at the prejunctional membrane (Werner 1960, Hubbard & Schmidt 1961). It seems that after acetylcholinesterase inhibition, acetylcholine can reach and excite presynaptic receptors on nerve endings not normally affected. As the most terminal part of the nerve ending is resistant to depolarization (Hubbard et al 1965, Blaber & Goode 1968) the cholinoceptors in question are probably located more centrally at the first node of Ranvier as illustrated in Figure 18.1. One of the physiological roles of junctional acetylcholinesterase may be to protect these receptors from effects of acetylcholine.

Repetitive firing following stimulus evoked action potentials disappears at stimulation frequencies more than 2 Hz and is not important in voluntary movements. The main effect of anticholinesterases on normal unblocked muscle is to cause paralysis partly by producing depolarizing block from a postsynaptic action of acetylcholine, and perhaps partly by a reduction in acetylcholine release which probably accounts for tetanic fade (Barnes & Duff 1953, Blaber & Bowman 1963a, Bowman 1980). It is only when neuromuscular transmission is impaired by drugs such as tubocurarine or in myasthenia gravis that anticholinesterases lead to facilitation.

Anticurare action

Whilst it is widely accepted that the anticurare action of anticholinesterase drugs is due to inhibition of acetylcholinesterase which allows the accumulation of

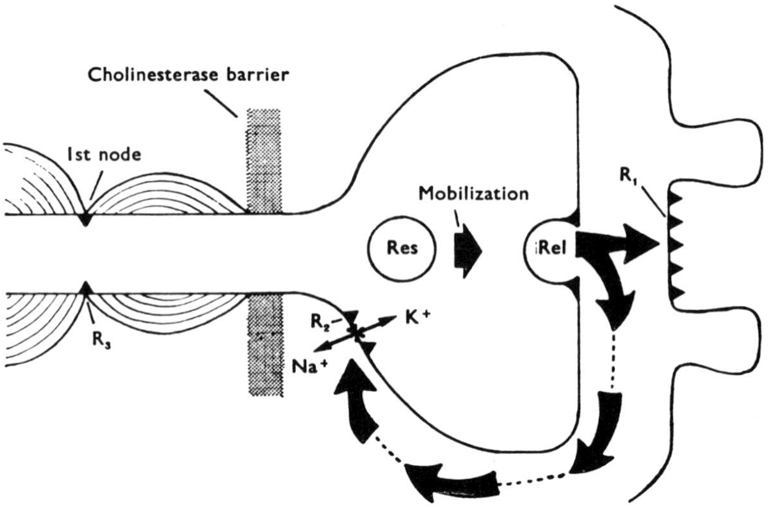

Fig 18.1 Postulated sites of cholinoceptors at the neuromuscular junction (W. C. Bowman). R_1 represents the post-junctional cholinoceptors that mediate the production of the epp when acetylcholine combines with them. R_2 represents hypothetical cholinoceptors on the nerve terminal membrane. Stimulation of these cholinoceptors by transmitter acetylcholine hastens mobilization of reserve acetylcholine (Res) into the readily releasable store (Rel), thereby maintaining transmitter output during high frequencies of stimulation. Block of the R_2 receptors results in tetanic fade. Different antagonists have different relative affinities for the R_1 and R_2 cholinoceptors. R_3 represents hypothetical cholinoceptors at the first node of Ranvier. These are normally protected from transmitter acetylcholine by a cholinesterase barrier, but they may be stimulated after cholinesterase inhibition producing localized depolarization that generates propogating action potentials which travel in both directions from the site of initiation.

transmitter in the synaptic gap, there is disagreement about the site or sites at which this additional acetylcholine exerts its anticurare effect (MacLagen 1976). Most workers subscribe to the view that anticurare action is a postsynaptic effect due to the increased concentration of acetylcholine competing with the antagonist for cholinoceptors. The other possible explanation involves a presynaptic mechanism resulting in an increase in the acetylcholine output from the nerve terminals, which would have exactly the same anticurare effect. This argument rests on whether it can be shown conclusively that anticholinesterase drugs are capable of increasing the quantal content of the end plate potential either by a direct presynaptic action or via a presynaptic action of the excess acetylcholine itself (Riker et al 1957, 1959, Blaber & Bowman 1959, Blaber & Christ 1967, Hobbiger 1976). Blaber (1970, 1972, 1973) showed that tubocurarine reduced the rate of refilling of the acetylcholine store in nerve terminals and demonstrated that edrophonium, in the cat, could reverse this tubocurarine induced reduction in the rate of refilling of the acetylcholine store.

Physostigmine

Physostigmine was originally obtained from the Calaber bean in West Africa and brought to England in 1840. In 1895 Jolly noted the resemblance between the signs of myasthenia and those of tubocurarine poisoning in animals and suggested that physostigmine (already known to antagonise tubocurarine) might be of therapeutic value. However it was nearly 40 years later before Mary Walker reported its successful use in myasthenia gravis in 1934, and then in 1935 reported that neostigmine was more effective. Physostigmine has been shown to antagonize non-depolarizing block in animals but the result was disappointing in humans (Baraka 1978). Its lipid solubility and consequent ability to cross the blood-brain barrier causing excitant effects is the reason for its application in the reversal of general anaesthesia. It is not used in an anticurare agent.

Neostigmine

This is the agent widely used in the UK for reversal of neuromuscular blockade. It is used in a dose range 2.5–5 mg. A number of isolated cases of cardiac arrest occurred following its use (Clutton Brock 1949, MacIntosh 1949) and these were attributed to the bradycardia associated with its muscarinic action. These reports led to the practice of always giving atropine prior to neostigmine, but Kemp & Morton (1962) demonstrated that in healthy patients a mixture of atropine 1.2 mg and neostigmine 2.5 mg did not cause bradycardia. This was attributed to the fact that atropine acted within 25 to 45 seconds whereas neostigmine took 100 seconds. Kjellberg & Tammisto (1970) confirmed these findings.

Pyridostigmine

Pyridostigmine is an analogue of neostigmine with one-quarter of its potency so that 10 mg pyridostigmine is equivalent to 2.5 mg neostigmine. Katz (1967b) concluded that it exhibited fewer muscarinic effects on the bowel and myocardium than neostigmine although Fogdall & Miller (1973) found there was no difference. It has been shown to have a slower onset and a longer duration of action than neostigmine as well as a greater therapeutic ratio (Miller et al 1974).

Edrophonium

Edrophonium has not been widely used as an anticurare agent in this country because of its apparently short duration of action, unreliable antagonism and the possibility of recurarization (Artusio et al 1950, MacFarlane et al 1950, Doughty & Wyllie 1952, Hunter 1952, Nastuk & Alexander 1954, Katz 1967, Sugai & Payne 1975). Some of these reports of unsustained and unreliable reversal may have been the result of inadequate dosage (10–20 mg) or imprecise/lack of monitoring of neuromuscular function. Recent studies measuring the twitch response suggest that in higher dosage (0.5–1.0 mg/kg) the duration of action of edrophonium is almost the same as neostigmine. In equiantagonistic doses the duration of antagonism during steady state 90% block of the twitch response was 66 minutes for edrophonium (0.5 mg/kg) and 76 minutes for neostigmine (0.04 mg/kg) (Cronelly et al 1982), while the pharmacokinetic profile of the two drugs has been shown to be very similar (Morris et

*'Curarization' — this implies paralysis with the non-depolarizing drug, D tubocurarine but again the term has crept into usage even when applied to drugs with a similar action.

al 1981). There has therefore been a revival of interest in edrophonium as an anticurare agent.

The importance of cholinesterase inhibition in the mechanism of action of edrophonium is unclear. The anticholinesterase activity of edrophonium has been shown to be less than that of neostigmine (Randall & Lehman 1950, Smith et al 1957) and muscarinic side-effects of edrophonium are less obvious which supports this finding. However, inhibition of acetylcholinesterase by a reversible inhibitor is probably not comparable to that produced by acylating anticholinesterases. As stated above, part of the anticurare action of edrophonium may involve an increase in the quantal release of acetylcholine. In the clinical situation Donati et al (1983) examined the ratio of the train of four when the first twitch was less than 70% of control during the antagonism of pancuronium blockade using neostigmine and edrophonium. They found the highest ratio after edrophonium, and concluded that it was a more effective antagonist at the presynaptic receptor than the other two drugs. If the train of four ratio reflects only presynaptic effects, then these results would support a presynaptic predominance for edrophonium. However, the results of dose response studies are confusing. Dose response curves for edrophonium during antagonism of a steady state tubocurarine induced neuromuscular block are not parallel to those obtained after neostigmine or pyridostigmine, suggesting different mechanisms of action (Cronelly et al 1982), but are parallel to those obtained with neostigmine after a bolus dose of pancuronium (Breen et al 1985). If these drugs have different mechanisms of action, then combining edrophonium and pyridostigmine or neostigmine might be expected to potentiate reversal. The possibility that combinations of anticholinesterases may work synergistically has been studied but so far results have been disappointing (Bevan et al 1984, Cronelly & Miller 1984).

Efficacy as anticurare agents

Large doses of edrophonium (0.5–1.4 mg/kg) produce adequate and sustained reversal of neuromuscular block provided that some spontaneous recovery of neuromuscular function has occurred. Bevan (1979), Kopman (1979), Ferguson et al (1980), Morris et al (1981) and Cronelly et al (1982) have demonstrated satisfactory reversal of pancuronium and tubocurarine blockade once the twitch response had recovered to 5–10% of control. This has also been noted following vecuronium (Baird et al 1982) and atracurium (Baird & Kerr 1983, Jones et al 1984).

As an anticurare agent edrophonium has a quicker onset of action than neostigmine and pyridostigmine (Ferguson et al 1980, Cronelly et al 1982, Jones et al 1984, Astley et al 1986). This may be due to the initial rapid release of acetylcholine from the motor nerve terminal or it may be related to the size of the molecule. Ramzan (1982) postulated that the difference in speed of onset of any two drugs was proportional to the rate of diffusion of the cation through the plasma, and since the molecular weight of edrophonium is 166 compared to 223 for neostigmine, it may diffuse more rapidly to its site of action. Bevan (1979) proposed that atropine should be administered 30–60 s before the edrophonium to block the undesirable muscarinic side-effects. However, these effects are less pronounced following the use of edrophonium than with neostigmine (Randall 1950, Baird et al 1982, Cronelly et al 1982). Whether this is due to the fact that edrophonium is not constantly in combination with the acetylcholinesterase enzyme or that its anticholinesterase properties are weak is not clear.

When attempts are made to reverse patients with no apparent recovery of neuromuscular function the outcome is often unsatisfactory and protracted. Neostigmine may be preferable to edrophonium under these circumstances. Katz (1967b) noticed that whereas neostigmine could reverse patients with no twitch response this was not always possible after edrophonium. He had used a small dose of edrophonium (10 mg) which may have accounted for his results, but more recent experiments (Rupp et al 1984) have confirmed this disappointing result with edrophonium when compared to the action of neostigmine. In our experiments we have monitored twitch and tetanic responses simultaneously during antagonism with edrophonium of atracurium induced neuromuscular blockade. We found that recovery of the twitch response after reversal with edrophonium, although longer than that with neostigmine, was still facilitated but that recovery of the tetanic response was unsustained (Fig 18.2). The recovery of the tetanic response of patients reversed in this way was not significantly different from control patients recovering spontaneously from the same dose of atracurium. The recovery of the tetanic response of patients reversed with neostigmine was significantly faster than the control group. One explanation of this failure may be that edrophonium depleted the acetylcholine stores as a result of increased prejunctional output and at high frequencies of stimulation mobilization could not be maintained.

In anaesthetized patients renal excretion accounts for 75% of the clearance of pyridostigmine, 70% of the clearance of edrophonium and 50% of the clearance of neostigmine (Conelly et al 1979, Morris et al 1981). Thus, in patients with impaired renal function excretion of these drugs is decreased and, in fact, this decrease has been shown to be greater than the corresponding decrease for pancuronium and tubocurarine (Miller et al 1977, Somogyii et al 1977). Reports of 'recurarization' in anephric patients are therefore probably not due to the muscle relaxant outlasting the antagonist.

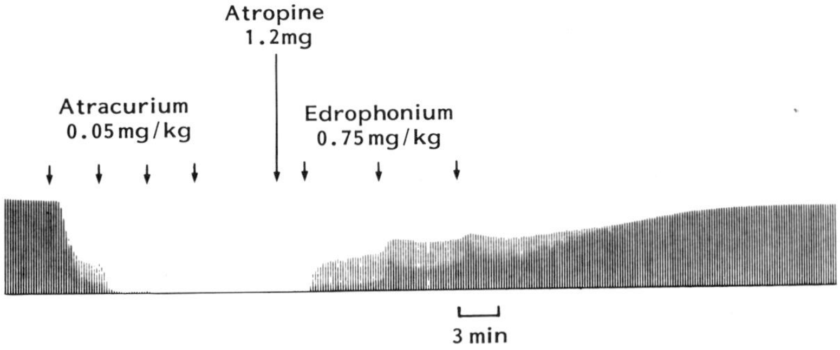

Fig 18.2 Tetanic response following neuromuscular blockade with incremental dose atracurium. The patient was reversed with edrophonium 0.75 mg/kg from 100% block of the tetanic response. Note the initial improvement in tetanic height and tetanic fade, followed immediately by worsening of both. The recovery of the tetanic response of patients reversed in this way did not differ significantly from control patients.

A certain degree of caution is necessary when using reversal agents. Perhaps the term 'recurarization' is not always correct as it is possible under certain circumstances to reintroduce neuromuscular block with anticholinesterases. The neuromuscular blocking properties of neostigmine have been known for many years (Briscoe 1936, Goodman & Gilman 1956, Blaber & Bowman 1963b, Payne et al 1980). If in the absence of neuromuscular monitoring neuromuscular function has recovered it is possible to reintroduce neuromuscular block with both neostigmine and edrophonium. The block so introduced following neostigmine can last for up to 20 minutes (Fig. 18.3). This is long enough to be clinically significant and may be the explanation for some reports of neostigmine resistant curarization. Payne et al (1980) found that although a single dose of 5 mg of neostigmine given to antagonize competitive neuromuscular block could result in neuromuscular block, it was more pronounced after two doses of 2.5 mg of neostigmine. In contrast, neuromuscular block reintroduced under the same conditions following edrophonium (Fig 18.4) is not as constant and is much shorter in duration (of the order of 3 minutes).

The reintroduction of neuromuscular block appears to depend upon the dose of anticholinesterase, the dose of muscle relaxant (more obvious with small doses), the individual relaxant (more likely after the shorter acting drugs) and the degree of spontaneous recovery already present when the anticholinesterase is administered. This neuromuscular block becomes more obvious at faster rates of stimulation (Briscoe 1937) and in practical terms means that it is only evident after tetanic

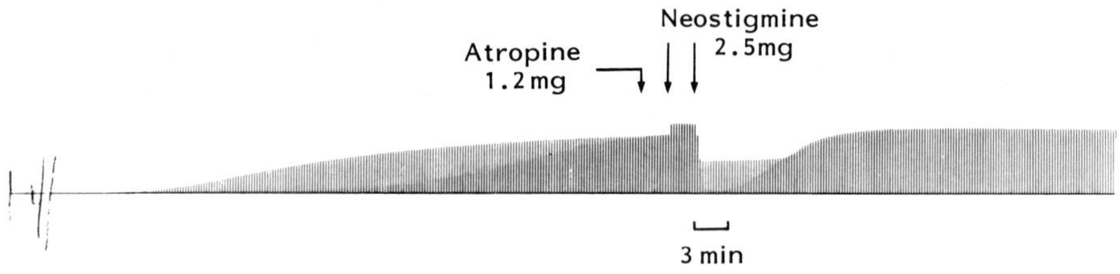

Fig 18.3 Tetanic response following neuromuscular blockade with 0.08 mg/kg of vecuronium. The patient was given neostigmine twice at a time when recovery was almost complete (note absence of tetanic fade). There was improvement of neuromuscular function after the first dose. After the second dose however tetanic height fell and tetanic fade was reintroduced which in this patient took longer than 15 min to recover.

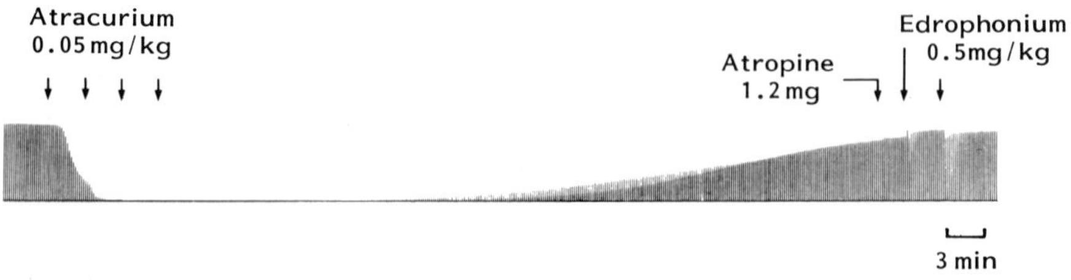

Fig 18.4 Tetanic response following neuromuscular block with incremental atracurium. This patient received edrophonium 0.5 mg/kg twice when recovery was almost complete. Note the initial and immediate facilitation after the first dose followed quickly by a fall in tetanic height associated with the reintroduction of fade. This deterioration is deeper and more persistant after the second dose, but still lasts less than 3 min.

stimulation so that if the twitch response is examined this effect is missed. Payne et al (1980) concluded that if recovery of the tetanic response had reached 50%, then a single dose of reversal agent should be sufficient to provide adequate reversal and further doses could result in block. The neuromuscular block seen following edrophonium is probably not clinically significant. We have failed to demonstrate neuromuscular block after pyridostigmine when given to reverse competitive neuromuscular blockade. The fact that fade is demonstrable after edrophonium suggests that in fact its mode of action may be similar to that of neostigmine.

The facilitatory drug 4-aminopyridine potentiates the effects of neostigmine and pyridostigmine in animals and man in doses smaller than those producing antagonism of neuromuscular blockade (Booij et al 1978, Miller et al 1979). Booij et al (1980) have reported the successful use of 4-aminopyridine alone in the reversal of vecuronium induced blockade. However, the central nervous stimulation that occurs may limit its use as a sole antagonist but if used in combination with an anticholinesterase it does reduce the atropine requirement (Miller et al 1979).

CONCLUSION

Following the recent introduction of two competitive neuromuscular blocking agents of medium duration, atracurium and vecuronium, antagonism of neuromuscular block can be achieved more quickly and reliably than by following block after drugs with a longer duration of action. However, the duration of action of three times the ED95 dose of both drugs has been shown to be approximately 1 hour (Agoston 1980, Payne & Hughes 1981, Basta 1982, Fragen 1982, Katz 1982), and therefore after short surgical procedures reversal is advisable. This is especially important if there is no recovery area, a situation that regrettably still exists in many hospitals (Lunn & Mushin 1982). Reversal is also advised after the use of longer acting agents. However, if neuromuscular monitoring indicates good recovery of function and there are trained staff to supervise the patient in the immediate post-operative period, then reversal after neuromuscular block with either atracurium or vecuronium is not obligatory as the offset of these two drugs in comparison with other competitive neuromuscular blocking agents is so rapid. Edrophonium acts more quickly than neostigmine, requires less atropine, and is associated with a smaller risk of reintroduction of block of any clinical significance, but is less effective when there is no apparent recovery of neuromuscular function. Neostigmine is more effective under these circumstances but its administration may result in neuromuscular block if repeated doses are given to a patient who has already recovered. Our preliminary results with pyridostigmine suggest that its efficacy as an anticurare agent lies between edrophonium and neostigmine, with less propensity to produce neuromuscular block in its own right.

Clinical assessment of the adequacy of neuromuscular function is notoriously inaccurate (Harrison 1978, Viby Mogensen et al 1979), but neuromuscular monitoring now offers the opportunity for a proper assessment of neuromuscular function. It is to be hoped that further advances in this field will enable the anaesthetist to reverse neuromuscular blockade quickly, without risk to the patient.

REFERENCES

Agoston S, Salt P, Newton D, Bencini A, Boomsma P, Erdmann W 1980 The neuromuscular blocking action of Org NC45 a new pancuronium derivative in anaesthetised patients. British Journal of Anaesthesia 52:53S
Ali H H, Kitz R J 1973 Evaluation of recovery from non-depolarizing neuromuscular block using a digital neuromuscular transmission analyser. Anaesthesia and Analgesia 52: 740–743
Ali H H, Savarese J J 1976 Monitoring of neuromuscular function. Anesthesiology 45: 216–242
Ali H H, Utting J E, Gray C 1970 Stimulus frequency in the detection of neuromuscular block in humans. British Journal of Anaesthesia 42: 967–977
Ali H H, Wilson R S, Savarese J J, Kitz R J 1975 The effect of tubocurarine on the indirectly elicited train of four muscle response and respiratory measurement in humans. British Journal of Anaesthesia 47: 570–573
Artusio J F, Riker W F, Wescoe W C 1950 Studies on the interrelationship of certain cholinergic compounds. Journal of Pharmacology and Experimental Therapeutics 100: 227–236
Astley B A, Hughes R, Payne J P 1986 Antagonism of atracurium induced neuromuscular blockade by neostigmine or edrophonium. British Journal of Anaesthesia 58: 1290–1295
Baird W L M, Bowman W C, Kerr W J 1982 Some actions of OrgNC45 and of edrophonium in the anaesthetised cat and in man. British Journal of Anaesthesia 54: 375–384
Baird W L M, Kerr W J 1983 Reversal of atracurium with edrophonium. A pilot study in man. British Journal of Anaesthesia 55: 63S
Baraka A 1978 Antagonism of neuromuscular block by physostigmine in man. British Journal of Anaesthesia 50: 1075–1076
Barnes J M, Duff J I 1953 The role of cholinesterase at the myoneural junction. British Journal of Pharmacology 8: 334–339
Basta S J et al 1982 Clinical pharmacology of atracurium besylate. A new nondepolarising muscle relaxant. Anesthesia and Analgesia 61: 723–729
Bevan D R 1979 Reversal of Pancuronium with edrophonium. Anaesthesia 34: 614–619
Bevan D R, Doherty W G, Breen P J, Donati F 1984 Mixtures of neostigmine and edrophonium are not synergistic. Anesthesiology 61: A298
Blaber L C 1970 The effect of facilitatory concentrations of decamethonium on the storage and release of transmitter at the neuromuscular junction of the cat. Journal of Pharmacology and Experimental Therapeutics 175: 664–672
Blaber L C 1972 The mechanism of the facilitatory action of edrophonium in the cat. British Journal of Pharmacology 46: 498–507
Blaber L C 1973 The prejunctional actions of some nondepolarising blocking drugs. British Journal of Pharmacology 47: 109–116
Blaber L C, Bowman W C 1959 A comparison between the effects of edrophonium and choline in the skeletal muscles of the cat. British Journal of Pharmacology 14: 456–466
Blaber L C, Bowman W C 1963a The effects of some drugs on the repetitive discharges produced in nerve and muscle by anticholinesterases. International Journal of Neuropharmacology 2: 1–16
Blaber L C, Bowman W C 1963b Studies on the repetitive discharges evoked in motor nerve and skeletal muscle after injections of anticholinesterase drugs. British Journal of Pharmacology 20: 326–344
Blaber L C, Christ D D 1967 The action of facilitatory drugs on the isolated tenuissimus muscles of the cat. International Journal of Neuropharmacology 6: 473–484
Blaber L C, Goode J W 1968 A comparison of the action of facilitatory and depolarising drugs at the mammalian motor nerve terminal. International Journal of Neuropharmacology 7: 429–440
Booij L H D J, Miller R D, Crul J F 1978 Neostigmine and 4-aminopyridine antagonism of lincomycin and pancuronium neuromuscular blockade. Anesthesia and Analgesia 57: 316–321
Booij L H D J, Van Der Pol F, Crul J F, Miller R D 1980 Antagonism of Org NC45 neuromuscular blockade by neostigmine, pyridostigmine and 4-aminopyridine. Anaesthesia and Analgesia 59: 31–34
Bowman W C 1980 Pharmacology of neuromuscular function. Wright, Bristol, ch 3 p 18
Boyd I A, Martin A R 1956 The endplate potential in mammalian muscle. Journal of Physiology 132: 74–91
Breen P J, Doherty W G, Donati F, Bevan D R 1985 The potencies of edrophonium and neostigmine as antagonists of pancuronium. Anaesthesia 40: 844
Briscoe G 1936 Shift in optimum rate of stimulation due to prostigmin. Journal of Physiology 86: 48P
Briscoe G 1937 Optimum stimulation rates for red and white skeletal mammalian muscles, and shift in rates produced by the eserine group. Journal of Physiology 90: 10P–11P
Brown G L, Dale H H, Feldberg W J 1936 Reactions of the normal mammalian muscle to acetylcholine and to eserine. Journal of Physiology 87: 394–425

Clutton Brock J 1949 Death following neostigmine. British Medical Journal 1: 1007
Cronelly R, Miller R D 1984 Onset and duration of edrophonium-pyridostigmine mixtures. Anesthesiology 61: A301
Cronelly R, Morris R B, Miller R D 1982 Edrophonium: duration of action and atropine requirement in humans during halothane anaesthesia. Anesthesiology 57: 261–266
Cronelly R, Stanski D R, Miller R D, Sheiner L B, Sohn Y J 1979 Renal function and the pharmacokinetics of neostigmine in anaesthetised man. Anesthesiology 51: 222–226
Donati F, Ferguson A, Bevan D R 1983 Twitch depression and train of four ratio after antagonism of pancuronium with edrophonium, pyridostigmine or pyridostigmine. Anesthesia and Analgesia 62: 314–316
Doughty A G, Wylie W D 1952 Antidotes to true curarising agents. British Journal of Anaesthesia 24: 66–80
Eccles J C, Katz B, Kuffler S W 1942 Effects of eserine on neuromuscular transmission. Journal of Neurophysiology 5: 211–230
Feng T P, Li T H 1941 Studies on the neuromuscular junction; a new aspect on the phenomena of eserine potentiation and post tetanic facilitation in mammalian muscles. Chinese Journal of Physiology 16: 37–56
Ferguson A, Egerszegi P, Bevan D R 1980 Neostigmine, pyridostigmine and edrophonium as antagonists of pancuronium. Anesthesiology 53: 390–394
Fogdall R P, Miller R D 1973 Antagonism of tubocurarine and pancuronium induced neuromuscular blockades by pyridostigmine in man. Anesthesiology 39: 504–509
Foldes F F, Monte A P, Brunn H M, Wolfson B 1961 Studies with muscle relaxants in unanaesthetised subjects. Anesthesiology 22: 230–236
Fragen R J, Robertson E N, Booij L H D J, Crul J F 1982 A comparison of vecuronium and atracurium in man. Anesthesiology 57: A253
Gal T J, Smith T C 1976 Partial paralysis with tubocurarine and the ventilatory response to carbon dioxide. Anaesthesiology 45: 22–28
Gissen A J, Katz R L 1969 Twitch, tetanus and post tetanic potentiation as indices of nerve muscle block in man. Anesthesiology 30: 481–487
Harrison G G 1978 Death attributable to anaesthesia. A 10 year survey (1967–1976). British Journal of Anaesthesia 50: 1041–1046
Hobbiger F 1976 Pharmacology of anticholinesterase drugs. In: Zaimis (ed) Handbook of Experimental Pharmacology. Springer-Verlag, Berlin vol 42: ch 4c, p 487
Hubbard J I, Schmidt R F 1961 Stimulation of the motor nerve terminals. Nature 191: 1103–1104
Hubbard J I, Schmidt R F, Yokota T 1965 The effect of acetylcholine upon mammalian motor nerve terminals. Journal of Physiology 181: 810–829
Hunter A 1952 Tensilon: a new anticurare agent. British Journal of Anaesthesia 24: 175–186
Johansen S H, Jorgensen M, Molbech S 1964 Effect of tubocurarine on respiratory and non respiratory muscle power in man. Journal of Applied Physiology 19: 990–994
Jolly F 1895 Pseudoparalysis myasthenica. Neurol. Zbl 14: 34
Jones R M, Pearce A C Williams J P 1984 Recovery characteristics following antagonism of atracurium with neostigmine or edrophonium. British Journal of Anaesthesia 56: 453–456
Katz R L 1967a Neuromuscular effects of tubocucarine, edrophonium and neostigmine in man. Anaesthesiology 28: 327–336
Katz R L 1967b Pyridostigmine (Mestinon) as an antagonist of tubocurarine. Anesthesiology 28: 528–534
Katz R L 1971 Clinical neuromuscular pharmacology of pancuronium. Anaesthesiology 34: 550–556
Katz R L, Stirt J, Murray A L, Lee C 1982 Neuromuscular effects of atracurium in man. Anaesthesia and Analgesia 61: 730–734
Kemp S W, Morton H J V 1962 The effect of atropine and neostigmine on the pulse rate of anaesthetised patients. Anaesthesia 17: 170–175
Kjellberg M, Tammisto T 1970 Heart rate changes after atropine and neostigmine given for the reversion of muscle paralysis. Acta Anaesthesiologies Scandinavica 14: 203
Kopman A 1979 Edrophonium antagonism of pancuronium induced neuromuscular blockade in man. Anesthesiology 51: 139–142
Lam H S, Cass N M, NG KC 1981 Electromyographic monitoring of neuromuscular block. British Journal of Anaesthesia 53: 1351–1356
Lunn J, Mushin W 1982 Mortality associated with anaesthesia. Nuffield Provincial Hospitals Trust
Macfarlane D W, Pelikan E W, Unna K R 1950 Evaluation of curarising drugs in man. Journal of Pharmacology and Experimental Therapeutics 100: 382–392
Macintosh R R 1949 Death following injection of neostigmine. British Medical Journal 1: 852

Maclagen J 1976 Competitive Neuromuscular Blocking Agents. In: Zaimis (ed) Handbook of Experimental Pharmacology. Springer Verlag, Berlin, 42: Ch 4b, p 421
Masland R L, Wigton R S 1940 Nerve activity accompanying fasciculation produced by prostigmin. Journal of Neurophysiology 3: 269–275
Meer C, Meeter E 1956 The mechanism of action of anticholinesterases II. The effect of DFP on the isolated rat phrenic nerve diaphragm preparation. A. Irreversible effects. Acta Physiologica et Pharmalogica Neerlandica 4: 454–471
Miller R D 1976 Antagonism of neuromuscular blockade. Anesthesiology 44: 318–330
Miller R D, Van Nyhuis L S, Eger E I Vitez T S, Way W L 1974 Comparative times to peak effect and durations of action of neostigmine and pyridostigmine. Anesthesiology 41: 27–33
Miller R D, Matteo R S, Benet L Z, Sohn Y J 1977 The pharmacokinetics of tubocurarine in man with and without renal failure. Journal of Pharmacology and Experimental Therapeutics 202: 1–7
Miller R D, Booij L H D J, Agoston S, Crul J F 1979 4 Aminopyridine potentiates neostigmine and pyridostigmine in man. Anesthesiology 50: 416–420
Morris R B, Cronelly R, Miller R D, Stanski D R, Fahey M R 1981 Pharmacokinetics of edrophonium and neostigmine when antagonising tubocurarine neuromuscular blockade in man. Anesthesiology 54: 399–402
Morris R B, Cronelly R, Miller R D, Stanski D R, Fahey M R 1981 Pharmacokinetics of edrophonium in anephric and renal transplant patients. British Journal of Anaesthesia 53: 1311–1313
Nastuk W L, Alexander J T 1954 The actions of 3 hydroxy phenyldimethylethylammonium (tensilon) on neuromuscular transmission in the frog. Journal of Pharmacology and Experimental Therapeutics 111: 302–328
Paton W D M, Waud D R 1967 The margin of safety of neuromuscular transmission. Journal of Physiology 191: 59–90
Payne J P, Hughes R 1981 Evaluation of atracurium in anaesthetised man. British Journal of Anaesthesia 53: 45–54
Payne J P, Hughes R, Al Azawi S 1980 Neuromuscular blockade by neostigmine in anaesthetised man. British Journal of Anaesthesia 52: 69–76
Ramzan I M 1982 Molecular weight of cation as a determinant of speed of onset of neuromuscular blockade. Anesthesiology 57: 247
Randall L O 1950 Anticurare action of phenolic quaternary ammonium salts. Journal of Pharmacology and Experimental Therapeutics 100: 83–93
Randall L O, Lehman G 1950 Pharmacological properties of some neostigmine analogues. Journal of Pharmacology and Experimental Therapeutics 99: 16–32
Riker W F, Roberts J, Standaert F G, Fujimori H 1957 The motor nerve terminal as the primary focus for drug induced facilitation of neuromuscular transmission. Journal of Pharmacology and Experimental Therapeutics 121: 286–312
Riker W F, Werner G, Roberts J, Kuperman A 1959 Pharmacologic evidence for the existence of a presynaptic event in neuromuscular transmission. Journal of Pharmacology and Experimental Therapeutics 125: 150–158
Riker W F, Wescoe W C 1946 The direct action of prostigmine on skeletal muscle. Its relationship to the choline esters. Journal of Pharmacology and Experimental Therapeutics 88: 58–66
Rupp S M, McChristian J W, Miller R D 1984 Neostigmine antagonises a profound neuromuscular block more rapidly than edrophonium. Anesthesiology 61: A297
Savarese J J, Ali H H 1977 Accurate prediction of individual metocurine dosage by clinical observation of the threshold of fade on the train of four stimulation. Meeting of the American Society of Anaesthetists. New Orleans (Abstract)
Smith C M, Mead J C, Unna K R 1957 Antagonism of tubocurarine III. Time course of action of pyridostigmine, neostigmine and edrophonium in vivo and in vitro. Journal of Pharmacology and Experimental Therapeutics 120: 215–228
Somogyi A A, Shanks C A, Triggs E J 1977 The effect of renal failure on the disposition and neuromuscular blocking action of pancuronium bromide. European Journal of Clinical Pharmacology 12: 23–29
Sugai N, Payne J P 1975 The skeletal muscle response to edrophonium during neuromuscular blockade by tubocurarine in anaesthetised man. British Journal of Anaesthesia 47: 1087–1092
Viby Mogensen J, Engbaek J, Jensen N H, Jorgensen B C, Ording H 1983 New developments in clinical monitoring of neuromuscular transmission: monitoring without equipment. Clinical experiences with Norcuron, Symposium. Geneva, p 66–71
Viby Mogensen J, Jorgensen B C, Ording H 1979 Residual curarisation in the recovery room. Anesthesiology 50: 539–541
Walker M B 1934 Treatment of myasthenia gravis with physostigmine. Lancet 1: 1200–1201

Walker M B 1935 Case showing effect of prostigmine on myasthenia gravis. Proceedings of the Royal Society of Medicine 28: 759–761

Walts L F, Levin N, Dillon J B 1970 Assessment of recovery from tubocurarine. Journal of the American Medical Association 213: 1894–1896

Werner G 1960 Neuromuscular facilitation and antidromic discharges in motor nerves and their relation to activity in motor nerve terminals. Journal Neurophysiology 23: 171–187

Williams N E, Webb S N, Calvey T N 1980 Differential effects of myoneural blocking drugs on neuromuscular transmission. British Journal of Anaesthesia 52: 1111–1114

Windsor J P W, Sebel P S, Flynn P J 1985 The neuromuscular transmission monitor. Anaesthesia 40: 146–151

Wright D L, Plummer D T 1973 Multiple forms of acetylcholinesterase from human erythrocytes. Journal of Biochemistry 133: 521–527

Wymore M L, Eisele J H 1978 Differential effects of tubocurarine on inspiratory muscles and two peripheral muscle groups in anaesthetised man. Anesthesiology 48: 360–362

19

L. Kaufman

Pain

INTRODUCTION

The discovery by Kosterlitz and Hughes in 1975 of endogenous peptides that bind to opiate receptors has produced a wealth of literature and started a new era of research accompanied by new terminology (Hughes 1983). It soon became clear that the original concept of one endogenous peptide, endorphin (endogenous morphine), was an over simplification and that many peptides and receptor sites were involved. The abundance of published literature, at times conflicting and intensely stimulating, may have overwhelmed clinicians wandering through the maze of detail. The concepts set out in this synopsis may already have been overtaken by more recent research studies.

Anatomical and physiological aspects of pain perception were reviewed by Jordan (1984), noting the importance of the periaqueductal grey area in the brain and the substantia gelatinosa, a semitranslucent area of grey matter that caps the posterior horn (Kitahata & Collins 1981, Yaksh 1981). Small diameter afferent fibres terminate in lamina one and two of the dorsal horn and this would include C fibres. Laminae one to five appear to accept afferents from A δ and C fibres. The substantia gelatinosa (lamina 2) has a high concentration of opioid receptors, endorphins and substance P and is the region where sensory impulses are modulated. Substance P (not P for pain) is released following stimulation of small primary afferent fibres and this is opposed by the action of endorphins. Intrathecal opiates inhibit the release of substance P. In contrast to local anaesthetics, spinal opioids do not produce motor blockade or hypotension as the sympathetic nerves also appear to be unaffected.

Yaksh & Rudy (1976) demonstrated that intrathecal opioids produced naloxone reversible analgesia in animals. The technique was applied to man for the relief of pain for inoperable carcinoma by Wang et al (1979). The opioid acts at the C and A δ afferent inputs to the 'wide dynamic range' (WDR) cells in the spinal cord which are associated with the transmission of pain. The spinal opioid appears to be particularly effective in suppressing noxious stimuli associated with C fibre stimulation and less effective in blocking A δ afferents which are readily affected by local anaesthetics. This appears to be confirmed clinically when spinal opioids reduce the pain associated with deep sensation but have a reduced effect on the pain of the skin incision which is mediated by A δ fibres. Homma et al (1983) demonstrated that the suppression of WDR neurones was dose dependent and that adrenaline was also capable of exerting a similar effect (Collins et al 1984). Adrenaline in a dose of 10 μg (a fifth of the dose used in previous experiments) applied to the cord had little effect on noxious stimulation but produced significant suppression of WDR neurones following fentanyl administered spinally 30 minutes previously. It was concluded that there was an interaction between α adrenergic drugs and spinal opiates, suggesting that the prolongation of action of the opioid was not due to the vasoconstrictor action of the adrenaline. The neural mechanisms of pain are outlined by Casey (1982) and by Mense (1983).

CLASSIFICATION OF RECEPTORS

Detailed reviews of opioid receptors and endorphins appeared in Anaesthesia Review 3 (Jordan 1985, Pinnock 1985). Martin et al (1976) suggested that there were three receptor sites which would explain some of the actions of opioids. The μ receptor was associated with analgesia, respiratory depression and small pupils. The μ receptor provided analgesia and sedation while the σ receptor was responsible for the psychological effects seen after drugs such as phencyclidine. Other studies suggested that enkephalins acted at δ receptor sites in the brain but the significance of this receptor at the moment appears to be speculative. Other receptors proposed included ϵ (epsilon) and τ, and other unidentified sites (Yaksh 1984a, Yaksh 1984b).

Morphine acts selectively at μ receptor sites which are are present in the cerebal cortex, in the periaquaductal grey region (PGR), and also in the dorsal horn. In addition to morphine, diamorphine, pethidine and fentanyl are agonists at μ receptors, as is the agonist/antagonist buprenorphine. Wood et al (1982) supported the concept of μ_1 receptors which mediated analgesia and regulation of cholinergic neurones, while μ_2 receptors were responsible for respiratory depression and dopaminergic neurones.

There are a high proportion of κ receptors in the spinal cord at which the peptide dynorphin appears to be active. The agonist/antagonist drugs such as pentazocine, nalbuphine and butorphanol have antagonist properties at μ sites and agonist properties at κ sites. For a guide to the structure and terminology of endogenous opioid peptoids see Cox (1982).

Yaksh (1983) demonstrated the presence of μ and δ receptor sites in the spinal cord of primates. He also showed that the onset and duration of action of opioids applied to the spinal cord was closely related to the lipid partition coefficient of the drug. Of the agents employed he showed that the order of potency was greater with beta endorphin, followed by morphine, L-methadone, pethidine and D-methadone. It was also noted that daily intrathecal morphine resulted in a loss of response over a 5–9 day period and sensitivity recurred after an opiate free interval of 7 days. Drugs with δ activity may be of value in patients who have become intolerant to intrathecal morphine. In further in vivo studies, Schmauss & Yaksh (1984) suggested that there were μ, δ and κ receptor sites in the spinal cord and proposed that there are μ/δ receptors for cutaneous thermal transmission and μ/κ receptors for visceral chemical transmission.

Tyers (1980) and Skingle & Tyers (1980) found that at least two opioid receptors were involved in the mediation of antinociception. Tests employing heat were specific for μ agonists, while tests employing pressure, chemical writhing or tooth pulp stimulation responded to both μ and κ agonists. Bryant et al (1983) suggested that buprenorphine and morphine produce analgesia by interacting with different opioid receptors and concluded that the predominant site of analgesia for buprenorphine was supraspinal. In man the epidural dose of buprenorphine was similar to that given intramuscularly, while in animal studies the intrathecal dose exceeded the parenteral dose. Hayes & Tyers (1983) found that μ receptor agonists produced their antinociceptive effects and side-effects by acting at the μ receptor. κ Receptor agonists appeared to produce little analgesia and the opioid side-effects are probably due to interaction with μ or other receptors.

Further detailed studies are still required to unravel the complexity of actions of opioids at receptor sites. Recent reviews include electrophysiology of opioids (Duggan & North 1984) and pharmacology of opioids (Martin 1984).

ENDOGENOUS OPIOIDS AND THE CARDIOVASCULAR SYSTEM

The cardiovascular effects of endogenous opioids have been reviewed extensively by Holaday (1983). The results are difficult to evaluate as there may be more than one type of opioid receptor involved and there may be secondary factors such as the peripheral action of catecholamines, histamine release or even other central transmitters. The state of consciousness of the animals may determine the outcome of experiments. In addition selectivity for specific receptors by opioids may not be absolute.

The intraventricular injection of enkaphalin analogues produce hypotension and bradycardia. Selective μ, δ and κ agonists injected into the anterior hypothalamus produced hypotension and bradycardia in low doses but had no effect on heart rate at higher doses (Pfeiffer et al 1983). Studies in man with intravenous infusions of DAMME (Met-enkephalin analogue) showed that it caused a fall in blood pressure by attenuating barorceptor function, an action medicated by μ receptors (Rubin et al 1983).

Interest in endogenous opioids and blood pressure suggested the possibility that they might be involved in circulatory failure associated with endotoxic shock. There are studies to suggest that pre-treatment with naloxone prevents the aftermath of endotoxic shock and that naloxone improves oxygenation, partly by improving haemodynamics and reducing shunting of the cardiac output, and partly by reversing the depressant effects of endogenous opioids (Mamazza et al 1984). The role of opioid antagonists in treatment remains speculative. Small doses of naloxone are ineffectual, while the results of larger doses may be influenced by the pH of naloxone which is highly acid (pH = 3). Other suggestions are that improvements in the circulation are due to the associated improvement in blood volume with intravenous fluids (see naloxone, p. 222).

INTRATHECAL MORPHINE

Intrathecal morphine has been studied in patients undergoing thoracotomy when 0.25 mg or 0.5 mg was injected at the end of operation. The duration of analgesia varied from 1 to 20 hours for the smaller dose and from 1 to 40 hours for the larger dose. The concentration of morphine in the CSF was high and dose dependant whereas the plasma concentration was low. The CSF concentration was higher than that seen after epidural administration of 6 mg of morphine (Nordberg et al 1984a).

Nordberg and colleagues also commented on the delayed onset of analgesia with spinal morphine. Post-operative pain relief could be prolonged using intrathecal cinchocaine and morphine compared with cinchocaine alone (Moore et al 1984a).

Moore et al (1984b) also measured the concentration in the CSF of morphine and heroin and found that after either 2 mg of intrathecal diamorphine or 2.5 mg of intrathecal morphine the concentration in the CSF was 4000 times greater than after the injection of 1 mg/kg of intravenous morphine. As diamorphine was more rapidly removed from the CSF than morphine because of its lipophilic properties they recommended that diamorphine was likely to be safer because of its shorter half-life.

Opioids are known to effect motility of the gastrointestinal tract. Animal studies have shown that intrathecal use of the drug appears to be species specific, affecting mice but not rats (Vaught et al 1983).

EPIDURAL MORPHINE

Pharmacokinetic aspects of epidural morphine analgesia have been studied by Nordberg et al (1983) who found that the technique produced dose dependent analgesia with concentrations of morphine much higher in the CSF than in the plasma. Although the elimination half-life for morphine was similar in the CSF and plasma, the long duration of morphine given epidurally seems to be dependent on a high concentration being present locally. In a further study Nordberg et al (1984) found that plasma morphine concentrations after epidural injection was similar to that found after intramuscular injections. Morphine reached a peak in the CSF after 135 ± 40 minutes and despite the high concentrations reached in the CSF it was calculated that only 2% of the drug administered epidurally was available to the CSF compartment. It is of interest that after 100 mg of intramuscular pethidine the drug can be detected within 18 minutes in the CSF reaching a maximum after 90 minutes. The transfer of pethidine from plasma in the CSF appears to occur very rapidly (Boreus et al 1983).

Other studies have compared plasma morphine concentrations of morphine following epidural morphine or diamorphine, assuming that diamorphine is a lipophilic form of morphine (Phillips et al 1984) (see p. 198). Plasma morphine concentrations were greater after epidural diamorphine than after epidural morphine, the mean peaks occurring at 5 and 10 minutes respectively. Similar results were reported with larger doses of the drugs by Watson et al (1984) who also calculated that the effects of epidural diacetyl morphine crossing the dura was 55% of that of morphine, presumably due to absorption of the heroin by epidural veins. Respiratory depression, particularly the rate, was noted only after epidural diacetyl morphine.

Respiration

Camporesi et al (1983) compared the respiratory response to CO_2 following 10 mg of morphine given either intravenously or epidurally. The maximum respiratory depression following intravenous injection occurred after 30 minutes which coincided with the peak level of morphine in the plasma. After epidural morphine, measurements of plasma levels, recorded 30 and 60 minutes later were significantly higher than after intravenous morphine. The degree and duration of respiratory depression was greater after epidural morphine, especially between the third and twenty-second hour. Respiratory rate was a poor indicator of impending apnoea. Kafer et al (1983) found that the maximum depression of ventilation in response to CO_2 occurred 1–2 hours following epidural injection followed by a further diminished response after 8 hours. They postulated two mechanisms for the biphasic depression of respiration. The early depression was due to absorption of morphine from the epidural veins and it then acted centrally, whereas the late phase was due to a rise in the segmental level of analgesia associated with the ascent of the morphine in the CSF towards the brain.

Physostigmine has been shown to reverse respiratory depressent effects of intravenous morphine by a possible central effect (Snir-Mor et al 1983). Shulman et al (1984) reported that 1 mg of physostigmine intravenously reversed the somnolence associated with the use of 5 mg of epidural morphine. They preferred the drug to naloxone when there was no apparent respiratory depression.

Adrenaline and epidural morphine

Bromage et al (1983) found that adrenaline 1:200 000 reduced the absorption of morphine from the epidural space by demonstrating that it reduced blood concentrations. With adrenaline, the onset of analgesia was quicker, it was more intense and had a longer duration of action. However, the incidence of side-effects such as pruritus, nausea, vomiting and difficulty of micturition were all increased. The ventilatory response to CO_2 was decreased between 6 and 16 hours. Bromage et al (1983) concluded that the use of adrenaline with epidural morphine intensified the action of the drug at cord and brainstem level. Rechtine et al (1984) reported excellent results of epidural morphine for preventing post-operative pain following lumbar laminectomy but that the addition of adrenaline appeared to have no beneficial effect.

DIACETYL MORPHINE (diamorphine: heroin)

The pharmacokinetics of diacetyl morphine have been studied in patients with chronic pain (Inturrisi et al 1984). The drug was either given intravenously (4–16 mg), intramuscularly (4 mg) or orally. Diacetyl morphine is rapidly metabolized in brain, kidney and liver, as well as blood, into 6-acetylmorphine and morphine, the maximum concentration being reached within minutes. The mean half-life of diamorphine was only 3 minutes. The onset of pain relief was rapid and coincided with the appearance of diamorphine and 6-acetylmorphine, but not morphine in the blood. 6-Acetylmorphine is equipotent with diamorphine but the former could not be measured in the blood stream following oral administration of diamorphine. Inturrisi et al (1984) concluded that oral diamorphine was an inefficient method of providing morphine for pain relief. Reference is also made to other studies showing that diamorphine was one and a half times more potent than morphine but only in female patients.

Apparently in some animals 6-acetylmorphine and morphine but not diamorphine are capable of being bound to opiate receptors but this may be species specific (Inturrisi et al 1985).

There are four distinct enzymes capable of hydrolysing diacetylmorphine to 6-monoacetylmorphine and morphine. Those in the plasma have little effect on degradation: the main enzymes involved are the RBC membrane enzyme at low concentrations and the RBC cytosolic (cytoplasmic) enzyme at high concentrations of diamorphine (Owen & Nakatsu 1983).

POST-OPERATIVE PAIN RELIEF

Pain relief following major abdominal surgery has in the main consisted of the administration of intramuscular injections of opiates at regular or even irregular intervals and often irrespective of the needs of the patients. Morphine may be withheld from patients even with intense pain for fear that a further injection given within 4 hours might cause profound respiratory depression. On the other hand intramuscular narcotics are given to patients without pain for night sedation, 'to settle the patient'. In a few centres, nerve block with local analgesic solutions are employed at the end of surgery to provide post-operative pain relief. This indeterminate approach has led to the quest for regimes to produce predictable and effective analgesia (Yaksh & Muller 1982, Bullingham 1983).

Spinal opioids (intrathecal and epidural)

A major contribution has been the introduction of epidural and spinal techniques using morphine, diacetylmorphine (heroin), buprenorphine and fentanyl (Cousins & Mather 1984). Stensteth et al (1985) reported on the use of epidural morphine in over a thousand patients after major surgery. An initial dose of 4 or 6 mg morphine was given with supplementary doses as necessary by catheter. Pain relief was satisfactory in 90% of patients. Respiratory depression was unusual and consisted mostly of reduction in respiratory rate which readily responded to naloxone. Nausea and vomiting occurred in 34% of patients, urinary retention in 42% of patients not having a urinary catheter, and pruritus in 11% of patients: this readily responded to naloxone. Mahnert et al (1983) reported flaccid paralysis of the legs following epidural morphine but the patient had been having heparin therapy.

The fear of pain following haemorrhoidectomy has deterred patients from seeking operation. This can be minimized by the surgeon infiltrating the haemorrhoids with local analgesia or performing a pudendal nerve block with either lignocaine or bupivacaine. Kuo (1984) found that a single epidural injection of 4 mg of morphine in 8 ml saline produced complete post-operative pain relief in 83% of his patients. Bailey & Sangwan (1985) found that 2.5 mg of diacetylmorphine in 10 ml saline given epidurally by the caudal route immediately after induction of anaesthesia produced better pain relief than 20 ml of 0.5% bupivacaine with a third of the patients requiring no further post-operative analgesia at all. The only urinary complications occurred with the bupivacaine patients.

Epidural morphine has been used in children and adolescents (Genski et al 1984) with a mean dose of 0.12 ± 0.03 mg/kg giving a mean duration of analgesia per dose of 10.8 ± 4.0 hours. The frequency of side-effects occurred when the dose was more than 0.1 mg/kg and increasing the dose did not prolong the duration of analgesia.

On demand low dose epidural morphine infusion has been used with a battery powered pump controlling a reservoir of morphine. Pain relief was effective in 100 patients without respiratory depression as assessed by blood gas analyses. 20% of the patients developed urinary retention (Chrubasik 1984).

Respiratory depression

The mechanism for this is still unclear. There have been suggestions that the morphine is absorbed via the epidural veins and then exerts a central action or it diffuses into the CSF and is carried rostrally. The breakdown products of morphine may also be active centrally. It may be dose related while the profound analgesia may reduce respiratory drive (Bullingham et al 1982, Cousins & Mather 1984). Jensen et al (1984) concluded that positioning the patient in 45° of head up elevation did not protect against respiratory depression following epidural morphine. Hammond (1984) reported on the successful use of nalbuphine to increase respiratory activity following the use of epidural diamorphine.

Respiratory function

It might have been expected that adequate post-operative pain relief would have resulted in an improvement in post-operative pulmonary function. Although pain relief was better with epidural morphine than those receiving intramuscular analgesia, there was no significant improvement in the epidural group in lung function tests as assessed by vital capacity (VC), forced expiratory volume over 1 second (FEV1) or functional residual capacity (FRC) (Bonnet et al 1984). In orthopaedic operations of the lower limb, pulmonary function was more affected following spinal bupivacaine and morphine compared with patients who had general anaesthesia with halothane. The FVC, the FRC and closing capacity (CC) were reduced in both groups. In the spinal group there was impaired gas distribution and V/Q mismatch, possibly due to hypoventilation (Hedenstierna & Lofstrom 1985).

Urinary function

There have been numerous reports of urinary retention following epidural morphine (see above). It has been suggested that there is an endogenous role for opioids in the lower urinary tract by decreasing detrusor pressure and increasing sphincteric tone. However, Husted et al (1985) agreed that epidural morphine did cause urinary retention, the effect occurring mainly in patients with abnormal detrusor function. Naloxone remains the treatment of choice.

Intrathecal diamorphine (heroin)

In a personal series of 250 cases given 2.5–5 mg intrathecal diamorphine in 4– 10 ml saline, without barbotage, the average duration of pain relief following major abdominal surgical procedure was 16 hours: 46 patients required no further analgesia in the first 24 hours, while a further 70 were pain-free beyond this time. Two patients had no post-operative narcotic analgesia whatsoever. In one control group when general anaesthesia was supplemented by intravenous fentanyl the first dose of analgesia was administered 1 hour post-operatively whereas in another control group given 10 mg of intravenous diamorphine, the first dose was given 4 hours post-operatively. There appears to be no direct relationship between the duration of analgesia and the patients' weight and height, dose of diacetyl-morphine or the volume injected. Age appears to be the only factor involved and is an indication for the use of smaller doses in the elderly.

Respiratory depression in the post-operative period was noted in elderly patients in the initial studies when patients were monitored with an impedance plethysmograph. Respiratory depression has seldom occurred since the technique of anaesthesia was modified to include minimal premedication, etomidate instead of thiopentone and atracurium (without reversal) instead of d-tubocurarine. Monitoring the end-tidal CO_2 confirms that apnoea at the end of operation is usually due to a low PCO_2. When intrathecal diamorphine was used for diagnostic or therapeutic purposes no instances of respiratory depression were noted.

In addition, the use of intrathecal diamorphine following induction of anaesthesia suppressed some of the endocrine responses to surgical stimulation, produced cardiovascular stability during operation and possibly contributed to improved patient well-being in the post-operative period (Child & Kaufman 1985). ADH levels rose with surgical stimulation, this being less in the intrathecal diamorphine group compared with the controls but the levels could be reduced in both groups by the use of intravenous bumetanide given at the beginning of surgery (Kaufman & Bailey 1986).

Barron & Strong (1984) used intrathecal diamorphine for total hip replacement and for spinal operations (laminectomy: spinal fusion — when the drug was injected by a surgeon under direct vision). The dose administered was in the range of 0.005–0.015 mg/kg but the duration of analgesia was not dose dependent. The total dose did not exceed 1 mg. There were no episodes of post-operative respiratory depression and the incidence of pruritus was low. In a series of 250 patients many had analgesia for more than 24 hours. (In an addendum, the series by Barron & Strong (1984) refers to 1000 patients).

Intravenous morphine

Marshall et al (1985) compared the use of continuous intravenous morphine with intramuscular morphine for the relief of post-operative pain following cholecystectomy. The patients receiving the intravenous infusion received as much supplementary morphine as the control group in the first 24 hours and considerably more in the 24 hour period when the intravenous infusion was discontinued. Side-effects, such as nausea and vomiting, were more common in the intravenous group.

Subcutaneous morphine

The introduction of small and reliable syringe pumps has led to a renewed interest in the use of subcutaneous infusions of morphine. Waldmann et al (1984) compared the blood levels of morphine sulphate given intravenously with that given subcutaneously via a 21-gauge butterfly needle inserted into the deltoid muscle. Using a method of assay which only measured morphine and not the metabolities they found at doses of

25 μg/kg per hour there was no significant difference in the serum levels made in the first 24 hours. The use of additional analgesics was the same for both groups of patients. The technique has been extended to provide pain relief following major abdominal operations and appears to be effective in a dose of 2–6 mg per hour without producing respiratory complications (B. Varley, personal communication).

CANCER PAIN RELIEF

The principles of management and relief of chronic pain are extensively reviewed by Brena & Chapman (1985). The review includes not only chapters on theories of pain and the philosophy of management but also discusses the use of nerve stimulation, nerve block, psychotherapy and drug therapy (Wall & Melzack 1984, Foley 1985). The aim of pain relief in cancer patients should be the continuous suppression of pain, the removal of the fear and memory of pain, while at the same time having an alert patient (Tuttle 1985). Doses of drugs should be adequate and administered before the effects of previous injections have worn off, while at the same time an attempt should be made to increase the interval between injections. Tuttle (1985) reviewed the place of the non-narcotic analgesics including acetylsalicylic acid, the use of antidepressants, as well as drugs used to prevent nausea and vomiting.

Oral morphine in cancer patients

There is a marked individual variation in the effectiveness of oral morphine administered to cancer patients. Sawe et al (1985) have studied the kinetics of morphine and the main metabolite, morphine-3-glucuronide and found the availability after oral administration varied between 30% and 69% and the plasma clearance rate ranged from 18.6 to 34 ml/kg per minute. In vivo studies were matched with in vitro studies from microsomes extracted from liver biopsy. The ratio of morphine-3-glucuronide to morphine reflects the extent of hepatic metabolism, but further studies are necessary to evaluate the usefulness of this ratio in the urine or plasma to predict the efficacy of hepatic metabolism of morphine.

Buccal morphine has been advocated by Bell et al (1985) in preference to intramuscular injection. Tablets containing 10 mg of morphine base given buccally were just as effective as intramuscular injection. The plasma levels were slightly lower following the buccal route but the decline in plasma level was slower compared with intramuscular injection.

Intravenous morphine

The safety and efficacy of continuously administered intravenous morphine for severe cancer pain has been studied by Citron et al (1984). The patients were given an initial bolus injection of 2–5 mg of morphine which was repeated at 10 minute intervals until the pain was relieved. Thereafter continuous intravenous morphine was administered with the hourly dose equal to the sum of the bolus doses. In some of the studies the mean dose was 20 mg per hour and this was increased by 33% if pain relief was inadequate and there were no signs of respiratory depression. In a small number of patients there was a reduction in PaO_2 and an increase in $PaCO_2$ which did not warrant alteration in the drug regime. Blood gas values tended to return to baseline levels despite an increase in the dose of morphine. The technique was considered to be safe and effective although somnolence and slowing of the respiratory rate were occasionally noted. The use of a respiratory monitor, such as an inductance or impedance plethysmograph, would be an additional safeguard. There have also been studies on patient controlled analgesia by continuous infusion; the literature has been reviewed by Graves et al (1983).

Epidural and spinal morphine

The differential effects of epidural morphine in the treatment of 55 patients with pain associated with cancer were reported by Arner & Arner (1985). The epidural catheter was tunnelled subcutaneously to the anterior abdominal wall and injections made through a micropore filter. The daily dose of morphine varied from 4–480 mg. Twenty-one patients became completely free from pain, the best results being obtained when the pain was continuous and deep seated in origin. Cutaneous pain appeared to be unaffected. This would confirm the view that opioids act on receptors mediated by C-fibres and not on A δ fibres which supply the skin.

The use of reservoirs have been described by Coombs et al (1982) where a reservoir is implanted under the skin, either on the interior abdominal wall or under the clavicle. The catheter may be silastic or stainless steel coated with fluoropolymers (Racz et al 1982). Penn et al (1984) have reported the use of epidural or intrathecal morphine using implanted pumps which were either of the constant rate of infusion type or were programmable. Wang (1985) found that long-term use of intrathecal morphine administered by catheter or implanted pump effectively relieved pain in 74% of the patients treated. There was no serious respiratory depression but somnolence, itching and sphincter disturbances were common. With long-term use there was mechanical failure of the pumps and tolerance to morphine developed. With intraspinal morphine, using implanted reservoirs, Coombs et al (1983) noted that patients were able to reduce their oral requirements of analgesics, although it was also noted that tolerance occurred as a significant increase in the dose of infused morphine was required.

REFERENCES

Arner S, Arner B 1985 Differential effects of epidural morphine in the treatment of cancer-related pain. Acta Anaesthesiologica Scandinavica 29: 32–36

Bailey P M, & Sangwan S 1985 Anaesthesia (in press)

Barron D W, Strong J E 1984 The safety and efficacy of intrathecal diamorphine. Pain 18: 279–285

Bell M D D, Murray G R, Mishra P, Calvey T N, Weldon G R, Williams N E 1985 Buccal morphine – the new route for analgesia? Lancet 1: 71–73

Bonnet F, Blery C, Satan M, Simonet O, Brage D, Gaudy J 1984 Effect of epidural morphine on post-operative pulmonary dysfunction. Acta Anaesthesiologica Scandinavica 28: 147–151

Boreus L O, Skoldefors E, Ehrnebo M 1983 Appearance of pethidine and norpethidine in cerebrospinal fluid of man following intramuscular injection of pethidine. Acta Anaesthesiologia Scandinavica 27: 222–225

Brena S F, Chapman S L 1985 Chronic pain: management principles. In: Clinics in Anaesthesiology. W B Saunders, London

Bromage P R, Camporesi E M, Durant P A, Neilsen C H 1983 Influence of epinephrine as an adjuvant to epidural morphine. Anaesthesiology 58: 257–262

Bryant R M, Olley J E, Tyers M B 1983 Antinociceptive action of morphine and buprenorphine given intrathecally in the conscious rat. British Journal of Pharmacology 78: 659–663

Bullingham R E S 1983 Opiate analgesic. In: Clinics in Anaesthesiology. W B Saunders, London

Bullingham R E S, McQuay H J, Moore R A 1982 Extradural and intrathecal narcotics. In: Atkinson R S, Langton-Hewer C (eds) Recent Advances in Anaesthesia and Analgesia No. 14 Churchill Livingstone, Edinburgh Ch 10, p 141–156

Camporesi E M, Nielsen C H, Bromage P R, Durant P A C 1983 Ventilatory CO_2 sensitivity after intravenous and epidural morphine in volunteers. Anesthesia and Analgesia 62: 633–640

Casey K L 1982 Neural mechanisms of pain: an overview. Acta Anaesthesiologica Scandinavica Suppl 74: 13–20

Child C, Kaufman L 1985 Effect of intrathecal diamorphine on the adrenocortical, hyperglycaemic and cardiovascular responses to major colonic surgery. British Journal of Anaesthesia 57: 389–393

Chrubasik J 1984 Epidural, on-demand, low-dose morphine infusion for postoperative pain. Lancet 1: 107

Citron M L, Johnston-Early A, Fossieck B E, Krasnow S H, Franklin R, Spagnolo S V, Cohen M H 1984 Safety and efficacy in continuous intravenous morphine for severe cancer pain. American Journal of Medicine 77: 199–204

Collins J G, Kitahata L M, Matsumoto M, Homma E, Suzukawa M 1984 Spinally administered epinephrine suppresses noxiously evoked activity of WDR neurons in the dorsal horn of the spinal cord. Anesthesiology 60: 269–275

Coombs D W, Saunders R L, Gaylor M, Pageau M G 1982 Epidural narcotic infusion reservoir: implantation technique and efficacy. Anesthesiology 56: 469–473

Coombs D W, Saunders R L, Gaylor M S et al 1983 Relief of continuous chronic pain by intraspinal narcotics infusion via an implanted reservoir. Journal of the American Medical Association 250: 2336–2339

Cousins M J, Mather L E 1984 Intrathecal and epidural administration of opioids. Anesthesiology 61: 276–310

Cox B M 1982 Endogenous opioid peptides: a guide to structures and terminology. Life Sciences 31: 1645–1658

Duggan A W, North R A 1984 Electrophysiology of opioids. Pharmacological Reviews 35: 219–281

Foley K M 1985 The treatment of cancer pain. New England Journal of Medicine 313: 84–95

Glenski J A, Warner M A, Dawson B, Kaufman B 1984 Postoperative use of epidurally administered morphine in children and adolescents. Mayo Clinic Proceedings 59: 531

Graves D A, Foster T S, Batenhorst R L, Bennett R L, Baumann T J 1983 Patient-controlled analgesia. Annals of Internal Medicine 99: 360–366

Hammond J E 1984 Reversal of opioid-associated late-onset respiratory depression by nalbuphine hydrochloride. Lancet 2: 1208

Hayes A G, Tyers M B 1983 Determination of receptors that mediate opiate side effects in the mouse. British Journal of Pharmacology 79: 731–736

Hedenstierna G, Lofstrom J 1985 Effect of anaesthesia on respiratory function after major lower extremity surgery. Acta Anesthesiologica Scandinavica 29: 55–60

Holaday J W 1983 Cardiovascular effects of endogenous opiates systems. Annual Review of Toxicology 23: 541–594

Hughes J (ed) 1983 Opioid peptides. British Medical Bulletin 39: 1–106

Homma E, Collins J G, Kitahata L M, Matsumoto M, Kawahara M 1983 Suppression of noxiously evoked WDR dorsal horn neuronal activity by spinally administered morphine. Anesthesiology 58: 232–236

Husted S, Djurhuus J C, Husegaard H C, Jepsen J, Mortensen 1985 Effect of postoperative extradural morphine on lower urinary tract function. Acta Anaesthesiologica Scandinavica 29: 183–185

Inturrisi C E, Max B M, Foley K M, Schultz M, Shin S U, Houde R W 1984 The pharmacokinetics of heroin in patients with chronic pain. New England Journal of Medicine 310: 1213–1217

Jordan C C 1984 Anatomical and physiological aspects of pain perception. In: Kaufman L (ed) Anaesthesia Review 2. Churchill Livingstone, Edinburgh

Jordan C C 1985 Opioid receptors. In: Kaufman L (ed) Anaesthesia Review 3. Churchill Livingstone, Edinburgh

Kafer E R, Brown J T, Scott D, Findlay J W A, Butz R F, Teeple E, Ghia J N 1983 Biphasic depression of ventilatory responses to CO_2 following epidural morphine. Anesthesiology 58: 418–427

Kaufman L, Bailey P M 1986 (in press)

Kitahata L M, Collins J G 1981 Spinal action of narcotic analgesics. Anesthesiology 54: 153–163

Kuo R J 1984 Epidural morphine for post-hemorrhoidectomy analgesia. Diseases of the Colon and Rectum 27: 529–530

Mamazza J, Hinchey E J, Chiu R C J 1984 The pulmonary effects of opiate blockade in septic shock. Journal of Surgical Research 36: 625–630

Marshall H, Porteous C, McMillan I, Macpherson S G, Nimmo W S 1985 Relief of pain by infusion of morphine after operation: does tolerance develop? British Medical Journal 291: 19–21

Martin W R 1984 Pharmacology of opioids. Pharmacological Reviews 35: 285–323

Martin W R, Eades C G, Thompson J A et al 1976 The effects of morphine and nalorphine-like drugs in the non-dependent and morphine-dependent chronic spinal dog. Journal of Pharmacology and Experimental Therapeutics 197: 517–532

Mense S 1983 Basic neurobiologic mechanisms of pain and analgesia. American Journal of Medicine 75(5A) 4–14

Mehnert J H, Dupont T J, Rose D H 1983 Intermittent epidural morphine instillation for control of postoperative pain. American Journal of Surgery 146: 145

Molke Jensen F, Madsen J B, Guldager H, Christensen A A, Eriksen H O 1984 Respiratory depression after epidural morphine in the postoperative period. Influence of posture. Acta Anaesthesiologica Scandinavica 28: 600–602

Moore A, Bullingham R, McQuay H, Allen M, Baldwin D, Cole A 1984a Spinal fluid kinetics of morphine and heroin. Clinical Pharmacology and Therapeutics 35: 40–45

Moore R A, Paterson G M C, Bullingham R E S, Allen M C, Baldwin D, McQuay H J 1984b Controlled comparison of intrathecal cinchocaine with intrathecal cinchocaine and morphine. British Journal of Anaesthesia 56: 837–841

Nordberg G, Hedner T, Mellstrand T, Dahlstrom B 1984a Pharmacokinetic aspects of intrathecal morphine analgesia. Anesthesiology 58: 345–551

Nordberg G E T, Hedner T, Mellstrand T, Dahlstrom B 1984a Pharmacokinetic aspects of intrathecal morphine analgesia. Anesthesiology 60: 448–454

Nordberg G, Hedner T, Mellstrand, Borg L 1984b Pharmacokinetics of epidural morphine in man. European Journal of Clinical Pharmacology 26: 233–237

Owen J A, Nakatsu K 1983 Diacetylmorphine (heroin) hydrolases in human blood. Canadian Journal of Physiology and Pharmacology 61: 870–875

Penn R D, Paice J A, Gottschalk W, Ivankovich A D 1984 Cancer pain relief using chronic morphine infusion. Journal of Neurosurgery 61: 302–306

Pfeiffer A, Feuerstein G, Kopin I J, Faden A I 1983 Cardiovascular and respiratory effects of mu-, delta- and kappa-opiate agonists microinjected into the anterior hypothalamic area of awake rats. Journal of Pharmacology and Experimental Therapeutics 225: 735–741

Phillips D M, Moore R A, Bullingham R E S, Allen M C, Baldwin A, Fisher A, Lloyd J W, McQuay H J 1984 Plasma morphine concentrations and clinical effects after thoracic extradural morphine or diamorphine. British Journal of Anaesthesia 56: 829–836

Pinnock C A 1985 Endorphins. In: Kaufman L (ed) Anaesthesia Review 3. Churchill Livingstone, Edinburgh

Racz G B, Sabonghy M, Gintaulas J, Kline W 1982 Intractable pain therapy using a new epidural catheter. Journal of the American Medical Association 248: 579–581

Rechtine G R, Cleveland C M R, Bohlman H H 1984 The use of epidural morphine to decrease postoperative pain in patients undergoing lumbar laminectomy. Journal of Bone and Joint Surgery 66: 113–116

Rubin P C, Howden C W, McLean K, Reid J L 1983 Endogenous opioids and baroreflex control in humans. Hypotension 5: 535–538

Sawe J, Kager L, et al 1985 Oral morphine in cancer patients: in vivo kinetics and in vitro hepatic glucuronidation. British Journal of Clinical Pharmacology 19: 495–501

Schmauss C, Yaksh T L 1984 In vivo studies on spinal opiate receptor systems mediating antinociception. II. Pharmacological profiles suggesting a differential association of mu, delta and kappa receptors with visceralchemical and cutaneous thermal stimuli in the rat. Journal of Pharmacology and Experimental Therapeutics 228: 1–12

Shulman M S, Sandler A, Brebner J 1984 The reversal of epidural morphine induced somnolence with physostigmine. Canadian Anaesthetic Society Journal 31: 678–680

Skingle M, Tyers M B 1980 Further studies on opiate receptors that mediate antinociception: tooth pulp stimulation in the dog. British Journal of Pharmacology 70: 323–327

Snir-mor I, Weinstock M, Davidson J T, Bahar M 1983 Physostigmine antagonizes morphine-induced respiratory depression in human subjects. Anesthesiology 59: 6–9

Stenseth R, Sellevold O, Breivik H 1985 Epidural morphine for postoperative pain: experience with 1085 patients. Acta Anaesthesiologica Scandinavica 29: 148–156

Tuttle C B 1985 Drug management of pain in cancer patients. Canadian Medical Association Journal 132: 121–134

Tyers M B 1980 A classification of opiate receptors that mediate antinociception in animals. British Journal of Pharmacology 69: 503–512
Vaught J L, Cowan A, Gmerek D E 1983 A species difference in the slowing effect of intrathecal morphine on gastrointestinal transit. European Journal of Pharmacology 94: 181–184
Wall P D, Melzack R 1984 Textbook of Pain. Churchill Livingstone, Edinburgh
Waldmann C S, Eason J R, Rambohul E, Hanson G C 1984 Serum morphine levels. Anaesthesia 39: 768–771
Wang J K 1985 Intrathecal morphine for intractable pain secondary to cancer of pelvic organs. Pain 21: 99–102
Wang J K, Nauss L A, Thomas J E 1979 Pain relief by intrathecally applied morphine in man. Anesthesiology 50: 149–151
Watson J, Moore A, McQuay H, Teddy P, Baldwin D, Allen M, Bullingham R 1984 Plasma morphine concentrations and analgesic effects of lumbar extradural morphine and heroin. Anesthesia and Analgesia 63: 629–634
Wood P L, Richard J W, Thakur M 1982 Mu opiate isoreceptors: differentiation with kappa agonists. Life Sciences 31: 2313–2317
Yaksh T L 1981 Spinal opiate analgesia: characteristics and principles of action. Pain 11: 293–346
Yaksh T L 1983 In vivo studies on spinal opiate receptor systems mediating antinociception. I. Mu and delta receptor profiles in the primate. Journal of Pharmacology and Experimental Therapeutics 226: 303–316
Yaksh T L 1984a Multiple opioid receptor systems in brain and spinal chord: Part I. European Journal of Anaesthesiology 1: 171–199
Yaksh T L 1984b Multiple opioid receptor systems in brain and spinal chord: Part II. European Journal of Anaesthesiology 1: 201–243
Yaksh T L, Rudy T A 1976 Analgesia mediated by a direct spinal action of narcotics. Science 192: 1357–1358
Yaksh T L, Muller H (ed) 1982 Spinal Opiate Analgesia — Experimental and Clinical Studies. Springer Verlag, Heidelberg

Update (1)

ABDOMINAL ANAESTHESIA

The influence of anaesthetic agents on the outcome of intestinal anastamoses has been reported in previous reviews (see Anaesthesia Review 1, 2, 3). The consensus of opinion is that the blood supply to the bowel, in particular the mucosa, is the critical factor and even in diverticular disease where the bowel is said to be made more irritable by drugs such as morphine and neostigmine the breakdown is minimal (Sangwan 1986). The use of atracurium has largely displaced the necessity for the use of atropine and neostigmine.

Recent animal studies by Tverskoy et al (1985) have confirmed earlier reports that halothane decreased vascular resistance and increased mesenteric blood flow. Enflurane produced little change but isoflurane increased splanchnic vascular resistance and decreased blood flow. The vasoconstriction was abolished by phentolamine, suggesting that the effect had been produced by circulating catecholamines.

Clonidine

Clonidine has been used successfully to treat five patients with pseudo intestinal obstruction following prolonged use or abuse of narcotic analgesics which inhibit gastrointestinal activity. Clonidine alleviates the symptoms of opiate withdrawal presumably by its central α_2 agonistic effects (Sandgren et al 1984).

APPARATUS

Oxygen masks

Hill et al (1984) found that at low inspiratory flow rates high volume Ventimasks and low volume Inspiron Accurox masks acted as fixed performance devices. Some

REFERENCES

Sandgren J E, McPhee M S, Greenberger N L 1984 Narcotic bowel syndrome treated with clonidine. Annals of Internal Medicine 101: 331–334

Sangwan S 1985 (in press)

Tverskoy M, Gelman S, Fowler K C, Bradley E L 1985 Intestinal circulation during inhalation anaesthesia. Anesthesiology 62: 462–469

variation occurred when peak inspiratory rate increased. They recommended that more consistent results were obtained with low volume masks and high oxygen flow rates.

Neonatal endotracheal tubes

The accurate placing of endotracheal tubes in the neonate requires skill as well as ingenuity in preventing them from becoming misplaced. Heller & Cotton (1985) have advocated the use of an endotracheal tube in which a fibre optic strand had been incorporated in the wall, allowing the tube to be visualized externally at will. The technique avoids the use of X-rays which are often used to check the position of the endotracheal tube.

Nebulizers

Douglas et al (1985) studied the flow rate of jet nebulizers which were being used to provide bronchodilator treatment with β-adrenergic agents (Rimiterol). It had been accepted that flow rates below 6 l/min produced droplets which were too large to be deposited in the tracheobronchial tract. However, the present study in chronic stable asthmatics showed that by reducing the flow rate from 8 l/min to 4 l/min the bronchodilator response was similar as assessed by FEV_1 and FVC.

Automatic blood pressure monitors

Johnson & Kerr (1985) have evaluated the accuracy of 5 non-invasive automatic blood pressure monitors. These included the Dinamap, the Narco and the Sentron which sense by oscillotonometry, the Copal which is semi-automatic and senses by auscultation and the Vitastat which can employ either method. Compared with intra-arterial recordings, the Copal and Sentron produced the best results. The Copal, being semi-automatic, is much cheaper than the fully automatic machines.

Pereira et al (1985) were critical of non-invasive methods of measurements, finding that oscillation tended to underestimate the intra-arterial systolic pressure while the diastolic pressure was inaccurate. They suggested that non-invasive methods of measurement of blood pressure were unsuitable for critically ill patients and for hypotensive anaesthesia. Arnold & McDevitt (1985), in studies of the indirect blood pressure measurement during intravenous isoprenaline infusions, found that the Dinamap recorder underestimated systolic pressure but overestimated diastolic pressure. The errors did not remain linear.

Van Egmond et al (1985) concluded that the Accutorr was a reasonably accurate oscillotonometer which is fully automated with an inflation phase of only 15–20 s and with a built in printer. A later model (2100 Datascope) incorporates the e.c.g. warning alarms which can be pre-set and can store data which can be displayed or printed at will. The Finapres is more accurate (derived from FINger Arterial PRESsure). Instead of an arm cuff there is a finger cuff which incorporates a photoplethysmograph measuring the absorption of the wavelength (infra-red) which is specific for arterial blood. Pressure readings were lower with the Finapres because of the distal position of the finger cuff. The intra-arterial method was considered the most accurate method of measurement.

REFERENCES

Arnold J M O, McDevitt D G 1985 Indirect blood pressure measurement during intravenous isoprenaline infusions. British Journal of Clinical Pharmacology 19: 114–116
Douglas J G, Leslie M J, Crompton G K, Grant I W B 1985 Is the flow rate used to drive a jet nebuliser clinically important? British Medical Journal 290: 29
Heller R M, Cotton R B 1985 Early experience with illuminated endotracheal tubes in premature and term infants. Pediatrics 75: 664–666
Hill S L, Barnes P K, Hollway T, Tennant R 1984 Fexed performance oxygen masks: an evaluation. British Medical Journal 288: 1261–1263
Johnson C J H, Kerr J H 1985 Automatic blood pressure monitors. A clinical evaluation of five models in adults. Anaesthesia 40: 471–478
Pereira E, Pry-Roberts C, Dagnino J, Anger C, Cooper G M, Hutton P 1985 Auscultatory measurement of arterial pressure during anaesthesia: a reassessment of the Korotkoff sounds. European Journal of Anaesthesiology 2: 11–20
Van Egmond J, Hasenbros M, Crul J F 1985 Invasive v. non-invasive measurement of arterial pressure. British Journal of Anaesthesia 57: 434–444

BLOOD TRANSFUSION

The increased use of blood components has led to more units of blood being supplied in concentrated form. Calkins et al (1982) have shown that the rapid administration of plasma reduced cells resulted in a 270% increase in plasma free haemoglobin. There was no correlation between flow rate and haemolysis. In addition to viscosity and flow rate, haemolysis may be influenced by pressure applied to the transfusion bag. They recommended that packed red cells should always be diluted with normal saline.

The National Blood Transfusion Service has recently introduced CPD red cell concentrates to which 100 ml of saline, adenine, glucose and mannitol (SAG-M) has been added. The saline dilutes the red cells, the adenine extends red cell storage, the glucose is for red cell metabolism and the mannitol reduces haemolysis. The shelf-life of the stored blood is up to 6 weeks. If more than 4 units of SAG-M blood are given, a bottle of plasma protein fraction (PPF) should be given simultaneously with the 5th unit which will also cover the 6th unit. Further PPF should be given to cover the 7th and 8th and a bottle for the 9th and 10th units. This will ensure there is not only adequate red cell replacement but also protein replenishment. In liver disease or in patients with a low plasma albumin, PPF should be administered with every 2 units of blood. (With the older type of CPD adenine suspended red cells, the routine use of PPF is unnecessary.)*

The use of blood substitutes has been outlined by Singer & Goldstone (1985). Kemner et al (1984) have drawn attention to the interaction between fluids used for

* These recommendations are taken from the National Blood Transfusion Service leaflet dated December 1984.

resuscitation with morphine. The half-life of morphine was prolonged when stroma free haemoglobin was administered, the effect being pH dependent and specific to morphine but not to codeine. The volume of distribution increased. There is also decreased binding of morphine to stroma free haemoglobin solutions compared with plasma. Fluosol DA 20% solution also prolonged the half-life of morphine by altering total body clearance. The dose of morphine administered to patients resuscitated with these solutions will need to be adjusted and possibly regulated by measuring serum concentrations.

There are possible problems associated with administering sodium lactate solutions (Hartmann's solution) through the same blood transfusion set as that used for whole blood. The calcium in the Hartmann's solution may inactivate the anticoagulant in the blood, leading to clot formation especially if the blood is warmed (Blagdon & Gibson 1985).

Derrington (1985) has commented on the disadvantages of microfilters. Apart from expense and the reduction in transfusion rate, haemolysis may occur with depth filters when pressure is applied to the transfusion bag. Proteins and white cells, present in solution in plasma, can pass through the filter and cause microaggregates in the lung. Derrington (1985) concluded that their routine use was not justified. On the other hand, microparticulate induced phlebitis was reduced by approximately two-thirds using a filter (0.22 μm) (Falchuk et al 1985).

REFERENCES

Blagdon J, Gibson T 1985 Potential hazard of clotting during blood transfusion using a blood warming pack. British Medical Journal 290: 1475–1476

Calkins J M, Vaughan R W, Cork R C, Barberii J, Eskelson C 1982 Effects of dilution, pressure, and apparatus on hemolysis and flow rate in transfusion, of packed erythrocytes. Anesthesia and Analgesia 61: 776–780

Derrington M C 1985 The present status of blood filtration. Anaesthesia 40: 334–347

Falchuk K H, Peterson L, McNeil B J 1985 Microparticulate-induced phlebitis: its prevention by in-line filtration. New England Journal of Medicine 312: 78–80

Kemner J M, Snodgrass W R, Worley S E, Hodges G R, Clark G M, Hignite C E 1984 Interaction of oxygen-carrying resuscitation fluids with morphine. Journal of Laboratory Clinical Medicine 104: 433–444

Singer C R J, Goldstone A H 1985 Recent advances in blood transfusion and blood products (1 & 2). In: Kaufman L (ed) Anaesthesia Review 3. Churchill Livingstone, Edinburgh, p 156–182

CARDIAC ARREST

Keenan & Boyan (1985) reported on the incidence of cardiac arrest over a 15 year period. Of the 27 cardiac arrests (incidence of 1.7 per 10 000), 14 patients subsequently died. A detailed analysis of the deaths show that the incidence was three times higher for children compared with adults and six times higher for emergencies compared with elective surgery. Inadequate ventilation including oesophageal intubation and displaced endotracheal tube were implicated in half the cardiac arrests while one-third resulted from overdose of inhalational agents. Progressive bradycardia was observed in 26 cases prior to the cardiac arrest. Eighteen of the arrests occurred during induction.

REFERENCES

Keenan R L, Boyan P 1985 Cardiac arrest due to anaesthesia. A study of incidence and causes. Journal of the American Medical Association 253: 2373–2377

OBSTETRICS

The physiology of the myometrium and uterine cervix have been reviewed in detail by Huszar & Naftolin (1984). The biochemical events associated with initiation of labour are also discussed, including factors affecting the myometrium and the cervix. The inhibition of premature labour is affected by β-adrenergic drugs and it has been suggested that calcium channel blocking agents might be equally effective. There is also the possibility of developing a prostaglandin synthesis inhibitor which does not cross the placental barrier.

Oxytocin release was inhibited by opioids in animal experiments and this was related to the intensity of analgesia. The order of potency was buprenorphine followed by morphine, pethidine, meptazinol and finally pentazocine. The close relationship between potency of analgesia and suppression of oxytocin release might explain the inhibition of labour during opioid analgesia (Clarke & Wright 1984).

Ritodrine

Marks & De Chazal (1984) reported on the successful use of epidural analgesia for caesarean section in a patient who developed ritodrine induced pulmonary oedema. Early in the pregnancy two episodes of supra-ventricular tachycardia were treated with verapamil. The pulmonary oedema appears to have been precipitated by propranolol given to control the heart rate.

Cano et al (1985) have confirmed the hypokalaemic action of ritrodrine. This effect has been ascribed to β-adrenergic stimulation (see Anaesthesia Review 2), but Cano et al (1985) found that the use of intravenous ritrodrine resulted in an increase in plasma insulin levels. There was also a significant fall in the serum calcium.

Curet et al (1984) studied the association between ruptured membranes, tocolytic therapy and respiratory distress syndrome (RDS) and found that although premature rupture of the membranes and isoxuprine individually lowered the incidence of RDS, there was an increased incidence of the complication when these factors were present together. They advised that β-adrenergic stimulating agents should not be administered to patients unless the membranes were intact.

Antacid therapy

The last confidential enquiry into maternal deaths (1982) still considered the skill of the anaesthetist to be the most important factor in the prevention of inhalation of gastric contents. H_2-receptor antagonists and antacids must still be considered as adjuncts and should not engender a false sense of security. There have been many studies on the use of drugs but little on improving technique. If antacids leave the stomach rapidly the results are ineffectual whereas if they leave slowly the gastric volume increases (O'Sullivan & Bullingham 1983). The duration of action of sodium citrate is short and may not last the duration of the surgical procedure (O'Sullivan et al 1984). Sodium citrate is no longer on the limited prescribing list as recommended by the DHSS. The most reliable regime of raising intragastric pH is the oral administration of ranitidine (150 mg) on the evening before operation and then again 2–4 hours prior to induction of anaesthesia. The intramuscular injection of metoclopramide (10 mg) 1–2 hours before induction decreases gastric fluid volume (O'Sullivan et al 1985).

In animal studies, Mizus et al (1985) showed that pre-treatment with aminophylline or isoprenaline prevented the increase in pulmonary artery pressure produced following the instillation of hydrochloric acid into the lungs. Isoprenaline was effective even after the acid was instilled. Isoprenaline and aminophylline also reduced the pulmonary vascular permeability following acid injury to the lung.

Anaesthesia

Bernstein et al (1985) recommended the use of ketamine as an alternative to thiopentone as an induction agent for caesarean section. Fetal Po_2, acid-base values and Apgar scores were comparable. The advantage of ketamine is that it produces amnesia and analgesia and maintains the blood pressure if there is severe bleeding.

Milsom et al (1985) compared the effects of epidural analgesia and general anaesthesia on maternal haemodynamics during caesarean section in fit patients. Many of the changes during epidural analgesia are associated with sympathetic blockade resulting in vasodilatation and a decrease in peripheral resistance, whereas those occurring during general anaesthesia may be ascribed to sympathetic stimulation occurring during intubation or due to the response to surgical manipulations under light anaesthesia. There was no difference in Apgar scores at 1 and 5 minutes or in umbilical vein pH with either technique. The study suggested that epidural analgesia might be preferred in patients with pre-eclamptic toxaemia.

Epidural analgesia may be associated with neonatal jaundice. Clark & Landaw (1985) were able to show that bupivacaine compared with mepivacaine and lignocaine was the most soluble, had the highest binding to protein and was the most potent in altering red blood cell viscosity. Bupivacaine was bound twice as much to neonatal red cells than to adult red cells. The reduced survival time of fetal red cells may lead to neonatal jaundice.

Pre-eclampsia

Plasma colloid osmotic pressure was lower in pre-eclamptic patients and was reduced during labour, reaching the lowest level between 16 and 18 hours following delivery (Zinaman et al 1985). They felt it was prudent to curtail the use of crystalloid solutions and resort to a colloid infusion instead.

Collins et al (1985) found that diuretics appeared to exert a favourable influence on blood pressure in pre-eclampsia but despite this there was very little improvement in post-natal survival.

A more encouraging approach has been suggested by Beaufils et al (1985). In order to prevent intravascular coagulation which often precedes pre-eclampsia, they administered low doses of aspirin (150 mg/d) and dipyridamole (300 mg/d) at the end of the first trimister. Although the patients treated were particularly prone to the possibility of pre-eclampsia, treatment appeared to prevent its occurrence by inhibiting platelet aggregation. (This was not measured during the trial. There were no complications to the mother or the fetus.)

Epilepsy in pregnancy

There are possible hazards during pregnancy of administering drugs for the control of epilepsy. Drugs may be cleared more rapidly during pregnancy and they may also cross the placental barrier. There is also the possibility of congenital malformations especially with valproic acid. A regime for the management of the pregnant epileptic has been outlined by Dalessio (1985), advocating the use of phenytoin or carbamazepine. The plasma levels should be monitored at regular intervals.

Vitamin K deficiency may develop in patients on phenytoin, phenobarbitone or primidone and may result in increased bleeding during labour. Even if vitamin K levels are normal in the mother they may be reduced in the newborn, leading to haemorrhagic disease. Treatment is with vitamin K or even freshly frozen plasma (Dalessio 1985).

Asthma

The alterations in pulmonary physiology during pregnancy have been summarized by Greenberger & Patterson (1985). There are reductions in residual volume and functional residual capacity and the alveolar-arterial oxygen gradient increases. During an asthmatic attack the minute volume has to increase and greater negative inspiratory pressures are required to ventilate obstructed bronchi. Maternal hypoxaemia would have a major effect on fetal oxygenation. Despite the possibility of teratogenetic effects of drugs (based on animal experiments), Greenberger & Patterson (1985) recommended the use of β-agonists such as terbutaline, metaproterenol and albuterol. These drugs act primarily at β_2 receptors which also produce uterine relaxation. Steroids may be necessary and it is suggested these are preferably given by inhalation. Hydrocortisone may be necessary during labour.

Phaeochromocytoma

Phaeochromocytoma during pregnancy presents risks to the mother and fetus. The diagnosis may be confused with pre-eclampsia. Venuto et al (1984) reported a patient who developed a phaeochromocytoma at 32 weeks. The blood pressure was controlled with prazosin and the baby delivered by elective caesarean section. The phaeochromocytoma was removed at a further operation 18 days later. Schenker & Granat (1982) reviewed the literature and concluded that before 20–24 weeks the tumour should be excised whereas after that period the pregnancy should be allowed to continue with the blood pressure controlled by adrenergic blocking agents. They recommended delivery by caesarean section and preferably removal of the tumour at the same operation.

Pain relief

Use of spinal opioids was referred to in Anaesthesia Review 3 (Ch. 12, 13). Animal experiments reported by Craft et al (1984) showed that epidural fentanyl had no effects on maternal or fetal arterial blood pressure, acid base status or on maternal central venous pressure, systemic and pulmonary vascular resistance, cardiac output and intrauterine pressure. Following the injection of 50 μg of fentanyl the maternal level reached a maximum at 60 minutes and the fetal at 45 minutes. After 100 μg of fentanyl the maximum maternal level was at 45 minutes and the fetal at 15 minutes. Measurements of β-endorphin levels during labour have shown these are significantly decreased following 1 mg of intrathecal morphine which also provided excellent pain relief (Abboud et al 1984a). In a further study Abboud et al (1984b) demonstrated that intrathecal morphine, 0.5 mg or 1 mg in 7.5% dextrose, provided excellent pain relief during labour. The onset of analgesia was from 15–60 minutes after injection and it lasted for 6–8 hours. Analgesia was less satisfactory when there was distension of the perineum either by the application of forceps or during the crowning of the fetal head. There was a high incidence of complications including pruritus, nausea and vomiting, urinary retention and drowsiness but these side-effects could be alleviated by naloxone which did not appear to affect analgesia. There was no significant maternal respiratory depression. In a personal series using intrathecal diamorphine, the onset of analgesia was rapid, there was no maternal or fetal respiratory depression and, although perineal distension required additional analgesia such as nitrous oxide and oxygen, patients experienced no perineal pain for up to 24 hours following episiotomy.

Intrathecal administration of small doses of morphine revealed only small amounts in the maternal blood. Following epidural morphine, however, there was a rapid uptake via the epidural venous plexus and blood concentrations approached that following intramuscular administration, producing levels likely to depress fetal respiration (Camporesi & Redick 1983).

REFERENCES

Abboud T K, Goebelsmann U, Raya J et al 1984a Effect of intrathecal morphine during labor on maternal plasma beta-endorphin levels. American Journal of Obstetrics and Gynecology 149: 709–710

Abboud T K, Shnider S M, Dailey P A et al 1984b Intrathecal administration of hyperbaric morphine for the relief of pain in labour. British Journal of Anaesthesia 56: 1351–1360

Beaufils M, Donsimoni R, Uzan S, Colau J C 1985 Prevention of pre-eclampsia by early antiplatelet therapy. Lancet 1: 840–842

Bernstein K, Gisselsson L, Jacobsson L, Ohrlander S 1985 Influence of two different anaesthetic agents on the newborn and the correlation between foetal oxygenation and induction-delivery time in elective caesarean section. Acta Anaesthesiologica Scandinavica 29: 157–160

Camporesi E M, Redick L F 1983 Clinical aspects of spinal narcotics: postoperative management and obstetric pain. In: R E S Bullingham (ed) Clinics in Anesthesiology. W B Saunders, London, Vol 1, p 57–70

Cano A, Tovar I, Parrilla J J, Abad L 1985 Metabolic disturbances during intravenous use of ritodrine: increased insulin levels and hypokalemia. Obstetrics and Gynecology 65: 356–360

Clark D A, Landaw S A 1985 Bupivacaine alters red blood cell properties: a possible explanation for neonatal jaundice associated with maternal anesthesia. Pediatric Research 19: 341–343

Clarke G, Wright D M 1984 A comparison of analgesia and suppression of oxytocin release by opiates. British Journal of Pharmacology 83: 799–806

Collins R, Yusuf S, Peto R 1985 Overview of randomised trials of diuretics in pregnancy. British Medical Journal 290: 17-23
Craft J B, Robichaux A G, Kim H-S, Thorpe D H, Mazel P, Woolf W A, Stolte A 1984 The maternal and fetal cardiovascular effects of epidural fentanyl in the sheep model. American Journal of Obstetrics and Gynecology 148: 1098-1104
Curet L B, Vijaya Rao A, Zachman R D, Morrison J C, Burkett G, Poole W K, Bauer C, Collaborative Group on Antenatal Steroid Therapy 1984 Association between ruptured membranes, tocolytic therapy, and respiratory distress syndrome. American Journal of Obstetrics and Gynecology 148: 263-368
Dalessio D J 1985 Current concepts: seizure disorders and pregnancy. New England Journal of Medicine 312: 559-563
Greenberger P A, Patterson R 1985 Current concepts: management of asthma during pregnancy. New England Journal of Medicine 312: 897-902
Huszar G, Naftolin F 1984 The myometrium and uterine cervix in normal and preterm labor. New England Journal of Medicine 311: 571-581
Marks R J, De Chazal R C S 1984 Ritodrine-induced pulmonary oedema in labour. Anaesthesia 39: 1012-1014
Milsom I, Forssman L, Biber B, Dottori O, Rydgren B, Sivertsson R 1985 Maternal haemodynamic changes during caesarean section: a comparison of epidural and general anaesthesia. Acta Anaesthesiologica Scandinavica 29: 161-167
Mizus I, Summer W, Farrukh I, Michael J R, Gurtner G H 1985 Isoproterenol or aminophylline attenuate pulmonary edema after acid lung injury. American Review of Respiratory Disease 131: 256-259
O'Sullivan G, Harrison B J, Bullingham R E S 1984 The use of radiotelemetry techniques for the in vivo assessment of antacids. Anaesthesia 39: 987-995
O'Sullivan G, Bullingham R E S 1983 Antacid prophylaxis in the pregnant patient. Anaesthesia 38: 998-999
O'Sullivan G, Sear J W, Bullingham R E S, Carrie L E S 1985 The effect of magnesium trisilicate mixture, metoclopramide and ranitidine on gastric pH, volume and serum gastrin. Anaesthesia 40: 246-253
Schenker J G, Granat M 1982 Phaeochromocytoma and pregnancy — an updated appraisal. Australian and New Zealand Journal of Obstetrics and Gynaecology 22: 1-10
Venuto R, Burstein P, Schnider R 1984 Pheochromocytoma: antepartum diagnosis and management with tumor resection in the puerperium. American Journal of Obstetrics and Gynecology 150: 431-432
Zinaman M, Rubin J, Lindheimer M D 1985 Serial plasma oncotic pressure levels and echoencephalography during and after delivery in severe pre-eclampsia. Lancet 1: 1245-1247

PHAEOCHROMOCYTOMA

In a recent review Bravo & Gifford (1984) considered the diagnosis, localization and management of phaeochromocytoma. They referred to the classic triad of sweating, tachycardia and headache which seemed to confirm the diagnosis in the majority of patients. However the presentation may vary (see Anaesthesia Review 1, 2, 3). Ganguly et al (1984) described a patient with adrenal phaeochromocytoma who initially was thought to have sick sinus syndrome requiring a pacemaker and who exhibited cyclic fluctuations of blood pressure. The hypertension was accompanied by bradycardia and the hypotension by tachycardia. The fluctuations in blood pressure were not controlled by phentolamine. As the patient had been previously treated with a diuretic, saline was infused which controlled the fluctuations of blood pressure.

A high proportion of Bravo & Gifford's patients (based on a study of 43 cases) had false negative results for urinary vanilmandelic acid and for metanephrines. Blood levels of catecholamines were raised but they are also raised in patients with hypertension: 4 of their patients with phaeochromocytonma had levels which fell within the range of values for patients with essential hypertension but none within the range for normotensives. Plasma catecholamines may be raised in patients with chronic renal failure (Darwish et al 1984). If the tests are not completely confirmatory, provocative tests include intravenous glucagon or suppression with clonidine. Bravo & Gifford (1984) considered that the concentration of total plasma catecholamines over 2000 pg/ml (11.82 mmol/l) to be diagnostic. The operative management consisted of the prior administration of phenoxybenzamine or prazosin. During operation phentolamine and sodium nitroprusside were used to control hypertension and propranolol to abolish arrhythmias.

Lenders et al (1985) reported on the use of nifedipine, a calcium channel blocker, in the treatment of phaeochromocytoma of the bladder. Nifedipine prevented the rise in blood pressure as well as the symptoms of headache and nausea during micturition despite a sharp increase in plasma catecholamine levels.

Catecholamines

Plasma potassium rises during muscular exercise and falls rapidly when exertion is stopped. Williams et al (1985) have confirmed that during exercise there are high plasma levels of noradrenaline and that the β-adrenergic receptors prevent the acute rises of plasma potassium during exercise, while α-adrenergic receptor stimulation augments hypokalaemia and prevents the fall in serum potassium when exercise stops.

The use of adrenaline in lignocaine anaesthetic solutions for dental analgesia causes a significant fall in serum potassium levels in young adults (Meechan & Rawlins 1985).

β-Adrenergic receptor stimulation increases cellular levels of potassium whereas α-adrenergic stimulation has the opposite effect (Williams et al 1984).

Plasma noradrenaline has been studied in patients with chronic congestive cardiac failure and it has been found that a single resting venous blood sample was the most satisfactory guide to prognosis. Heart rate, plasma renin, serum sodium and stroke volume index were of less value than the level of noradrenaline in determining prognosis. The level is also higher in patients who died from progressive heart failure than in those who died suddenly (Cohn et al 1984).

Studies on leucocytes from normal volunteers have shown that noradrenaline depresses membrane sodium pump activity. This effect is suppressed by propranolol implying that the effect is mediated by β receptors. There may be implications in this study in patients with hypertension (Riozzi et al 1984).

β-Adrenergic blocking drugs

Biochemical and physiological aspects of adrenergic receptors are considered by Lefkowitz et al (1984), while the biochemical mechanisms of β-adrenergic receptor regulation are reviewed by Stiles et al (1984). Age appears to affect adrenoceptor function and there is evidence that there is diminished responsiveness to β receptor stimulation although this effect is less marked at the α-adrenergic receptor (Kelly & O'Malley 1984). Metoprolol alters the cardiorespiratory response to exercise with greater utilization of oxygen and creatine phosphate stores (Hughson 1984).

Paradoxical hypertension may develop following repair of coarctation of the aorta and this can be prevented by the administration of propranolol for 2 weeks prior to surgery and for 1 week in the post-operative period. Following resection of the aneurysm there are increased concentrations of plasma noradrenaline and plasma renin. Compared with patients treated for coarctation without β-blockers, the patients given propranolol had not only reduced blood pressure but also decreased plasma renin. There were no differences in the level of plasma noradrenaline (Gidding et al 1985).

Drug interactions with β-blockers have been summarized by Beeley (1984). Enzyme inducing drugs increase the clearance of β-blockers such as propranolol and metoprolol which are lipid soluble and readily metabolized. β-Blockers may affect other drugs by reducing hepatic blood flow. Although propranolol lowers the clearance of lignocaine by decreasing hepatic blood flow by 25%, the main cause of reduced clearance is due to the inhibition of hepatic enzymes which metabolize lignocaine (Bax et al 1985). There are also interactions with antiarrhythmic drugs, while recovery from hypoglycaemia may be prolonged in diabetics on treatment.

REFERENCES

Bax N D S, Tucker G T, Lennard M S, Woods H F 1985 The impairment of lignocaine clearance by propranolol — major contribution from enzyme inhibition. British Journal of Clinical Pharmacology 19: 597–603

Beeley L 1984 Drug interactions and β-blockers. British Medical Journal 289: 1330–1331

Bravo E L, Gifford R W 1984 Current concepts: pheochromocytoma: diagnosis, localization and management. New England Journal of Medicine 311: 1298–1303

Cohn L N, Levine T B, Olivari M T et al 1984 Plasma norephinephrine as a guide to prognosis in patients with chronic congestive heart failure. New England Journal of Medicine 311: 819–823

Darwish R, Elias A N, Vaziri N D, Pahl M, Powers D, Stokes J D 1984 Plasma and urinary catecholamines and their metabolites in chronic renal failure. Archives of Internal Medicine 144: 69

Ganguly A, Grim C E, Weinberger M H, Henry D P 1984 Rapid cyclic fluctuations of blood pressure associated with an adrenal pheochromocytoma. Hypertension 6: 281–284

Gidding S S, Rocchini A P, Beekman R et al 1985 Therapeutic effect of propranolol on paradoxical hypertension after repair of coarctation of the aorta. New England Journal of Medicine 312: 1224–1228

Hughson R L 1984 Alterations in the oxygen deficit-oxygen debt relationships with β-adrenergic receptor blockade in man. Journal of Physiology 349: 375–387

Kelly J, O'Malley K 1984 Adrenoceptor function and ageing. Clinical Science 66: 509–515

Lenders J W M, Sluiter H E, Thien T 1985 Treatment of a phaeochromocytoma of the urinary bladder with nifedipine. British Medical Journal 290: 1624–1625

Lefkowitz R J, Caron M G, Stiles G L 1984 Mechanisms of membrane-receptor regulation: biochemical, physiological and clinical insights derived from studies of the adrenergic receptors. New England Journal of Medicine 310: 1570–1579

Meechan J G, Rawlins M D 1985 The effect of adrenaline in lignocaine anaesthetic solutions on serum potassium levels. Proceedings of the British Pharmacological Society, p C39

Riozzi A, Heagerty A M, Bing R F, Thurston H, Swales J D 1984 Noradrenaline: a circulating inhibitor of sodium transport. British Medical Journal 289: 1025–1027

Stiles G L, Caron M G, Lefkowitz R J 1984 β-adrenergic receptors: biochemical mechanisms of physiological regulation. Physiological Reviews 64: 661–743

Williams M E, Gervino E V, Rosa R M et al 1985 Catecholamine modulation of rapid potassium shifts during exercise. New England Journal of Medicine 312: 823–827

Williams M E, Rosa R M, Silva P, Brown R S, Epstein F H 1984 Impairment of extrarenal potassium disposal by α-adrenergic stimulation. New England Journal of Medicine 311: 145–149

L. Kaufman

Update (2)

ALLERGY

Induction agents may be associated with allergic type responses. Recently thiopentone has been implicated in immune haemolytic anaemia and renal failure. A patient acquired an antibody against thiopentone and the I antigen on the red cell membrane appeared to be the receptor site for the thiopentone antibody complex (Habibi et al 1985). The patient had undergone two previous operations with thiopentone as the induction agent without mishap but on this occasion haemoglobinuria resulted post-operatively. Later acute intravascular haemolysis and renal failure occurred. Detailed blood studies confirmed the presence of a specific antibody against thiopentone.

Harle et al (1984), using choline-sepharose assay, were able to detect IgE antibodies to suxamethonium in patients who recently had severe anaphylactoid reactions after the drug was administered. There is likely to be cross sensitivity to other drugs such as d-tubocurarine and alcuronium (Fisher & Baldo 1983).

REFERENCES

Fisher M, Baldo B 1983 Adverse reactions to alcuronium. An Australian disease? Medical Journal of Australia 1: 630–632

Habibi B, Basty R, Chodez S, Prunat A 1985 Thiopental-related immune hemolytic anemia and renal failure: specific involvement of red-cell antigen I. New England Journal of Medicine 312: 353–355

Harle D G, Baldo B A, Fisher M M 1984 Detection of IgE antibodies to suxamethonium after anaphylactoid reactions during anaesthesia. Lancet 1: 930–932

ANAESTHETIC AGENTS

Midazolam

Midazolam (Hypnovel), a recently introduced benzodiazepine, seemed a reasonable alternative to diazepam but Byatt et al (1984) reported accumulation of the drug after repeated doses leading to prolonged respiratory depression and prolonged unconsciousness. Although midazolam was used with other drugs such as papaverine or chloral hydrate, the prolonged period of recovery may be misinterpreted and a neurological cause sought for the failure to regain consciousness.

Etomidate

Duthie et al (1985) found that a single dose of etomidate produced no clinically significant adrenocortical suppression in patients undergoing minor surgical procedures. However there was some inhibition of 11-β-hydroxylase activity. During the first hour of anaesthesia (nitrous oxide, oxygen and halothane), the plasma cortisol fell transiently but this also occurred in the control group of patients who were given thiopentone. In a further study Moore et al (1985) investigated the peri-operative endocrine effects of etomidate infusion during hysterectomy: they too concluded that etomidate suppressed only adrenocortical function without producing any obvious clinical adverse effects. They even suggested that etomidate might be a novel means of producing stress free anaesthesia (misnomer: the stress of surgery is still present, the response to surgical stimuli is suppressed). Bailey (1986) has confirmed the drop in plasma cortisol levels, reaching a maximum of 20% 30 minutes after induction with etomidate.

Atropine

The effect of low doses of atropine on gastrointestinal secretions has shown that acid and pepsin secretion are readily inhibited. Patients with duodenal ulcer require 2–4 times as much to produce the same effect. The maximum increase in heart rate following atropine was much less in patients with duodenal ulcer (Hirschowitz et al 1984). Hyoscine has a greater affinity apparently for the muscarinic receptor compared with atropine (Cohen & Haberman 1984). Atropine also inhibited secretion of growth hormone (Taylor et al 1985).

REFERENCES

Bailey P 1986 (in press)
Byatt C M, Lewis L D, Dawling S, Cochrane G M 1984 Accumulation of midazolam after repeated dosage in patients receiving mechanical ventilation in an intensive care unit. British Medical Journal 289: 799–800
Cohen S, Haberman F 1984 The molal volumes of atropine and hyoscine in relation to their respective potencies. British Journal of Pharmacology 83: 807–811
Duthie D J R, Fraser R, Nimmo W S 1985 Effect of induction of anaesthesia with etomidate on corticosteroid synthesis in man. British Journal of Anaesthesia 57: 156
Hirschowitz B I, Molina E, Ou Tim L, Helman C 1984 Effects of very low doses of atropine on basal acid and pepsin secretion, gastrin and heart rate in normals and DU. Digestive Diseases and Science 29: 790–796
Moore R A, Allen M C, Wood P J, Rees L H, Sear J W 1985 Peri-operative endocrine effects of etomidate. Anaesthesia 40: 124–130
Taylor B J, Smith P J, Brook C G D 1985 Inhibition of physiological growth hormone secretion by atropine. Clinical Endocrinology 22: 497–501

ANALGESIC AGENTS

Fentanyl

Fentanyl is frequently used to provide analgesia during the course of surgery. It had been claimed that it had little effect on cardiovascular stability, but recent reports (Lowenstein & Philbin 1983) have shown that this only appears to be so in the presence of pancuronium which predisposes to tachycardia. Caution must be exerted when using other muscle relaxants such as d-tubocurarine and atracurium. During cardiopulmonary bypass, serum concentrations of fentanyl fall but rise when lung ventilation and perfusion are restarted. This would indicate that fentanyl is sequestered in the lungs during bypass surgery (Bentley et al 1983).

Bidwai et al (1976) reported that large doses of fentanyl (1 ml/kg) decreased urinary output, presumably as a result of ADH release. This effect could be antagonized by nitrous oxide. However Ecoffey et al (1984) noted that fentanyl caused a marked fall in blood pressure, a factor known to release ADH, but despite this fentanyl suppressed the ADH response to osmotic and hypotensive stimuli.

Alfentanil

The advantages of alfentanil have been discussed by Stanski & Hug (1982). Alfentanil has a smaller volume of distribution, clearance and terminal half-life (Bower & Hull 1982). It is less lipid soluble than fentanyl.

In elderly patients over the age of 65 years plasma clearance was reduced and the plasma terminal half-life prolonged compared with a group of young adults, following the administration of 50 μg/kg (Helmers et al 1984). These changes are probably due to a reduction in hepatic metabolism. Two cases of unexpected respiratory depression have been reported by Sebel et al (1984) following alfentanil infusion and which responded to intravenous naloxone.

In animal studies high dose alfentanil resulted in an increase in left ventricular end diastolic pressure (D'Aubioul et al 1984). They also noted that there was a marked increase in heart rate and A-V dissociation and despite this they concluded that alfentanil was safe in animals provided they were artificially ventilated.

Alfentanil, in an initial dose of 150 μg/kg followed by a continuous infusion of 3 μg/kg per minute, suppressed intra-operative plasma cortisol and glucose concentrations in only the first 3 hours of the post-operative period (Moller et al 1985). Although there was cardiovascular stability during operation, the high incidence of nausea and vomiting and the frequency of respiratory depression made the technique unacceptable. In addition Moller et al (1985) concluded that the inhibition of the endocrine response to surgery was too limited in duration to contribute to a reduction in post-operative morbidity.

Morphine

Care is necessary in the use of intravenous morphine for sedation in patients with decreased renal function. Ball et al (1985) reported on reduced morphine clearance in patients with renal impairment and warned of the dangers of mistaking cerebral damage for overdose of morphine especially in patients in intensive care situations. However, despite this potential hazard, sleep time in patients in intensive care units following major abdominal surgery was less than 2 hours per night following high dose morphine anaesthesia. Sleep time was measured by continuously recording the electroencephalogram, electrooculogram and electromyogram (Aurell & Elmqvist 1985).

In addition Rodriguez et al (1983) favoured the use of intravenous morphine (initial dose of 1 or 4 mg/kg followed by an infusion of 0.2 or 0.5 mg/kg per hour) to reduce post-operative metabolic rate. This was in a study of patients who became hypothermic during surgical procedures and the use of morphine, although significantly increasing the rewarming period, produced a significant reduction in shivering, heat loss and myocardial work while at the same time maintained cardiovascular function.

Laska et al (1984) noted that caffeine potentiated the action of mild analgesics and in animal studies this had been confirmed for morphine (Misra et al 1985). The mode of action of caffeine is unknown and may involve pharmacokinetic or dispositional factors. Naloxone still reverses the analgesia. The clinical implications of this are still to be evaluated.

REFERENCES

D'Aubioul J, Van Gerven W, Van de Water A, Xhonneux R, Reneman R S 1984 Cardiovascular and some respiratory effects of high doses of alfentanil in dogs. European Journal of Pharmacology 100: 79–84

Aurell J, Elmqvist D 1985 Sleep in the surgical intensive care unit: continuous polygraphic recording of sleep in nine patients receiving postoperative care. British Medical Journal 290: 1029–1032

Ball M, Moore R A, Fisher F, McQuay H J, Allen M C, Sear J 1985 Renal failure and the use of morphine in intensive care. Lancet 1: 784–786

Bentley J B, Conahan T J, Cork R C, 1983 Fentanyl sequestration in lungs during cardiopulmonary bypass. Clinical Pharmacology and Therapeutics 34: 703–706

Bidwai A V, Liu W S, Stanley T H, Bidwal V, Loeser E A, Shaw C L 1976 Canadian Anaesthetists Society Journal 23: 296–302

Bower S, Hull C J 1982 Comparative pharacokinetics of fentanyl and alfentanil. British Journal of Anaesthesia 54: 871–877

Ecoffey C, Simon D, Samil K, Diraison P M, Poggi J, Noviant Y, Ardaillou R 1984 Antidiuretic hormone response to osmotic stimulus under fentanyl anaesthesia. Acta Anaesthesiologica Scandinavica 28: 245–248

Helmers H, Van Per A, Woestenborghs R, Noorduin H, Heykants J 1984 Alfentanil kinetics in the elderly. Clinical Pharmacology and Therapeutics 36: 239–243

Laska E M, Sunshine A, Mueller F, Elvers W B, Siegel C, Rubin A 1984 Enhancement of analgesic efficacy of acetaminophen, aspirin and their combination with caffeine: caffeine as an analgesic adjuvant. Journal of the American Medical Association 251: 1711–1718

Lowenstein E, Philbin M 1983 Narcotic anaesthesia. In: Bullingham R E S (ed) Clinics in Anaesthesiology. WB Saunders, London. p 5–15

Misra A L, Pontani R B, Vadlamani N L 1985 Potentiation of morphine analgesia by caffeine. British Journal of Pharmacology 84: 789–791

Moller I W, Krantz T et al 1985 Effect of alfentanil anaesthesia on the adrenocortical and hyperglycaemic response to abdominal surgery. British Journal of Anaesthesia 54: 591–594

Rodriguez J L, Weissman C et al 1983 Morphine and postoperative rewarming in critically ill patients. Circulation 68: 1238–1246

Sebel P S, Lalor J M, Flynn P J, Simpson B A 1984 Respiratory depression after alfentanil infusion. British Medical Journal 289: 1581–1582

Stanski D R, Hug C C 1982 Alfentanil — a kinetically predictable narcotic analgesic. Anaesthesiology 57: 435–437

CIMETIDINE

Cimetidine may influence the action of other drugs such as diazepam, propranolol and local anaesthetic agents by impairing microsomal oxidation in the liver. However in a controlled study by Greenblatt et al (1984), in patients who were given cimetidine and diazepam, plasma concentrations of diazepam and desmethyldiazepam were elevated compared to controls but the increase was of minimal clinical importance. Greenblatt et al (1984) added a note of caution on their findings as the patients that they studied were under 50 years of age. The use of cimetidine and diazepam in the elderly and in patients with medical disorders such as liver disease or chronic respiratory disease may result in increased drowsiness and sedation.

The kinetics of cimetidine has been studied by Ziemniak et al (1984) in patients suffering from shock from burns. Cimetidine is often administered to burns patients to prevent stress gastric ulcers. During the early period of resuscitation with intravenous fluids there was decreased renal clearance of cimetidine but an increase in non-renal clearance. The latter may be due to increased oxidative metabolism in the liver associated with the hypermetabolic state following major burns. The increased clearance of cimetidine was related to the extent of the burn (Martyn et al 1985).

REFERENCES

Greenblatt D J, Abernethy D R, Morse D S, Harmatz J S, Shader R I 1984 Clinical importance of the interaction of diazepam and cimetidine. New England Journal of Medicine 310: 1639–1643

Martyn J A J, Greenblatt D J, Abernethy D R 1985 Increased cimetidine clearance in burn patients. Journal of the American Medical Association 253: 1288–1291

Ziemniak J A, Watson W A, Saffle J R, Smith I L, Russo J, Warden G D, Schentag J J 1984 Cimetidine kinetics during resuscitation from burn shock. Clinical Pharmacology and Therapeutics 36: 228–233

DOMPERIDONE

Four cases of cardiac arrest have been reported following intravenous administration of domperidone. In three of the patients hypokalaemia was present. It was felt that domperidone may precipitate fatal cardiac arrhythmias when given in dose to suppress the emetic effects of cytotoxic drugs (Roussak et al 1984).

REFERENCES

Roussak J B, Carey P, Parry H 1984 Cardiac arrest after treatment with intravenous domperidone. British Medical Journal 289: 1579

ENDOCRINE RESPONSE TO STRESS

Naloxone and experimental shock

Evans et al (1984a) devised a model in animals to assess endotoxic shock. They found that naloxone increased the survival rate of experimental shock in the animal. It caused only limited and transient increases in mean arterial pressure with little effect on the cardiac index. Peripheral resistance rose but substantial increases in the mean arterial pressure were produced if there was volume replacement. The findings suggested that naloxone had a myocardial action (Evans et al 1984a). However DeMaria et al (1985) found that 0.4–1.2 mg of naloxone given intravenously was ineffectual in maintaining the blood pressure in septic shock in man.

The use of opioid antagonists, not only in septic and cardiogenic shock but also in chronic obstructive pulmonary disease and mental illness, has been reviewed by McNicholas & Martin (1984). Although endogenous opioids do not appear to be involved in the regulation of respiration in man they did have effects on respiratory function tests in chronic asthmatic patients. Al-Damluji et al (1983) administered 8 mg of naloxone at midnight (i.e. 24:00) and this was followed by a continuous infusion of 5.6 mg per hour until 10:00 on two successive nights. The peak expiratory flow rate (PEFR), FEV_1 and FVC which were measured at 06:00 were unchanged but between 08:00 and 20:00 on the day following the first infusion there was a significant improvement in PEFR and FEV_1; the explanation for this was unclear. There is a possibility that this could be due to the increase in ACTH and cortisol that occurs following the use of naloxone.

Naloxone failed to antagonize the respiratory depressant effects of midazolam (Forster et al 1983) but it did appear to interact with halothane when assessing the effect of morphine on the heart rate response to noxious stimuli (Kissin et al 1984).

Steroids

Steroids, including dexamethesone or methylprednisolone, improved shock reversal if administered within 4 hours of shock and thereafter it did not improve the survival rate (Sprung et al 1984).

Endocrine response

The endocrine and metabolic responses to surgery have been reviewed by Kehlet (1984) and Hall (1985). Christenson et al (1982) reported that even elective surgery was followed by a pronounced feeling of fatigue lasting for at least a month in about a third of the patients. Christenson & Kehlet (1984) found that the fatigued patients had a pronounced loss in weight in the triceps and upper arm muscle circumference and had reduced levels of serum transferrin. The pre-operative measurement of various parameters including electrolytes, lymphocytes, minerals and albumin were unhelpful in determining which patients would become fatigued. They have suggested that it might be possible to increase pre-operative nutrition and advocated regional analgesia to inhibit the afferent impulses suppressing the endocrine metabolic response to surgery.

Plasma β-endorphin levels have been measured in patients undergoing elective major surgery under anaesthesia with nitrous oxide, oxygen and halothane (the muscle relaxant was not identified). McIntosh et al (1985) found that there was a true circadian rhythm pre-operatively of β-endorphin levels and this was altered or even abolished for up to 72 hours. The plasma level or β-endorphin was significantly elevated following surgery.

Moore (1984) while not commenting on muscle fatigue noticed that there was less depression in lymphocytes following epidural analgesia compared with general anaesthesia. Hall (1985), however, stressed the limitations of current techniques of suppressing the endocrine response to surgical stimulation by inhibition of afferent stimulation, the use of high dose opioid analgesia or by the infusion of hormones such as insulin or adrenoceptor blocking agents. Hall (1985) reported excellent analgesia and suppression of plasma cortisol following epidural diamorphine but no effect on circulating glucose, lactate, pyruvate or non-esterified fatty acid (NEFA). However, Child & Kaufman (1985) found that the intrathecal administration of diamorphine was far superior than intravenous fentanyl in that the hyperglycaemic response to stimulation was delayed and the adrenocortical response was significantly depressed both during and following major abdominal surgery. In the intrathecal group of patients there were no significant cardiovascular responses to the incision. Analgesia following operation was required at 0.97 ± 0.2 hours in the fentanyl group of patients but only after 17.27 ± 3.4 hours in the patients who had intrathecal diamorphine. Although intrathecal opiates do not appear to affect autonomic afferent stimulation, the cardiovascular and hormonal responses appear to be suppressed.

Hjortso et al (1985) compared patients undergoing major abdominal surgery receiving fentanyl during operation and morphine post-operatively with a group of patients receiving extradural analgesia initially with etidocaine and later with morphine. Although pain relief was significantly better in the extradural group, the regime failed to prevent the increase in urine excretion of cortisol, adrenaline, noradrenaline and nitrogen. They concluded that the relief of pain had little influence on the endocrine response to stimulation during abdominal surgery. Hakanson et al (1985) concluded that thoracic extradural morphine was less effective than thoracic extradural bupivacaine in suppressing metabolic responses to upper abdominal surgery. In an earlier study Moller et al (1984) concluded that spinal anaesthesia with tetracaine had only a transient inhibitory effect on the endocrine response to surgery and it was related to the level of sensory loss produced by the local anaesthetic solution. Epidural analgesia with etidocaine also failed to modify post-operative depression of delayed hypersensitivity (Hjortso et al 1984).

Korinek et al (1985) compared extradural morphine with extradural bupivacaine and found in the latter group that plasma ADH was unchanged in the post-operative period whereas in those patients receiving extradural morphine there was the delayed but step-wise increase in plasma ADH, indicating that the morphine has reached the brainstem. A recent study by Kaufman & Bailey (1986), on the other hand, showed that the rise in ADH following surgical stimulation was less in patients given intrathecal diamorphine compared with controls. Bumetanide (0.0075 mg/kg) appeared to prevent the release of ADH. They also confirmed that the urinary output did not appear to be related to ADH levels.

A recent study of the endocrine response to surgery in patients undergoing hysterectomy has shown that isoflurane failed to suppress the rise in blood glucose levels during surgery and in the post-operative period. Adrenaline and noradrenaline levels increased significantly. There was an initial fall in cortisol levels which may have been due to the etomidate, but 1 hour following the end of surgery the levels had tended to rise again (Rolly et al 1984).

Nitrogen balance

Burns et al (1981) claimed that naftidrofuryl reduced the urinary excretion of nitrogen following surgical procedures in a study limited to the first 2 days following operation. Jackson et al (1984), who studied the negative nitrogen loss for a period of 5 days, were unable to substantiate these results. The blood lactate concentration was lower than in the control groups. This may have been due to the selection of the groups or associated with the intravenous therapy.

The post-operative negative nitrogen balance following elective surgery may be reduced by the pre-operative infusion of 5 mg/kg per minute of glucose. This regime reduced the excretion of urea and 3-methylhistidine, suggesting not only a reduction in protein breakdown but a possible improvement in protein synthesis for the first 24 hours following operation (Crowe et al 1984).

Bessey et al (1984) simulated the metabolic response to injury by infusing volunteers with cortisol, glucagon and epinephrine and were able to produce negative nitrogen balance, potassium loss, hyperglycaemia, hyperinsulinaemia, insulin resistance, sodium retention and leukocytosis. None of the hormones given individually produced the same effect as the administration of all three hormones together. Glucose and insulin concentrations rose, suggesting some degree of insulin resistance.

There is still debate as to the choice of fluid for resuscitation following severe shock or even to reduce the negative nitrogen loss following surgery. Smith & Norman (1982) found that in the animal model a mixture of crystalloid and colloid produced better results than either given alone. Plasma renin and plasma aldersterone reached high levels in burn patients treated with low volume colloids during resuscitation. The highest levels were reached 5 days following the burn. Clinical deterioration occurred in two patients who had secondary peaks of these hormone levels 7–14 days after the accident (Griffiths et al 1983).

Catecholamines

Catecholamine levels have been measured in man in response to maximal stress. In intensive care situations there are moderate elevations of plasma noradrenaline up to 1.37 ng/ml, whereas acute stress such as occurs during cardiac arrest may result in levels reaching 35.9 ng/ml. Patients in intensive care units developed plasma levels of noradrenaline which were twice as great as normal resting controls but the level rose 32 times following cardiac arrest. With close monitoring it is possible to survive plasma adrenaline concentrations as high as 273 ng/ml (Wortsman et al 1984). From animal studies Tilders et al (1985) found that argine vasopressin (AVP) was involved in activating the pituitary–adrenal system, possibly by potentiating the effects of corticotrophin releasing hormone (CRF).

Opioids

Pfeiffer & Herz (1984) have reviewed the endocrine actions of opioids, drawing attention to their widespread effects and variation according to species. In rats opioids stimulate ACTH and corticosterone secretion whereas in man there is inhibition. In both species naloxone stimulates the release of ACTH. Oxytocin and vasopressin release are inhibited by opioids at posterior pituitary level in animals, the effects being reversed by naloxone. There is an action at pancreatic level increasing levels of insulin and glucagon, an effect which may not be reversed by naloxone in man. Bouloux et al (1985) have shown that the enkephalin (DAMME) depressed noradrenaline and adrenaline levels, reducing their release in response to hypoglycaemia. Naloxone had no effect on basal plasma catecholamine levels but caused a significant increase in adrenaline response to hypoglycaemia. DAMME and naloxone had no effect on the blood glucose response to hypoglycaemia induced by insulin (see Ch. 19).

Thus it can be seen that the hormonal and metabolic responses to stress and surgical stimulation are complex. The results may be influenced by the extent and duration of surgery, laboratory measurements and the timing of sampling as well as the technique of anaesthesia. Etomidate caused a 20% reduction in cortisol levels, a factor which may effect the subsequent rise. The various hormones may interact and it is speculative to extrapolate results from animal experiments. The philosophical debate as to whether suppression of the endocrine response to trauma and surgical stimulation is beneficial remains unresolved.

REFERENCES

Al-Damluji S, Thompson P J, Citrone K M, Turner-Warwick M 1983 Effect of naloxone on circadian rhythms in lung function. Thorax 38: 914–918

Bessey P Q, Watters J M, Aoki T T, Wilmore D W 1984 Combined hormonal infusion simulates the metabolic response to injury. Annals of Surgery 200: 264–281

Blandford R L, Burden A C 1984 Abnormalities of cardiac conduction in diabetics. British Medical Journal 289: 1659

Bouloux P-M G, Grossman A, Lytras N, Besser G M 1985 Evidence for the participation of endogenous opioids in the sympathoadrenal response to hypoglycaemia in man. Clinical Endocrinology 22: 49–56

Burns H J G, Galloway D J, Ledingham I McA 1981 Effect of naftidrofuryl on the metabolic response to surgery. British Medical Journal 283: 7–8

Child C S, Kaufman L 1985 Effects of intrathecal diamorphine on the adrenocortical, hyperglycaemic and cardiovascular responses to major colonic surgery. British Journal of Anaesthesia 57: 389–393

Christensen T, Kehlet H 1984 Postoperative fatigue and changes in nutritional status. British Journal of Surgery 71: 473–476

Christensen T, Bendix T, Kehlet H 1982 Fatigue and cardiorespiratory function following abdominal surgery. British Journal of Surgery 69: 417–419

Crowe P J, Dennison A, Royle G T 1984 The effect of pre-operative glucose loading on postoperative nitrogen metabolism. British Journal of Surgery 71: 635–637

DeMaria A, Effernan J J, Grindlinger G A, Craven D E, McIntosh T K, McCabe W R 1985 Naloxone versus placebo in treatment of septic shock. Lancet 1: 1363–1365

Evans S F, Hinds C J, Varley J G 1984a A new canine model of endotoxin shock. British Journal of Pharmacology 83: 433–442

Evans S F, Hinds C J, Varley J G 1984b Effects of intravascular volume expansion on the cardiovascular response to naloxone in a canine model of severe endotoxin shock. British Journal of Pharmacology 83: 443–448

Forster A, Morel D, Bachmann M, Gemperle M 1983 Respiratory depressant effects of different doses of midazolam and lack of reversal with naloxone — a double-blind randomized study. Anesthesia and Analgesia 62: 920–924

Griffiths R W, Millar J G B, Albano J, Shakespeare P G, 1983 Observations on the activity of the renin-angiotensin-aldosterone (RAA) system after low volume colloid resuscitation for burn injury. Annals of the Royal College of Surgeons of England 65: 212–215

Hakanson E, Rutberg H, Jorfeldt K L, Martensson J 1985 Effects of the extradural administration of morphine or bupivacaine, on the metabolic response to upper abdominal surgery.British Journal of Anaesthesia 57: 394–399

Hall G M 1985 The anaesthetic modification of the endocrine and metabolic response to surgery. Annals of the Royal College of Surgeons of England 67: 25–29

Hjortso N-C, Andersen T, Frosig F, Neumann P, Rogon E, Kehlet H 1984 Failure of epidural analgesia to modify postoperative depression of delayed hypersensitivity. Acta Anaesthesiologica Scandinavica 28: 128–131

Hjortson N-C, Christensen N J, Kehlet H 1985 Effects of the extradural administration of local

anaesthetic agents and morphine on the urinary excretion of cortisol, catecholamines and nitrogen following abdominal surgery. British Journal of Anaesthesia 57: 400–406
Jackson J M, Khawaja H T, Weaver P C, Talbot S T, Lee H A 1984 Naftidrofuryl and the nitrogen, carbohydrate, and lipid responses to moderate surgery. British Medical Journal 289: 581–586
Kaufman L, Bailey P M 1986 (in press)
Kehlet H 1984 Epidural analgesia and the endocrine-metabolic response to surgery. Update and perspectives. Acta Anaesthesiologica Scandinavica 28: 125–127
Kissin I, Kerr C R, Smith L R 1984 Effect of morphine on the heart rate response to noxious stimulation: interaction with halothane and naloxone. Pain 18: 351–358
Korinek A M, Languille M, Bonnet F, Thibonnier M, Sasano P, Lienhart, A, Viars P 1985 Effects of postoperative extradural morphine on ADH secretion. British Journal of Anaesthesia 57: 407–411
McIntosh T K, Bush H L, Palter M, Hay J R, Aun F, Yeston N S, Egdahl R H 1985 Prolonged disruption of beta-endorphin dynamics following surgery. Journal of Surgical Research 38: 210–215
McNicholas L F, Martin W R 1984 New and experimental therapeutic roles for naloxone and related opioid antagonists. Drugs 27: 81–93
Moller I W, Hjortso E, Krantz T, Wandall E, Kehlet H 1984 The modifying effect of spinal anaesthesia on intra- and postoperative adrenocortical and hyperglycaemic response to surgery. Acta Anaesthesiologica Scandanivica 28: 266–269
Moore T C 1984 Anesthesia associated with depression in lymphocyte traffic: less with regional anesthesia than with general anesthesia in sheep. American Journal of Surgery 148: 71–76
Pfeiffer A, Herz A 1984 Endocrine actions of opioids. Hormone Metabolic Research 16: 286–397
Rolly G, Versichelen L, Moerman E 1984 Cardiovascular, metabolic and hormonal changes during isoflurane N_2O anaesthesia. European Journal of Anaesthesiology 1: 327–334
Smith J A R, Norman J N 1982 The fluid of choice for resuscitation of severe shock. British Journal of Surgery 69: 702–705
Sprung C L, Caralis P V, Marcial E H et al 1984 The effects of high-dose corticosteroids in patients with septic shock. The New England Journal of Medicine 311: 1137–1143
Tilders F J H, Berkenbosch F, Vermes I, Linton E A, Smelik P G 1985 Rise of epinephrine and vasopressin in the control of the pituitary-adrenal response to stress. Federation Proceedings 44: 155–160
Wortsman J, Frank S, Cryer P E 1984 Adrenomedullary response to maximal stress in humans. American Journal of Medicine 77: 779–784

MUSCLE RELAXANTS

Atracurium

Bell et al (1984) reported on the use of atracurium in five patients with myasthenia gravis who were having thymectomy. An initial dose of 0.1 mg/kg was administered followed by incremental doses which were reversed at the end of surgery with atropine and neostigmine.

A patient with myasthenia gravis being treated with pyridostigmine and neostigmine orally had a laparotomy for resection of colon for diverticular disease (personal series). Only 10 mg of atracurium were administered for an operation lasting 2.5 hours. The relaxant was not reversed, there was no post-operative respiratory insufficiency and the oral anticholinesterase drugs were not required post-operatively.

REFERENCES

Bell C F, Florence A M, Hunter J M, Jones R S, Utting J E 1984 Atracurium in the myasthenic patient. Anaesthesia 39: 961–968

SLEEP APNEA SYNDROME (SAS)

This subject has been reviewed by Apps(1983) and Partridge (1984). The paraphysiology of sleep apnea and its causes has also been reviewed by Cherniack

(1984). In a further study by Guilleminault et al (1983) of 400 patients with SAS, 48% were found to have cardiac arrhythmias during sleep. These included ventricular tachycardia, sinus arrest for up to 13 seconds and second degree atrioventricular block. Nearly 20% had premature ventricular contractions. The arrhythmias usually occurred during a fit of obstructive apnea. Tracheotomy was performed in 50 patients after which SAS disappeared as well as the significant cardiac arrhythmias (ventricular ectopic beats still occurred).

The frequency of ventricular arrhythmias is reduced during sleep but this increases in patients with neurological disorders associated particularly with cerebrovascular disease (Rosenberg et al 1983). SAS was present in 30% of patients with essential hypertension (Lavie et al 1984).

SAS is often associated with obesity but Onal et al (1985) have shown that there are significant correlations between daytime measurements of pulmonary volume and inspiratory airway conductance and the severity of sleep induced apnea. Airway resistance appears to contribute to SAS but there are still central neurological factors.

The apnea of SAS may be considered to be central, obstructive or have a mixture of these components. In the post-operative period use of drugs in the course of anaesthesia may give rise to a situation similar to SAS in that they can cause respiratory depression and, unless the airway is protected, respiratory obstruction may ensue. There is also the possibility of patients with unrecognized SAS presenting for operation.

REFERENCES

Apps M C P 1983 Sleep-disordered breathing. British Journal of Hospital Medicine 30: 339–347

Cherniack N S 1984 Sleep apnea and its causes. Journal of Clinical Investigation 73: 1501–1506

Guilleminault C, Connolly S J, Winkle R A 1983 Cardiac arrhythmia and conduction disturbances during sleep in 400 patients with sleep apnea syndrome. American Journal of Cardiology 52: 490–494

Lavie P, Ben-Yosef R, Rubin A-H E 1984 Prevalence of sleep apnea syndrome among patients with essential hypertension. American Heart Journal 108: 373–376

Onal E, Leech J A, Lopata M 1985 Relationship between pulmonary function and sleep-induced respiratory abnormalities. Chest 87: 437–441

Partridge M R 1984 Sleep apnea syndromes. In: Kaufman L (ed) Anaesthesia Review 2 Churchill Livingstone, Edinburgh, p 10–20

Rosenberg M J, Uretz E, Denes P 1983 Sleep and ventricular arrhythmias. American Heart Journal 106: 703–709

Index